STEROID RECEPTORS,
METABOLISM
AND PROSTATIC CANCER

STEROID RECEPTORS, METABOLISM AND PROSTATIC CANCER

Proceedings of a
Workshop of the Society
of Urologic Oncology and Endocrinology
Amsterdam, 27–28 April, 1979

Editors: F. H. Schröder and H. J. de Voogt

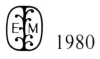 1980

Excerpta Medica, Amsterdam-Oxford-Princeton

International Congress Series No 494
ISBN Excerpta Medica 90 219 9379 1
ISBN Elsevier North-Holland 0444 90119 1

Publisher:
Excerpta Medica
305 Keizersgracht
1000 BC Amsterdam
P.O. Box 1126

Sole Distributors for the USA and Canada:
Elsevier North-Holland Inc.
52 Vanderbilt Avenue
New York, N.Y. 10017

Printed in The Netherlands by Casparie, Heerhugowaard

Table of Contents

Welcome Address

H. J. de Voogt
Department of Urology, University Hospital, Leiden, The Netherlands

Ladies and Gentlemen,

First of all I would like to extend a cordial welcome to all of you who have accepted our invitation and taken the trouble to travel, some over long distances, to be here today to present what I look forward to as some very interesting papers, or to listen to these and take an active part in the discussions.

Amongst you there is a small group of dedicated biochemists and urologists from different parts of Europe, which has met in the past on several occasions in Leiden and Hamburg. These were rather informal meetings where, in a friendly atmosphere, we could exchange our ideas and experiences on the matter of steroid receptors in prostatic tissue.

From the programme it might be concluded that a European Prostate Cancer Research Group actually exists, but this is not so. However, we have been thinking about bringing such a group into being — if not today then in the near future.

It has always been a pleasure for me to organize these meetings and I got the impression from many of you that you wanted to continue them. However, on the one hand due to the burden of my daily work I did not see an opportunity to continue on my own, while on the other I thought that it might be much more informative to invite other research workers whom we knew of through their publications, personal acquaintance or meetings. I felt we could learn much more in this way and probably even set out lines or paths along which our future research efforts might be directed. I must say that we were aware of the fact that we may have overlooked quite a few people of whom we did not know.

At one point I had the opportunity to discuss this with Schering and indirectly with Prof. Neumann, and I was very glad when they gave me their support in organizing this meeting, which is what I had in mind. Through their generosity we were able to invite people from more remote places in Europe as well as from the U.S. and Canada. Once again, I am very glad that you all reacted favourably to the proposals that I was able to work out together with Prof. Schröder and Dr Teulings, with whom a scientific committee was formed.

From the beginning we have said that, though it seems to be a much more formal meeting, with official presentations, it should still remain and have the nature of a workshop, which means that there must be ample time for discussion, as well as informal get-togethers during breaks for coffee and meals.

You will therefore find that after each presentation there is a short time for questions which should be more technical or simply clarify points. After each session there is a longer period for more general discussions and I have asked the chairmen of the sessions to look after this very carefully.

Much to my regret I have to tell you that Prof. Mainwaring unfortunately had to cancel his attendance at the last moment. For that reason we had to change the programme: in his place Prof. Neumann will speak. This will give more time for discussion in Saturday morning programme.

With this I officially declare this workshop open and wish you all a good meeting.

I
RECENT ADVANCES ON
THE METABOLISM AND MECHANISM OF ACTION
OF STEROIDS IN THE PROSTATE

Combined effects of testosterone, estradiol and hydrocortisone on rat ventral prostate in organ culture

T. Feyel-Cabanes, M. T. Picard-Groyer, S. Weiller, E. E. Baulieu and P. Robel
Research Unit on Molecular Metabolism and the Physiopathology of Steroids, Bicêtre Hospital, Bicêtre, France

Introduction

It is widely accepted that the development of benign prostatic hypertrophy (BPH) requires the presence of testes. BPH has rarely if ever been reported in men castrated in youth or as young adults. However, once BPH has developed to a degree where urinary obstruction is present, the testes seem less important. If elderly men with advanced BPH are castrated, relief of bladder neck obstruction is variable. Some regression of epithelial elements occurs, but the stromal elements of BPH nodules are not affected. The point to be emphasized is that each cell type in the prostate does not necessarily respond in equivalent fashion to sex steroid hormones [1].

The ageing process is, indeed, accompanied by changes in circulating sex hormones. The concentration of circulating testosterone (both total and unbound) is decreased in older men. The concentration of circulating estradiol is almost unchanged. Hence the ratio of unbound estradiol/unbound testosterone appears to be significantly increased in such men [2].

Prostatic hypertrophy resembling the human disease never occurs spontaneously in the rat ventral prostate, nor can it be induced in organ culture by physiological concentrations of testosterone. Indeed when culture takes place in Medium 199 without supplementation, and in the absence of hormone, epithelial cells regress but stromal components are not affected and even tend to proliferate. Testosterone maintains the epithelial cells and prevents the increase of perialveolar and interstitial stroma [3]. We show in this paper that estradiol in conjunction with androgen induces simultaneous hypertrophy of epithelial and stromal elements [4, 5].

Materials and methods

Chemicals

Estradiol, testosterone and hydrocortisone were obtained from Roussel-Uclaf, France. Medium 199 was obtained from Flow Laboratories Ltd.,

Scotland. Methyl-^{3}H thymidine was from the Radiochemical Centre, Amersham, England.

Animals

Male Wistar rats were obtained from Iffa Credo. St Germain sur l'Arbresle, France, and sacrificed at 7 weeks of age.

Organ culture

Explants of ventral prostate were cultured in serum-free medium as previously described [3]. After a 24-hour preincubation in hormone-free medium to eliminate any interference by endogenous hormones the explants were transferred to medium containing estradiol, testosterone or hydrocortisone either alone or in combination. Hormones were added to the medium in propylene glycol. Control cultures in hormone-free medium received an equal volume of solvent. After 72 hours all explants were transferred into similar fresh media for a further 72 hours. For each treatment examined a minimum of 10 explants from different animals were cultured. Methyl-^{3}H thymidine (0.2 Ci/mmol, 4 μCi per ml) was added to some cultures 22 hours after the transfer to fresh medium.

Light microscopy and autoradiography

Explants were fixed in Bouin's aqueous fixative and cut into 5-μm sections. The preparations were covered with Ilford L4 nuclear emulsion. After a two week exposure at 4°C the emulsions were developed in D 19 B (Kodak) and fixed. Sections were stained with hematoxylin eosin. Other sections were stained with periodic acid-Schiff to reveal the mucopolysaccharides. For evaluation of alkaline phosphatase according to Gomori [6] explants were fixed in 80% ethanol at 0°C.

Results

Several concentrations of testosterone (1−100 nM), estradiol (1−1,000 nM), and hydrocortisone (10−1,000 nM) were used alone or in combination. Representative experiments semi-quantitatively evaluating hormonal effects on ventral prostate epithelial and stromal elements are summarized in figure 1.

At all concentrations of testosterone $\geqslant$ 1 nM the prostatic explants were maintained in a state comparable to that observed before culture, confirming preceding observations [3] (Figure 2). The glandular epithelium mainly consisted of tall columnar cells, showing well developed rough endoplasmic reticulum, supranuclear Golgi area, secretory granules and microvilli under electron microscopic examination (data not shown). The perialveolar sheath was composed of 1 or 2 layers of smooth muscular cells and of fibroblasts [7].

The interalveolar stroma was reduced to a few dispersed fibroblasts and macrophages. Periodic acid-Schiff and alkaline-phosphatase staining predominated in the epithelial cells [4], whereas thymidine labelling was almost exclusively restricted to perialveolar and interstitial fibroblasts (Figure 3).

In the absence of testosterone alveolar diameter was reduced, the epithe-

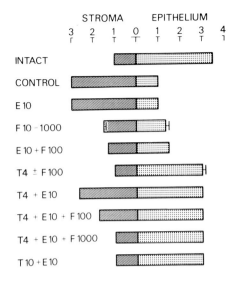

Fig. 1. Effects of testosterone (T), estradiol (E), and hydrocortisone (F) on rat ventral prostate epithelium and stroma. The numbers following T, E or F are the concentrations of hormones used and are expressed in nM. The arbitrary scales apply to light microscopic, periodic acid-Schiff and alkaline phosphatase staining data, as follows: Epithelium: 4 = fully maintained, 3 = maintained (predominant columnar cells), 2 = partly maintained (predominant cuboidal cells), 1 = not maintained (predominant flat cells). Stroma: 1 = completely regressed, 2 = partly regressed, 3 = not regressed.

lium was atrophic and its cells flattened, with disappearance of secretory granules and microvilli and, in addition, exhibition of dense bodies. In contrast the perialveolar sheath was thickened; retracted muscular cells showed 'holly-leaf' spines and signs of micropinocytosis. Moreover, the stroma was well developed, with many fibroblasts and active macrophages readily visible together with a dense network of collagen fibers. Periodic acid-Schiff and alkaline phosphatase stains were predominant in the stromal cells, mainly fibroblasts. Thymidine labelling of the nuclei of the same cells also tended to increase.

Regardless of the concentration used, estradiol alone did not alter the morphologic, staining and labelling characteristics observed without hormone.

When estradiol (> 0.1 nM) was added to physiological concentrations of testosterone (1 or 4 nM), the epithelium was well developed and more stimulated than with testosterone alone. In particular, thymidine labelling of nuclei was markedly increased.

However, interstitial tissue was also developed almost as much as in the absence of hormones or in the presence of estradiol alone. All features observed separately in androgen-stimulated epithelial cells and in no-hormone or estradiol-exposed stromal cells were observed when testosterone (1 to 4 nM) and estradiol (1 to 1,000 nM) were present together.

This was no longer the case when estradiol (1 nM to 1,000 nM) was added to supraphysiological concentrations of testosterone (10 nM and more). The latter again provoked a typical androgenic stimulation of epithelial cells, but the stroma was unresponsive to estradiol. Biochemical parameters were

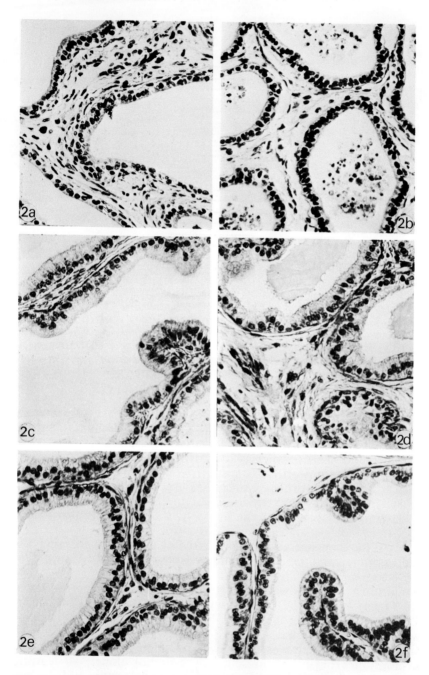

Fig. 2. Light microscopy of 7-day cultures (T. Feyel-Cabanes). a, without hormone; b, 10 nM estradiol; c, 4 nM testosterone; d, 4 nM testosterone with 10 nM estradiol; e, 100 nM testosterone; f, 100 nM testosterone with 100 nM estradiol. × 300. (from [5]).

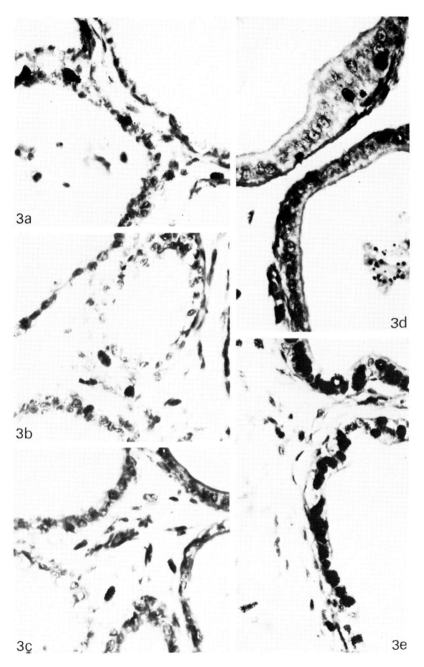

Fig. 3. ^3H *thymidine-autoradiography of 7-day cultures (S. Weiller). a, without hormone; b, 10 nM estradiol; c, 100 nM hydrocortisone; d, 4 nM testosterone; e, 4 nM testosterone with 10 nM estradiol.* × *500.*

also similar to those observed with testosterone alone.

Several experiments were made with 1 to 4 nM testosterone in presence of 1,000 nM cyproterone acetate, a classic antiandrogen [8, 9]. Even at such large concentrations cyproterone acetate had no androgenic activity, but counteracted very markedly testosterone effects on epithelial and stromal cells. Preliminary observations were made with combinations of lower testosterone concentrations (0.01 and 0.1 nM), which only partially maintain epithelial cells, and estradiol (10 to 1,000 nM). Here again no full antiandrogenic action of estradiol was observed, since the stroma was increased as in control cultures without hormone, whereas epithelial cells were more maintained than by testosterone alone. Diethylstilboestrol, a non-steroidal oestrogen (0.1 to 1,000 nM), was also substituted for estradiol. Even at the highest concentration used it displayed no antagonistic effect on androgen-dependent inhibition of stromal development. Finally, tamoxifen, an anti-oestrogen with mixed oestrogenic agonist and antagonist activity in the rat uterus [10] and purely antagonist activity in the chick oviduct [11], was used alone (1 to 100 nM), in the presence of testosterone (1 nM) or of estradiol (1 to 10 nM), and in the presence of both testosterone (4 nM) and estradiol (1 to 10 nM). Tamoxifen showed no effect on its own and did not modify the effects of testosterone and estradiol when used separately or in combination.

Glucocorticoids are known to modify the growth parameters of fibroblasts in tissue culture and, at least under certain conditions, to inhibit cell growth, glucose uptake and protein synthesis, in particular the synthesis of collagen [12, 13]. When added to rat ventral prostate explant cultures, hydrocortisone (10 to 1,000 nM) prevented the increase of stroma observed in control cultures, whereas the stimulation of epithelial cells was minimal, if it occurred at all. The staining of connective tissue with periodic acid-Schiff was also greatly decreased, and thymidine incorporation into nuclear deoxyribonucleic acid (DNA) was greatly reduced. Hydrocortisone did not significantly modify the responsiveness of the cultured explants to testosterone. In contrast, when hydrocortisone (100 to 1,000 nM) was combined with estradiol (10 to 100 nM), with or without testosterone (4 nM), stroma was as regressed as in cultures with testosterone alone.

Discussion

The effects of estradiol alone or associated with testosterone have been studied in seminal vesicles and prostate in several species. These *in vivo* observations have been difficult to interpret due to complex indirect hormonal changes. However, such hormone treatments of castrated or prepubertal animals caused an increase of the muscular and stromal components of the accessory sexual glands [14–23]. The present *in vitro* experiments essentially confirm observations *in vivo*. The use of organ culture in completely defined, serum-deprived medium allowed operation at known concentrations of both hormones and the exclusion of extra-prostatic factors.

The effects of testosterone on ventral prostate can be reproduced partly in an *in vitro* culture system [3]. In the absence of hormone, the regression observed is similar to that after castration. The mechanism for the striking increase in smooth muscle cells, fibroblasts and other stromal cells in culture without testosterone, whether estradiol is present or not, is unknown. Testosterone can apparently repress this increase when present at physiological concentrations but cannot do so when estradiol is present at the same time. This antitestosterone effect of estradiol is observed only on stroma and not on epithelial cells, which remain fully stimulated. However, at supraphysiological concentrations testosterone overrides the antagonistic effect of any concentration of estradiol and the stroma remains repressed by the androgen. These results suggest a greater sensivity of stromal than epithelial cells to the antiandrogenic effects of estradiol.

Several authors have suggested the presence of oestrogen receptor in rat ventral prostate [24, 25]. Oestrogen receptor has recently been unequivocally identified (M. Ginsburg and I. Jung-Testas, personal communication) although in small amounts (less than 10% of the concentration of androgen receptor). However the oestrogenic effects on rat ventral prostate observed in organ culture do not show the hormone specificity of oestrogen receptors. Diethylstilboestrol, which displays oestrogenic activity and high binding affinity for oestrogen receptors (Table) [26], could not replace estradiol, at least in the range of concentrations tested and tamoxifen, an antioestrogen acting at the oestrogen receptor level in several systems [10, 11, 27], did not antagonize estradiol action nor did it display any estradiol-like activity. We suggest it is possible that estradiol acts via the androgen receptor because it binds to this receptor with high affinity [28] while both diethylstilboestrol and tamoxifen show only negligible affinity (Table). This could explain the relatively large concentration of estradiol needed. If the estradiol effect takes place at the androgen receptor level, it still has to be found out whether androgen receptor in epithelial or stromal cells or both is concerned. Autoradiographic experiments have shown that androgen receptors are located mainly if not exclusively in epithelial cells of rat ventral prostate [28, 29, 30]. Therefore, it is not impossible that the inhibitory effect of testosterone on interstitial stroma and, consequently, estradiol activity is indirect. It must also be kept in mind that a full antiandrogenic response is difficult to obtain with estradiol, in contrast to cyproterone acetate. Estradiol in fact enhances testosterone action on epithelial cells, an effect never observed with pure antiandrogens.

Estradiol inhibits testosterone 5α-reductase. Selective inhibition by natural oestrogens such as estradiol as opposed to the synthetic oestrogen diethylstilboestrol could explain the difference observed between the 2 oestrogens. However, both compounds have been shown to give similar inhibition of prostatic 5α-reductase [3]. Moreover, testosterone is more effective in repressing stromal growth than its metabolite androstanolone [3].

Table   Affinity of natural and synthetic hormones for receptors

	Affinity for	
	Oestrogen receptor	Androgen receptor
Estradiol	++++	++
Diethylstilboestrol	++++	±
Tamoxifen	++	±
Androstanolone or testosterone	±	++++

Composite table summarizing the affinity of different compounds for known androgen and oestrogen receptors [26, 28]. ++++: Dissociation constant (K_D) $\sim$ 0.1 nM; ++: $K_D \simeq$ 10 nM; ±: $K_D \geqslant$ 1 μM.

Until now the rat prostate has not been considered suitable for the study of human prostatic disease. In particular, no morphological abnormalities, spontaneous or experimentally induced, have been observed that resemble human BPH. It is, therefore, extremely interesting that the hormones and organ culture technique used here allow explants to be obtained in which the epithelial and stromal cells are developed simultaneously as in the disease, and the possible role of oestrogen/androgen imbalance in the resumption of prostate growth is stressed.

This culture system might also be used to screen hormonal combinations for effectiveness in the medical treatment of human BPH.

Acknowledgments

We thank Jean Secchi for his very valuable help, and Heather Mullis, Martine Rossillon and Christine Barrier for the preparation of the manuscript. The financial assistance of INSERM, the Centre National de la Recherche Scientifique (CNRS) and the faculty of Medicine Paris-Sud is acknowledged.

References

1. Hechter, O. (1976): Reflections on the NIH Workshop on BPH. In: *Benign Prostatic Hyperplasia*, p. 269. Editors: J. T. Grayhack, J. D. Wilson, and M. J. Scherbenske. DHEW Publication N° (NIH) 76–1113.
2. Vermeulen, A. (1976): Testicular hormonal secretion and aging in males. In: *Benign Prostatic Hyperplasia*, p. 269. Editors: J. T. Grayhack, J. D. Wilson and M. J. Scherbenske. DHEW Publication N° (NIH) 76–1113.
3. Baulieu, E. E., Le Goascogne, C., Groyer, A., Feyel-Cabanes, T. and Robel, P. (1975): Morphological and biochemical parameters of androgen effects on rat ventral prostate in organ culture. *Vitam. Horm. 33*, 1.
4. Feyel-Cabanes, T., Robel, P. and Baulieu, E. E. (1977): Effets conjoints de la testostérone et de l'oestradiol sur le lobe ventral de la prostate de rat en culture organotypique. *Comptes Rendus de l'Académie des Sciences, Paris (Série D), 285,* 1119.
5. Feyel-Cabanes, T., Secchi, J., Robel, P. and Baulieu, E. E. (1978): Combined effects of testosterone and estradiol on rat ventral prostate in organ culture. *Cancer Res., 38,* 4126.
6. Gomori, G. (1946): The study of enzymes in tissue sections. *Am. J. Clin. Pathol., 16,* 347.
7. Flickinger, C. J. (1972): The fine structure of the interstitial tissue of rat prostate. *Am. J. Anat., 134,* 107.
8. Neumann, F., von Berswordt-Wallrabe, R., Elger, W., Steinbeck, H., Hahn, J. D. and Kramer, M. (1970): Aspects of androgen-dependent events as studied by antiandrogens. In: *Recent Progress in Hormone Research*, Vol. XXVI, p. 337. Editor: E. B. Astwood. Academic Press, New York.
9. Santti, R. S. and Johannsson, R. (1973): Some biochemical effects of insulin and steroid hormones on the rat prostate in organ culture. *Exp. Cell Res., 77,* 111.
10. Harper, M. J. K. and Walpole, A. L. (1967): A new derivative of triphenylethylene: effect on implantation and mode of action in rats. *J. Reprod. Fertil., 13,* 101.
11. Sutherland, R., Mester, J. and Baulieu, E. E. (1977): Tamoxifen is a potent 'pure' anti-oestrogen in chick oviduct. *Nature, (London), 267,* 434.
12. Pratt, W. B. and Aronow, L. (1966): The effect of glucocorticoids on protein and nucleic acid synthesis in mouse fibroblasts growing *in vitro. J. Biol. Chem., 241,* 5244.
13. Cutroneo, K. R. and Counts, D. F. (1975): Antiflammatory steroids and collagen metabolism: glucocorticoid mediated alterations of prolyl hydroxylase activity and collagen synthesis. *Mol. Pharmacol., 11,* 632.

14. Freud. J. (1933): Conditions of hypertrophy of the seminal vesicles in rats. *Biochem. J., 27,* 1438.
15. Courrier, R. and Gros, G. (1934): Action de la folliculine chez le singe mâle impubère. Modification des annexes. *Comptes Rendus de la Société de Biologie, 118,* 686.
16. Korenchewsky, V. and Dennison, M. (1935): Histological changes in the organs of rats injected with oestrone alone or simultaneously with oestrone and testicular hormone. *J. Pathol. Bacteriol., 41,* 323.
17. Overholser, M. and Nelson, W. (1935): The effect of estrin and male hormone injected separately and simultaneously upon the smooth muscle and epithelium of the seminal vesicle in the albino rat. *Anat. Rec., 62,* 247.
18. Huggins, C. and Johnson-Clark, P. (1940): Quantitative studies of prostatic secretion. II. The effect of castration and of estrogen injection on the normal and on the hyperplastic prostate glands of dogs. *J. Exp. Med., 72,* 747.
19. Emmens, C. W. and Parker, A. S. (1947): Effect of exogenous estrogens on the male mammal. *Vitam. Horm., 5,* 233.
20. Bern, H. A. (1951): Estrogen and alkaline phosphatase activity in the genital tract of the male mouse. *Endocrinology, 48,* 25.
21. Price, D. and Williams-Ashman, H. G. (1971): The accessory reproductive glands of mammals. In: *Sex and Internal Secretions,* Vol. I, p. 366. Editor: W. C. Young. The Williams and Wilkins Co., Baltimore.
22. Tisell, L. E. (1971): The growth of the ventral prostate, the dorsolateral prostate, the coagulating glands and the seminal vesicles in castrated adrenalectomized rats injected with oestradiol and/or cortisone. *Acta Endocrinol. (Copenhagen), 68,* 485.
23. Neumann, F., Richter, K. D. and Penge, J. (1975): Animal models in the study of antiprostatic drugs. *Vitam. Horm., 33,* 103.
24. Armstrong, E. G. and Bashirelahi, N. (1974): A specific binding protein for 17β-estradiol in retired breeder rat ventral prostate. *Biochem. Biophys. Res. Commun., 61,* 628.
25. Van Beurden-Lamers, W. M. O., Brinkmann, A. O., Mulder, E. and Van der Molen, J. (1974): High affinity binding of oestradiol-17β by cytosols from testis interstitial tissue, pituitary, adrenal, liver, and accessory glands of the male rat. *Biochem. J., 140,* 495.
26. Baulieu, E. E., Atger, M., Best-Belpomme, M., Corvol, P., Courvalin, J. C., Mester, J., Milgrom, E., Robel, P., Rochefort, H. and De Catalogne, D. (1975): Steroid hormone receptors. *Vitam. Horm., 33,* 649.
27. Jordan, V. C., Dix, C. J., Rowsby, L., and Prestwich, G. (1977): Studies on the mechanism of action of the non-steroidal anti-oestrogen tamoxifen (ICI 46,474) in the rat. *Mol. Cell. Endocrinol., 7,* 177.
28. Blondeau, J. P., Corpéchot, C., Le Goascogne, C., Baulieu, E. E. and Robel, P. (1975): Androgen receptors in the rat ventral prostate and their hormonal control. *Vitam. Horm., 33,* 319.
29. Tveter, K. J. and Attramadal, A. (1969): Autoradiographic localization of androgen in the rat ventral prostate. *Endocrinology, 85,* 350.
30. Sar, M., Liao, S. and Stumpf, W. E. (1970): Nuclear concentration of androgens in rat seminal vesicles and prostate demonstrated by dry-mount autoradiography. *Endocrinology, 86,* 1008.
31. Nozu, K. and Tamaoki, B. I. (1974): Characteristics of the nuclear and microsomal steroid Δ^4-5α-hydrogenase of the rat prostate. *Acta Endocrinol. (Copenhagen), 76,* 608.

Discussion

M. Bruchovsky (Edmonton, Canada): What dose of hydrocortisone and cyproterone acetate would you use to treat prostatic hyperplasia?

P. Robel: I don't know. In organ culture, the effective concentrations would be 100—1,000 nM hydrocortisone and 1,000—10,000 nM cyproterone acetate.

F. Rommerts (Rotterdam, The Netherlands): You showed effects of 1 nM estradiol on these tissue cultures. Did you try lower concentrations?

P. Robel: Yes. 0.1 nM estradiol was the smallest effective concentration.

Androgen-sensitive protein in rat ventral prostate: a specific intracellular protein and a secretory protein

S. Liao, C. Chen, R. Loor and R. A. Hiipakka
The Ben May Laboratory for Cancer Research and the Department of Bio-chemistry, University of Chicago, Chicago, Illinois, U.S.A.

During the last 10 years we have been engaged in studies of four proteins in the rat ventral prostate (Table I). These include a high-affinity androgen-binding receptor protein which upon binding to an active androgen can tightly associate with nuclear chromatin. Such an interaction appears to involve one or more nuclear proteins, which have been called nuclear acceptors. The receptor-acceptor interaction is believed to cause a change in the pattern of ribonucleic acid (RNA) synthesis that can be utilized in the protein-synthesizing system.

In this article, we summarize briefly our recent work on the other two proteins (Table I) which are stimulated by androgens in rats. One of these is a major prostate protein which we named α-protein [1]. The androgen effect on the synthesis of this protein is, however, sluggish and the response appears to be secondary to other events augmented by androgens. In contrast, the synthesis of a specific spermine-binding protein which we found two years ago [2] is very sensitive to androgenic manipulation of the experimental animals. This protein may be one of the earliest proteins induced in the prostate after androgen is given to castrated rats.

The spermine-binding protein was discovered during our study of the mechanism involved in the rapid androgen stimulation of the activity of the initiation factor required for protein synthesis [3, 4]. Protein binding of polyamine was studied since initiation factor activity is highly sensitive to low concentrations of polyamines, especially spermine [5]. When the whole prostate cytosol preparation was incubated with ^{3}H-spermine and the mixture analysed by gradient centrifugation (Figure 1), a distinct radioactive peak was found in the vicinity of 3 S [2]. Trypsin or chymotrypsin, but not pancreatic ribonuclease (RNAse) or deoxyribonuclease (DNAse) reduced the formation of the 3 S radioactive complex. This 3 S protein is not present in blood and only the ventral prostate among the many organs we studied is rich in this polyamine-binding component. The protein appears to localize intracellularly: it is not detected in prostate fluid. The spermine-binding protein has been purified to homogeneity from the prostate cytosol by salt fractionation, by chromatography on diethylaminoethyl (DEAE)-cellulose,

Table I Four proteins involved in the androgen-mediated growth of rat ventral prostate.

Protein	Representative ligands	Precipitated by ammonium sulphate (% saturation)	Approx. % of cytosol protein	Eluted from DEAE-cellulose by	Sedimentation Low KCl	Sedimentation High KCl	Heat stability of ligand binding at 50–60°C	Binding to chromatin
α-Protein	DHT (Ka:10^7M^{-1}) testosterone progesterone estradiol	50–70	20–30	0.2M KCl	3–4S	3–4S	Relatively stable	No
β-Protein	DHT (Ka:10^{11}M^{-1}) and other androgens	0–40	0.002	0.05M KCl	3–4S 7–8S Aggreg.	3–4S	Unstable	Tight
Nuclear acceptor protein	Androgen-receptor complex, DNA	80	Not applicable	Not determined	Not determined		Relatively unstable	Tight
Spermine binding protein	Spermine (Ka:10^7M^{-1}) thermine	55–70	0.5–1.0	0.3M KCl	3S	3S	Unstable	No

Sephadex G-200, spermine-Sepharose, phosphocellulose, and concanavalin A-Sepharose columns, and by gradient centrifugation [6].

The molecular weight of this protein is about 30,000. It binds spermine noncovalently and without prior metabolism. Among many amines which we have tested, only spermine and thermine, a tetramine with one less carbon than spermine, can bind well to the protein. Spermidine is a weak binder, whereas diamines of various sizes are not very effective. The dissociation constant for spermine is of the order of 0.1 μM, which is much lower than its concentration ($\sim$ 7 mM) in the rat ventral prostate [7].

After castration the spermine-binding activity of the prostate protein fractions decreases to approximately one-half in about one day. Antiandrogens such as cyproterone or flutamide also reduce the activity. A more rapid reduction was seen when normal rats were injected with cycloheximide, an inhibitor of protein synthesis. The half-life of the spermine-binding activity estimated from such an experiment was about 3.5 hours [8]. Injection of androstanolone (DHT) into castrated rats significantly elevated this activity within 30 minutes. The activity returned to the normal level within a few hours after androgen administration.

The androgen effect was considerably less pronounced when castrated rats were injected with a large dose of cycloheximide or dactinomycin. The androgen effect may therefore be dependent on synthesis of new RNA or protein which is needed for induction either of the binding protein or of other factors that can affect the binding activity [8].

The biological significance of the spermine binding activity is not clear. It is conceivable that secretion as well as intracellular translocation or compartmentalization of polyamines is dependent on their binding to certain cellular proteins. Conversely, spermine may assist intracellular relocalization of certain acidic proteins. Thus, androgen may mediate a number of cellular processes which are affected by spermine or by the binding protein.

We found α-protein during cellular fractionation of the steroid binding proteins in rat ventral prostate [1]. Unlike the receptor protein (β-protein) for androgen, α-protein binds androgens weakly. It also binds progestogens and oestrogens, but not glucocorticosteroids. Whereas the androgen-receptor complex readily binds to prostate nuclear chromatin, the androgen-α-protein complex cannot bind tightly to the nuclear chromatin. The most interesting property of α-protein is that it can, with or without an androgen attached, inhibit the androgen-receptor complex from binding to nuclear chromatin [1]. This inhibition is not mimicked by serum albumin or by other major proteins in the prostate. The inhibition does not appear to cause irreversible destruction of the receptor complex or of the nuclear acceptor site [9].

Besides its inhibitory action α-protein can release androgen-receptor complex already attached to nuclear chromatin. To show this we first allowed radioactive receptor complex to bind to prostate nuclei. The nuclei were then washed for removal of excess receptor complex and incubated again either with or without inhibitor (Table II). At a low concentration of the inhibitor (experiment I), a significant loss of radioactivity occurred at 20°C but not at 0°C. At a high concentration of the inhibitor (experiment II) release of radioactivity from chromatin was evident even at 0°C but more obvious at 20°C. Without inhibitor there was no temperature-dependent loss of radioactivity from chromatin. By gradient centrifugation we found that all radioactivity released from the nuclei was associated with a protein that sedimented as 3 S.

Table II Effect of inhibitor on the temperature-dependent release of the radioactive androgen-receptor complex from the nuclear chromatin.

Initial mixture for receptor retention	Second incubation		Radioactive complex retained (counts per minute)	Inhibition (%)
	Additional inhibitor (mg)	Temperature (°C)		
		Experiment I		
Complete	0.0	0	1,083	–
+ Inhibitor	0.0	0	751	31
Complete	1.3	0	1,048	3
Complete	1.3	20	784	28
		Experiment II		
Complete	0.0	0	1,432	–
+ Inhibitor	0.0	0	672	53
Complete	3.0	0	1,114	23
Complete	0.0	20	1,498	–
+ Inhibitor	0.0	20	639	56
Complete	3.0	20	914	39

The prostate cell nuclei were incubated with ^{3}H-DHT-receptor complex (10,000 counts per minute in experiment I and 15,000 in experiment II) in the absence (complete) or presence of inhibitor (1.3 mg in experiment I and 3.0 mg in experiment II) and washed. The washed nuclei were incubated again with or without inhibitor at 0°C or 20°C for 20 minutes and the radioactive receptor complex retained and extractable with 0.4 KCl was measured [9].

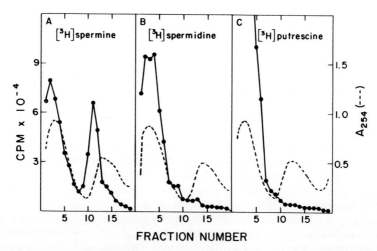

Fig. 1.   Specific spermine binding by a 3 S cytosol protein of the rat ventral prostate. The cytosol was mixed with the radioactive amine (2 µCi) shown and analysed by gradient centrifugation in a linear sucrose gradient (5–20% sucrose containing 20 mM trometamol(tris)-HCl, pH 7.5). Centrifugation was performed with a Spinco SW-56 rotor at 54,000 revolutions per minute at 0–2°C for 20 hours. Fractions (0.2 ml each) were collected and numbered from the top of the centrifuge tube. CPM = counts per minute. (This experiment was performed by Dr. T. Liang in our laboratory.)

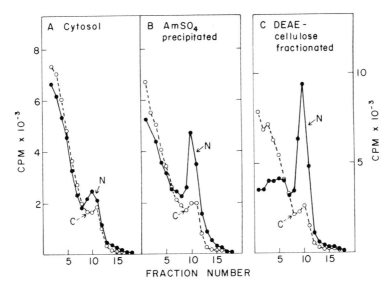

Fig. 2. Effect of castration on the ^{14}C-spermine-binding activity of cytosol proteins. Castration was performed 40 hours prior to the experiment. Ventral prostates from normal (N) or castrated (C) rats (5 rats/group) were homogenized and the cytosol protein fractions isolated. For measurement of polyamine-binding activity, ^{14}C-spermine (0.05 μCi) and edetic acid (EDTA) (final concentration: 4 mM) in 0.2 ml were added to the incubation mixture. 0.2 ml of the mixture was analysed by gradient centrifugation as shown in figure 1, except that the sucrose gradient medium contained 40 mM glycine buffer, pH 8.7. The amounts of protein used were 300 μg cytosol protein in A, 113 μg ammonium sulphate (50–75% saturation)-precipitated protein in B and 30 μg DEAE-cellulose column fractionated protein in C (from Liang et al. [2]).

α-Protein has also been studied more recently by Lea *et al.* [10] and by Heyns *et al.* [11, 12], who referred to it as 'prostate binding protein'. In agreement with these studies, we found that the protein has two major subunits (A and B), each of which contains two subcomponents [13]. The larger subcomponent (molecular weight (mw): 15,000) is a glycopolypeptide which may be a common component in both subunits A and B. No carbohydrate was found in the smaller subcomponents (mw: 10,000 and 14,000, respectively, in A and B). We have purified all components and have determined their amino acid compositions and other chemical properties.

The inhibitory activity of α-protein on chromatin binding of androgen-receptor complex can be mimicked by subunit A, but not by subunit B. The major active component appears to be the small acidic component (mw: 11,000) of subunit A [13]. Although there is no evidence that α-protein or the subunit component can actually regulate the receptor-chromatin interaction in intact prostate cells, the possibility that certain protein factors control binding of receptor to chromatin or promote the release of receptor from the nuclei may be worthy of consideration. Such a protein factor may play a role in maintaining hormonal response at a normal level.

Besides the possibility that a protein factor regulates receptor-chromatin interaction we have suggested that, in the target cells, steroid-receptor complexes may bind to nuclear RNA or to ribonucleoprotein particles (RNP) and may be recycled back to the cytoplasm [14–17]. Receptor binding of

RNA or RNP may be important in protecting RNA from nuclease attack, or in the processing and utilization of RNA needed for protein synthesis.

As a part of our effort to determine the feasibility of such a process we have studied the capacity of many synthetic and natural RNAs to liberate the DHT- and estradiol-receptor complexes from chromatin or deoxyribonucleic acid (DNA). Preliminary investigation has indicated that RNAs with certain nucleotide compositions were far better than others in carrying out this function. Additional studies are needed to show whether this specificity is due to the primary nucleotide sequences or to the secondary and tertiary structure of RNA or RNP.

The studies described above indicate that the nuclear chromatin-receptor interaction is a dynamic process which may be tied directly to the subcellular action of the steroid receptor and may be regulated by cellular factors. We believe that further exploration in this area is important for an understanding of the molecular process involved in hormonal regulation of growth and function of the target cells.

Acknowledgments

This study was supported by Grant BC-151 from the American Cancer Society, Inc., and Grants AM-09461 and HD-07110 from the U.S. National Institutes of Health.

References

1. Fang, S. and Liao, S. (1971): Androgen receptors: steroid- and tissue-specific retention of a 17β-hydroxy-5α-androstan-3-one protein complex by cell nuclei of ventral prostate. *J. Biol. Chem., 246,* 16.
2. Liang, T., Mezzetti, G., Chen, C. and Liao, S. (1978): Selective polyamine-binding proteins: spermine binding by an androgen-sensitive phosphoprotein. *Biochim. Biophys. Acta, 542,* 430.
3. Liang, T. and Liao, S. (1975): A very rapid effect of androgen on the initiation of protein synthesis in the prostate. *Proc. Natl. Acad. Sci. U.S.A., 72,* 706.
4. Liang, T., Castaneda, E. and Liao, S. (1977): Androgen and initiation of protein synthesis in the prostate: binding of Met-tRNA$_f$^{Met} to cytosol initiation factor and ribosomal subunit particles. *J. Biol. Chem., 252,* 5692.
5. Hung, S. C., Liang, T., Gluesing, L. M. and Liao, S. (1976): On the factors effecting the initiation of protein synthesis in the rat ventral prostate: androgens, polyamines, and conjugated protein. *J. Steroid Biochem., 7,* 1001.
6. Mezzetti, G., Loor, R. and Liao, S. (1979): Androgen-sensitive spermine binding protein of rat ventral prostate: purification of the protein and characterization of the hormonal effect. In preparation.
7. Pegg, A. E., Lockwood, D. H. and Williams-Ashman, H. G. (1970): Concentration of putrescine and polyamines and their enzymic synthesis during synthesis androgen-induced prostate growth. *Biochem. J., 117,* 17.
8. Loor, R. M., Mezzetti, G., Chen, C. and Liao, S. (1979): A specific spermine-binding protein in the rat prostate: purification and rapid induction by androgen. *Fed. Proc., 38,* 410.
9. Shyr, C.-I. and Liao, S. (1978): A protein factor that inhibits binding and promotes the release of the androgen-receptor complex. *Proc. Natl. Acad. Sci., U.S.A., 75,* 5969.
10. Lea, O. A., Petrusz, P. and French, F. S. (1977): Prostatein: a dihydrotestosterone binding protein secreted by the rat ventral prostate. *Endocrinology (Suppl.), 100,* 217 (abstract).
11. Heyns, W., Peeters, B. and Mous, J. (1977): Influence of androgens on the concen-

tration of prostatic binding protein (PBP) and its mRNA in rat prostate. *Biochem. Biophys. Res. Commun., 77*, 1492.
12. Heyns, W., Peeters, B., Mous, J., Rombauts, W. and DeMoor, P. (1978): Purification and characterization of prostatic binding protein and its subunits. *Eur. J. Biochem., 89*, 181.
13. Chen, C., Hiipakka, R. A. and Liao, S. (1979): Prostate α-protein: subunit structure, polyamine binding, and inhibition of nuclear chromatin binding of androgen-receptor complex. *J. Steroid Biochem.,* (in press).
14. Liao, S. and Fang, S. (1969): Receptor proteins for androgens and the mode of action of androgens on gene transcription in ventral prostate. *Vitam. Horm., 27*, 17.
15. Liao, S., Tymoczko, J. L., Howell, D. K., Lin, A. H., Shao, T. C. and Liang, T. (1973): Interaction of ribonucleoprotein particles and sex steroid-receptor complexes: a model for receptor cycling and possible function. In: *Endocrinology*, p. 404. Editor: R. O. Scow. Amsterdam, Excerpta Medica.
16. Liao, S., Liang, T. and Tymoczko, J. L. (1973): Ribonucleoprotein binding of steroid-'receptor' complexes. *Nature, New Biol., 241*, 211.
17. Liang, T. and Liao, S. (1974): Association of the uterine 17β-estradiol-receptor complex with ribonucleoprotein *in vivo* and *in vitro. J. Biol. Chem., 249*, 4671.

Discussion

N. Bruchovsky (Edmonton, Canada): Following castration nuclear content of androgen receptor decreases. Is there any evidence that the fall is caused by inhibitory fraction (α-protein), as might be suggested by a post-castration increase in α-protein, either in cytoplasm or the nucleus?

S. Liao: After castration, the α-protein content of the rat ventral prostate appears to decrease at a rate similar to the rate of reduction in the amounts of total tissue proteins in the prostate. The decrease in the nuclear content of androgen receptor after castration may be due to the loss of androgen from the prostate rather than to increase in α-protein.

M. E. Harper (Cardiff, U.K.): Have you measured your spermine-binding protein in other tissues? I am wondering whether this protein is specifically involved in the growth-processes of the prostate alone. It is possible that the prostate cell, which produces spermine in large quantities, needs to bind this compound which, because of its high binding affinity to RNA might interfere with the essential changes in conformation needed for the functioning of various species of RNA.

S. Liao: The polyamine contents in the rat ventral prostate are very high (~ 7 nM). Polyamines may bind to nucleic acids and play important roles in the functions and metabolism of nucleic acids. We do not know, however, how much spermine is actually in the prostate cell or bound to spermine-binding protein. Among ten rat tissues we have checked, only the ventral prostate is rich in this protein. Liver or spleen may have proteins that can bind spermine but they do not seem to be the same protein. We are trying to raise antibody against the binding protein to see whether the protein is prostate specific.

H. J. van der Molen (Rotterdam, The Netherlands): How should we visualize the time schedule of the events which you postulate to occur under the influence of the α-protein? Is there sufficient time for RNA synthesis for the α-protein and for the spermine-binding protein when the effect on the sper-mine-binding protein is so fast?

S. Liao: The androgen effect on the spermine-binding protein is seen about 30 minutes after androgen injection. This is about the length of time required for newly-synthesized RNA to be processed and transported out of the cell nucleus for utilization. The androgen effect on α-protein is a very slow phenomenon and can be seen only several hours after androgen is injected into the castrated rats. If α-protein really plays a role in suppressing nuclear function it probably can do so only after the prostate cell is well-grown and can make and accumulate a large quantity of α-protein.

H. J. van der Molen: Is spermine-binding protein specific to the rat or does it also occur in other species?

S. Liao: We do not know this yet. We will look into this in the near future.

P. M. D. Robel (Bicêtre, France): How do the subunits A and B of α-protein and the subunits of prostate-binding protein compare?

S. Liao: We believe the A and B subunits of α-protein are the same as the F and S subunits of prostate-binding protein studied by Dr. Heyns and his co-workers. Since both groups have antibodies it can easily be checked. We are also determining amino acid sequences of some of the subunit components.

F. Rommerts (Rotterdam, The Netherlands): What is the rationale for the use of glutaraldehyde for fixation of the spermine to the binding pro-tein? How can you prevent the spermine-binding protein complex being bound to other proteins by glutaraldehyde fixation?

S. Liao: We have compared the experimental results obtained by gradient centrifugation and by glutaraldehyde fixation and found that they are very similar in terms of hormonal effect, stability, molecular weight, and many other properties. Apparently glutaraldehyde does not fix spermine to other prostate proteins that do not have a reasonably high affinity to spermine. Glutaraldehyde fixation of ligands to specific binding proteins has been seen in many other cases.

F. H. Schröder (Rotterdam, The Netherlands): Do you have evidence that the amounts of α-protein and spermine receptor protein in the prostate cells are sufficient to play a role in the normal function of these cells?

S. Liao: It is not possible to answer this question since we do not really know the cellular functions of these proteins. Both proteins are present mainly in the cytosol fraction (α-protein, 20–30%; spermine-binding pro-tein, 0.5–1.0%) but they may be compartmentalized in the prostate. α-Pro-tein is a secretory protein. It is present in the prostate fluid and the endo-plasmic reticulum space. Whether an active component of this protein can enter the cell nucleus to regulate the receptor-chromatin interaction is not clear.

K.-D. Voigt (Hamburg, FRG): Your data, I think, are very important, as they allow speculation concerning independent paths of androgen action in target organs. I would therefore like to ask whether it would be conceivable that the spermine receptor complex gets all the transcriptional levels or whether it is also translocated to the nucleus and induces transcriptional events.

S. Liao: This is certainly an important point which we would like to pursue further. We attached radioactive iodine to the spermine-binding protein and studied its interaction with nuclei or chromatin *in vitro* but the iodinated protein was not able to bind tightly to the nuclear components. This does not eliminate the possibility that the protein may play an important role at the nuclear level. The spermine-protein complex may enter nuclei and affect the function of a nuclear protein or an enzyme (such as protein kinase of RNA polymerase) without being tightly bound to it.

Action of anti-androgens on accessory sexual glands

F. Neumann*, K. D. Richter**, B. Schenck***, U. Tunn**** and Th. Senge****
*Research Laboratories of Schering AG, Berlin (West) and Bergkamen; **Universität Münster, Münster; ***Bergmannsheil Bochum, Bochum; and ****Ruhr-Universität Bochum, Marien-Hospital, Herne, Federal Republic of Germany

The accessory sex glands represent classical target organs for androgens and thus also for anti-androgens. As in androgen deprivation following surgical castration, treatment with anti-androgens leads to loss of function and atrophy. In contrast to substances such as oestrogens, which exert an inhibitory effect on testicular androgen biosynthesis via inhibition of gonadotrophin secretion, and particularly luteinizing hormone (LH) secretion, anti-androgens act at cellular level by competition [1–3]. Anti-androgens, unlike oestrogens, are, therefore, also capable of inhibiting the action of exogenously-administered androgens. The agonist/antagonist ratio is relatively favourable. To achieve 50% inhibition of the stimulant action of testosterone propionate, about 3 to 10 times the equivalent amount of cyproterone acetate is required. A tenfold preponderance of the anti-androgen produces almost 100% inhibition of the androgen effect. Figure 1 shows the response of the seminal vesicles of adult, sexually mature rats after 12 days' treatment with increasing doses of cyproterone acetate. A dose-dependent weight decrease occurs. A dose of 3.0 mg/rat/day causes weight reduction of approximately 50%. Figure 2 shows the result of an analogous experiment in dogs, conducted over a 6-month period. The first column indicates the prostate weights of the intact dogs. The dogs in Group 2 were castrated and underwent replacement with an androstanolone metabolite ($3\alpha,17\beta$-androstanediol). The dogs in Group 3 received $3\alpha,17\beta$-androstanediol and cyproterone acetate. It can be seen that the action of the androgen is completely abolished (see also Figures 3 and 4). A decrease in desoxyribonucleic acid (DNA) and ribonucleic acid (RNA) occurs (Figure 5). RNA exhibits the greater reduction. This can be illustrated clearly by forming the DNA/RNA quotient (Figure 6). Figure 7A shows the histology of a highly secretory canine prostate. The animals in question are again castrated dogs which have undergone replacement with $3\alpha,17\beta$-androstanediol. Figure 7B shows the picture following additional administration of cyproterone acetate. Figures 8A and 8B show the same in semithin layer sections. It can be seen that the androgen effect is completely abolished. Total atrophy, particularly of the epithelial portion, results. The influence of anti-androgens causes a loss of

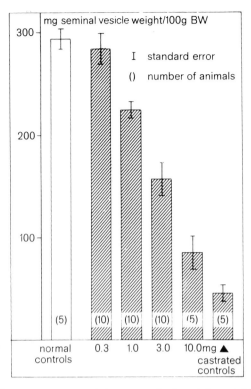

Fig. 1. Influence of cyproterone acetate on seminal vesicle weight of normal male rats (subc. administration for 12 days). BW = body weight.

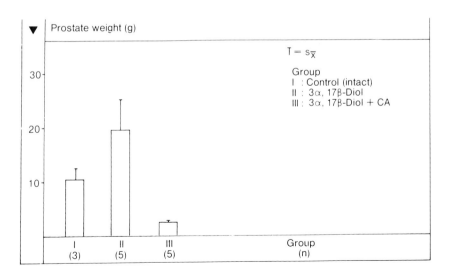

Fig. 2. Effect of 3α,17β-androstanediol and cyproterone acetate on prostate weight in the castrated dog. Duration of treatment: 6 months. Injections were given 3 × weekly. Weekly dose: 3α,17β-androstanediol: 25 mg; cyproterone acetate: 600 mg.

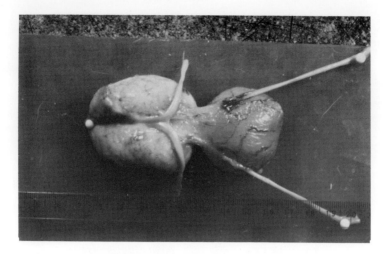

Fig. 3.   Prostate of a castrated dog after 6 months of treatment with 3α,17β-androstanediol (25 mg weekly). Note the prostate hyperplasia.

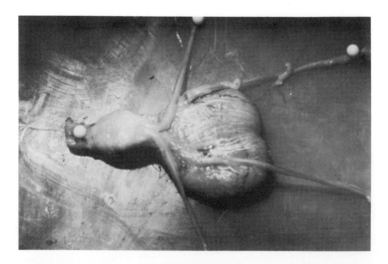

Fig. 4.   Prostate of a castrated dog after 6 months of treatment with 3α,17β-androstanediol (25 mg weekly) and cyproterone acetate (600 mg weekly). Note the total atrophy of the prostate.

the characteristic enzymes and component substances, such as acid phosphatase, aminopeptidase and zinc. Figure 9 shows the zinc content in normal canine prostate, in the prostate of castrated dogs with 3α,17β-androstanediol replacement and also, in Group III, in dogs which received cyproterone acetate in addition. Zinc was measured by means of atomic absorption. The zinc content is seen to decrease by the power of ten under the influence of the anti-androgen. By means of histochemical methods it can be shown that acid phosphatase disappears completely (Figures 10A and B). Zinc can also be demonstrated very well by histochemistry, as is proved by Figure 11A. This

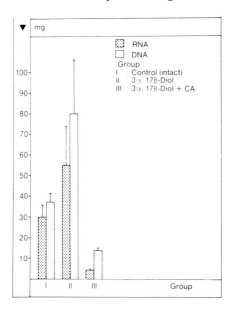

Fig. 5. RNA and DNA content of prostate in the castrated dog after 6-months' s.c. treat-ment with 3α,17β-androstanediol and cyproterone acetate. Weekly dose: 3α,17β-andro-stanediol: 25 mg; cyproterone acetate: 600 mg.

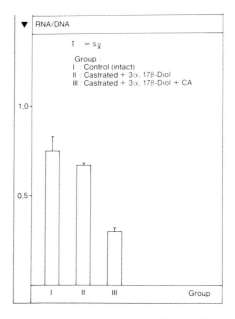

Fig. 6. RNA/DNA-ratio of prostate in the castrated dog after 6-months' treatment with 3α,17β-androstanediol and cyproterone acetate. Weekly dose: 3α,17β-androstanediol: 25 mg; cyproterone acetate: 600 mg.

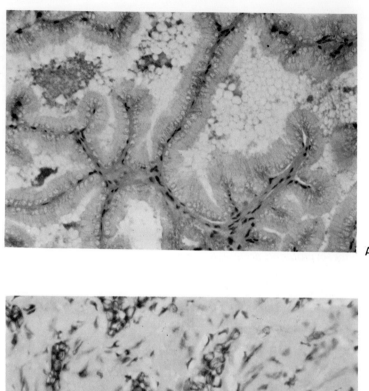

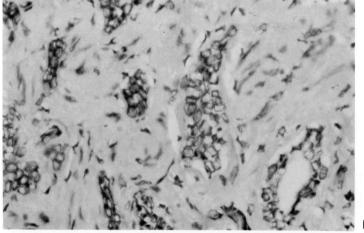

Fig. 7.   Prostate of castrated dogs, A) after 6 months of treatment with 3α,17β-androstane-
diol (25 mg weekly), and B) after 6 months of treatment with 3α,17β-androstanediol (25
mg weekly) and cyproterone acetate (600 mg weekly). Staining: Goldner. Magnification:
a) ca. 120 ×; b) ca. 300 ×.

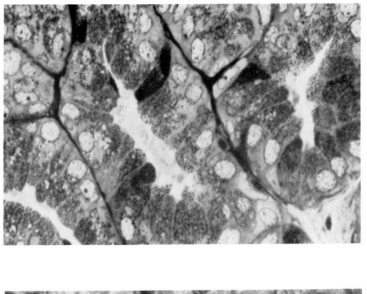

A

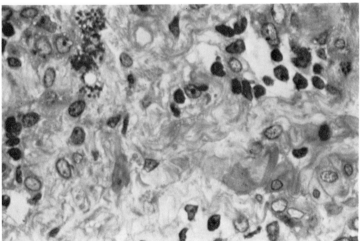

B

Fig. 8. Prostate of castrated dogs (semithin sections), A) after 6 months of treatment with 3α,17β-androstanediol (25 mg weekly) and B) after 6 months of treatment with 3α,17β-androstanediol (25 mg weekly) and cyproterone acetate (600 mg weekly). Staining: Laczkó. Magnification: a) ca. 1200 ×; b) ca. 1200 ×.

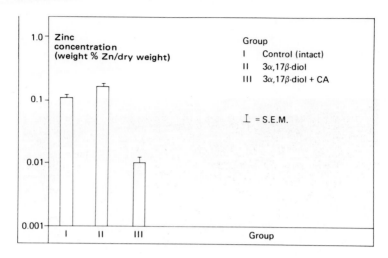

Fig. 9. Zinc concentration of the prostate in the castrated dog after 6-months' treatment with 3α,17β-androstanediol and cyproterone acetate. Weekly dose: 3α,17β-androstanediol: 25 mg; cyproterone acetate: 600 mg.

again shows a canine prostate after 6 months' treatment with the androstanolone metabolite. When cyproterone acetate is administered simultaneously, the histochemical reaction is negative (Figure 11B).

The effectiveness of different anti-androgens depends not only on structure, but also on whether they are so-called 'pure' anti-androgens or anti-androgens of the cyproterone acetate type [1, 4, 5]. Cyproterone acetate, in addition to its anti-androgenic properties, possesses pronounced progestational and thus antigonadotrophic properties [6, 7]. A typical 'pure' anti-androgen is the nonsteroidal compound flutamide. 'Pure' anti-androgens also inhibit the negative feedback effect of androgens at neural (hypothalamic) control centres. An androgen deficit at the periphery is stimulated centrally and consequently an increased gonadotrophin secretion and thus also increased testosterone secretion occurs. Increased LH secretion leads to hyperplasia of the interstitial cells. Figure 12 shows schematically the normal feedback mechanism, figure 13 the feedback mechanism following administration of a 'pure' anti-androgen of the flutamide type. Figure 14 illustrates, by reference to an experiment in intact, sexually mature rats, how, after treatment with flutamide, the LH and, in a parallel manner, the serum testosterone concentrations increase dose-dependently. As a result of increased testosterone secretion, the effects of the anti-androgen become more or less attenuated as time progresses. Anti-androgens of the cyproterone acetate type with additional progestational and thus antigonadotrophic properties behave in a different manner. There is no gonadotrophin stimulation, and therefore also no stimulation of androgen biosynthesis. The hormone levels (LH, testosterone) tend, in fact, to be slightly reduced following treatment with cyproterone acetate, but are never increased. This seems to us to be an important aspect for therapy with anti-androgens. The occurrence of Leydig cell hyperplasia must be expected when non-castrates are treated with 'pure' anti-androgens.

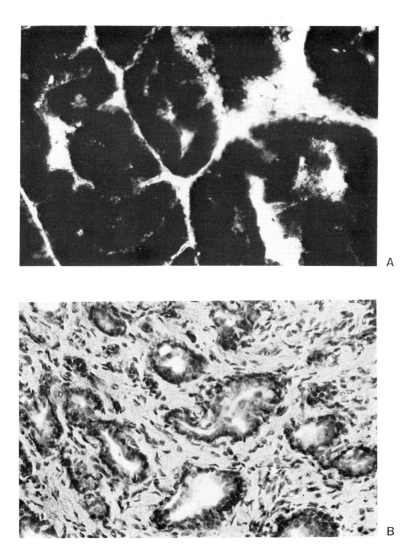

Fig. 10. Prostate of castrated dogs (acid phosphatase), A) after 6 months of treatment with 3α,17β-androstanediol (25 mg weekly) and B) after 6 months of treatment with 3α,17β-androstanediol (25 mg weekly) and cyproterone acetate (600 mg weekly). Magnification: a) 600 ×; b) 300 ×.

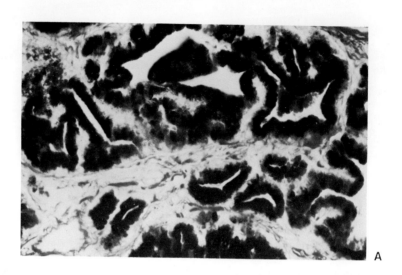

A

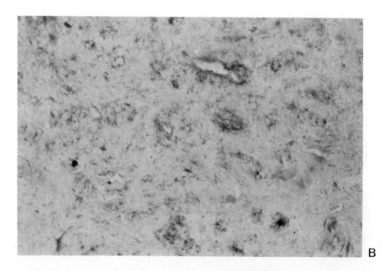

B

Fig. 11. Prostate of castrated dogs (zinc content), A) after 6 months of treatment with 3α,17β-androstanediol (25 mg weekly) and B) after 6 months of treatment with 3α,17β-androstanediol (25 mg weekly) and cyproterone acetate (600 mg weekly). Magnification: a) ca. 600 ×; b) ca. 300 ×.

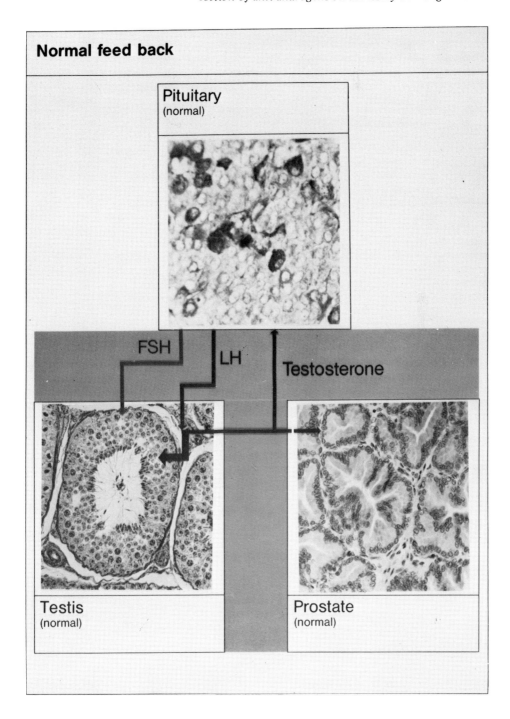

Fig. 12. Normal feedback mechanism.

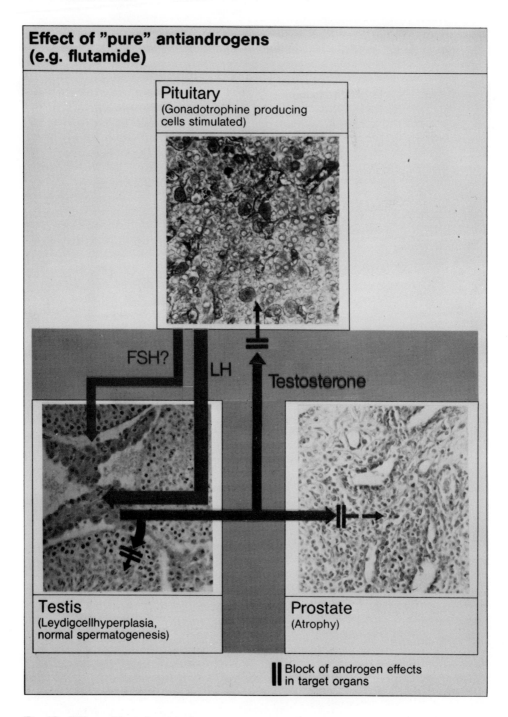

Effect of "pure" antiandrogens (e.g. flutamide)

Pituitary
(Gonadotrophine producing cells stimulated)

FSH?   LH   Testosterone

Testis
(Leydigcellhyperplasia, normal spermatogenesis)

Prostate
(Atrophy)

‖ Block of androgen effects in target organs

Fig. 13. Effect of 'pure' anti-androgen on feedback mechanism.

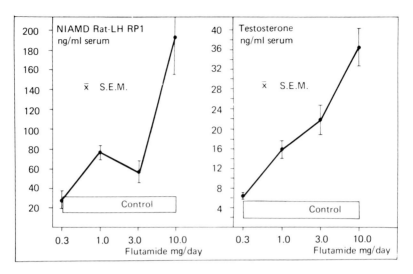

Fig. 14. Serum LH and testosterone levels of adult male rats after 6 weeks of treatment with various doses of flutamide.

Anti-androgens inhibit the function of the 'healthy' prostate. The extent to which prostatic carcinoma is androgen-dependent and, consequently, the extent to which the 'therapeutic' influence of anti-androgens appears advisable and justified is a more difficult question to answer. Hardly any experimental models exist by means of which this question could be examined [8]. With a few exceptions, it has not as yet proved possible to induce prostatic carcinomas by appropriate hormone treatment (androgens). One of the exceptions is a spontaneously occurring adenocarcinoma (R-3227) in the Copenhagen rat. This was first discussed and subsequently reported by Dunning [9]. These tumours were maintained successfully over many generations by transplantation in genetically compatible hosts. It only grows well in intact male rats, less well in females. It does not grow at all in castrated animals [9–13]. Castration of tumour-bearing animals does not result in cure, however; only a prolongation of survival time has been observed [14]. A second exception concerns adenocarcinomas of the dorsal prostate of NB rats following chronic treatment with testosterone propionate or testosterone propionate + estrone [15]. These tumours were likewise transplantable, although all transplantations, with the exception of one tumour, were autonomous. One tumour proved to be oestrogen-dependent and grew only in host animals undergoing oestrogen replacement. The oestrogen-dependency of these tumours is an argument against the utilizability of this model. Adenocarcinomas occasionally occur spontaneously in dogs [16]. The occurrence of adenocarcinomas in the prostate which is present in the female mastomys has also been reported [17]. Mastomys is a virtually undomesticated species of rodent indigenous to Africa. No studies have yet, to our knowledge, been conducted with this model. Our own investigations have, however, shown the prostates of female mastomys to be less androgen-dependent than the prostates of male animals.

Prostatic tumours induced with hydrocarbons generally no longer showed any hormone dependency. In our opinion both facts still apply as regards the

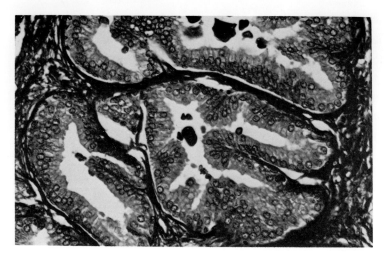

Fig. 15. Human prostate hyperplasia. Staining: Azan. Magnification: 190 ✕.

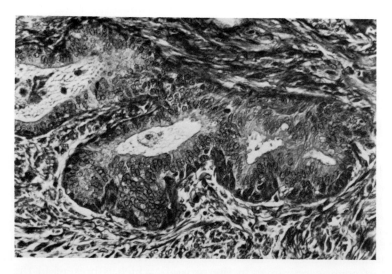

Fig. 16. Treatment of the host animal with testosterone propionate. Staining: Azan. Magnification: 190 ✕.

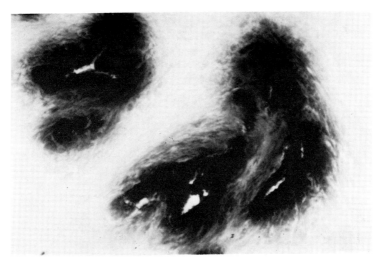

Fig. 17. Treatment of the host animal with testosterone propionate. Note the acid phosphatase activity. Magnification: 190 ×.

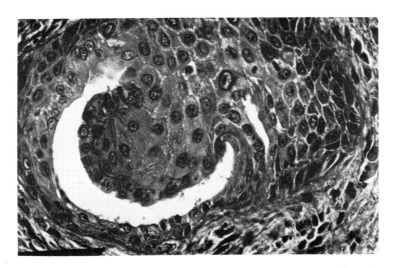

Fig. 18. Treatment of the host animal with testosterone propionate. Note the squamous metaplasia. Staining: Azan. Magnification: 190 ×.

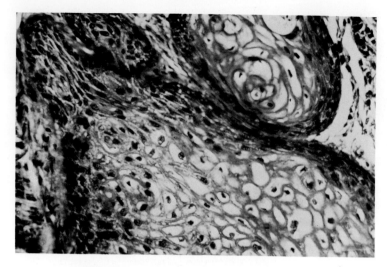

Fig. 19.   Treatment of the host animal with testosterone propionate and cyproterone
acetate. Note the bloated type of degeneration and the pyknosis in the metaplastic
epithelium. Staining: Azan. Magnification: 190 X.

heterologous transplantation of human prostatic carcinomas (e.g., in nude
mice) [8].

Heterotransplantation of human prostatic adenomas has proved to be a
usable model; it was at least possible to demonstrate hormone(androgen)-
dependency [18]. Naturally, the conclusions which this model allows as
regards the effectiveness of a hormone or drug in prostatic carcinomas are
limited. This method is based on the technique developed by Forsberg and
Ingemanson for heterotransplantation of human cervical epithelium into
newborn rats [19]. Immunosuppression is effected by treatment with anti-
lymphocytic serum. As a rule, the duration of the experiment is 14 days to
3 weeks. The viability of the implants is checked by means of histological
and enzyme histochemical methods [20].

Another parameter is the demonstration of active DNA synthesis [21].
Transplants of this kind will even grow without androgen replacement,
although secretory activity is very low. After replacement with testosterone
propionate or androstanolone, the transplants show the typical differentiation already known from prostatic hyperplasia (Figures 15 and 16). The key
enzymes, such as acid phosphatase and zinc, are also demonstrable (Figure
17). Metaplastic changes can be observed almost regularly in the transplants.
The changes in question are of the squamous metaplasia type (Figure 18).
It is interesting to note that this metaplasia reacts to treatment with cyproterone acetate with hydropic degeneration (Figure 19). Prostatic carcinoma
patients on oestrogen therapy are known to display very similar signs of
degeneration in the neoplastic areas of the carcinomatous tissue [22–27]. It
can be concluded from this, with due caution, that cyproterone acetate is
effective in prostatic carcinoma. We know from a controlled multi-centre
study still in progress that, under therapy with cyproterone acetate, distinct
signs of regression have often been observed in punch biopsies [28]. (In this
collaborative study, cyproterone acetate in injection form is being tested

against a depot oestrogen. Only freshly diagnosed cases have been included. Castration is not performed. Punch biopsy material is evaluated centrally by Professor Dhom.) On the other hand, prostatic carcinoma is known to be only partially and intermittently androgen-dependent. Anti-androgens can only be expected to be effective if androgen-dependency is still present.

Facts and considerations in support of the use of anti-androgen therapy in prostatic carcinoma

An assessment of this kind must take into account advantages and disadvantages as compared to oestrogen therapy and orchiectomy. Oestrogens cause a substantial increase in prolactin secretion. Data available to us show the increase of serum prolactin concentrations under cyproterone acetate to be either minimal or absent.

A number of studies have shown that prolactin intensifies the action of androgens on RNA synthesis in the prostate [29]. Androgen uptake into the prostate is also increased by prolactin [30]. Oestrogen therapy causes as marked a reduction of androgen concentrations as orchiectomy, although secretion of the adrenal androgens, above all androstenedione and dehydroepiandrosterone, is unimpaired. A series of studies has revealed that adrenal hyperplasia can even occur on oestrogen therapy and following orchiectomy, and that secretion of adrenal androgens may even be increased [31]. The increased secretion of androgens of adrenal origin is caused by intensified adrenocorticotrophic hormone (ACTH) secretion or greater responsiveness of the adrenal cortex to ACTH. Anti-androgens inhibit the effect of adrenal androgens. ACTH secretion and responsiveness of the adrenal cortex to ACTH is not affected or tends to be lessened.

The loss of responsiveness to oestrogens observed in long-term therapy could be attributable to desensitization of neural centres at which oestrogens exert their negative feedback in respect of gonadotrophin inhibition. Because of their different mechanism of action, however, anti-androgens are very unlikely to display this tendency in therapeutic use. This may be the reason why a number of patients who have developed resistance to oestrogens have reacted to cyproterone acetate with remissions. A form of treatment alternating oestrogens with anti-androgens might indeed be worth trying.

A direct action of oestrogens on the carcinoma cells is controversial. In animal experiments, oestrogens have been found to exert an antimitotic effect virtually only at high doses. Since the oestrogen doses used clinically are relatively low, it is unlikely that they can exert a direct effect on the prostate or the carcinoma cells.

The serious (particularly cardiovascular) side effects of oestrogens do not occur with cyproterone acetate.

We hope that, on conclusion of the controlled multi-centre study (1980?), we shall be in a position to state whether anti-androgens represent a viable alternative to other methods of endocrine therapy of prostatic carcinoma.

References

1. Neumann, F. and Steinbeck, H. (1974): Antiandrogens. In: *Handbook of Experimental Pharmacology*, Vol. 35/2, Chapter VI, pp. 235–484. Editors: O. Eichler, A. Farah, H. Herken and A. D. Welch. Springer Verlag, Berlin, Heidelberg, New York.

2. Mainwaring, W. I. P., Ed. (1977): *The Mechanism of Action of Androgens. Monographs on Endocrinology*, Vol. 10, Springer Verlag, Berlin, Heidelberg, New York.
3. Bruchovsky, N. (1979): Molekularer Wirkungsmechanismus von Androgenen und Antiandrogenen. In: *Androgenisierungserscheinungen bei der Frau*, pp. 7–21. Editors: J. Hammerstein, U. Lachnit-Fixson, F. Neumann and G. Plewig. Excerpta Medica, Amsterdam.
4. Neumann, F., Gräf, K.-J., Hasan, S. H., Schenck, B. and Steinbeck, H. (1977): Central actions of antiandrogens. In: *Androgens and Antiandrogens*, pp. 163–176. Editors: L. Martini and M. Motta. Raven Press, New York.
5. Neumann, F. and Schenck, B. (1976): New antiandrogens and their mode of action. *J. Reprod. Fertil., Suppl. 24*, 129–149.
6. Neumann, F., Elger, W., Nishino, Y. and Steinbeck, H. (1977): Probleme der Dosisfindung: Sexualhormone. *Arzneimittel-Forschung (Drug Research), 27, 2a*, 296–318.
7. Neumann, F., Schleusener, A. and Albring, M. (1979): Pharmakologie der Antiandrogene. In: *Androgenisierungserscheinungen bei der Frau*, pp. 149–194. Editors: J. Hammerstein, U. Lachnit-Fixson, F. Neumann and G. Plewig. Excerpta Medica, Amsterdam.
8. Neumann, F., Richter, K.-D. and Senge, Th. (1975): Animal models in the study of antiprostatic drugs. *Vitam. Horm. (N.Y.), 33*, 103–135.
9. Dunning, W. F. (1963): Prostate cancer in the rat. *Natl. Cancer Inst., Monograph. 12*, 351–369.
10. Voigt, W. and Dunning, W. F. (1974): In vivo metabolism of testosterone-^{3}H in R-3327, and androgen-sensitive rat prostatic cancers of Copenhagen rats. *Cancer Res., 34*, 1447–1450.
11. Voigt, W., Feldman, M. and Dunning, W. F. (1975): 5α-Dihydrotestosterone-binding proteins and androgen sensitivity in prostatic cancers of Copenhagen rats. *Cancer Res., 35*, 1840–1846.
12. Smolev, J. K., Coffey, D. S. and Scott, W. W. (1977): Experimental models for the study of prostatic adenocarcinoma. *J. Urol., 118*, 216–220.
13. Smolev, J. K., Heston, W. D. W., Scott, W. W. and Coffey, D. S. (1977): Characterization of the Dunning R 3327H prostatic adenocarcinoma: an appropriate animal model for prostatic cancer. *Cancer Treat. Rep., 61*, 273–287.
14. Weissman, R. M., Coffey, D. S. and Scott, W. W. (1978): *The effects of castration on survival of animals with prostatic cancer.* American Urology Society, p. 53 (Discussion).
15. Noble, R. L. (1977): Sex steroids as a cause of adenocarcinoma of the dorsal prostate in NB rats, and their influence on the growth of transplants. *Oncology, 3.*
16. Dixon, F. J. and Moore, R. A. (1952): *Atlas of Tumor Pathology*, Section VIII, Fascicles 31 b and 32. Armed Forces Institute of Pathology, Washington.
17. Snell, K. C. and Stewart, H. L. (1965): Adenocarcinoma and proliferative hyperplasia of the prostate gland in female rattus (Mastomys) natalensis. *J. Nat. Cancer Inst., 35*, 7–9.
18. Senge, T., Richter, K. D. and Reis, H. E. (1973): Der Einfluss von Sexualsteroiden auf Prostataadenomheterotransplantate. *Verh. Dtsch. Ges. Urologie, 24*, 234–235.
19. Forsberg, J. G. and Ingemanson, C. A. (1967): Successful growth of human columnar cervical epithelium grafted into neonatal rats. *Acta Obstet. Gynecol. Scand., 46*, 581–590.
20. Richter, K. D., Senge, T. and Reis, H. E. (1971): Morphologisches und cytochemisches Verhalten von menschlichem Prostatagewebe nach Heterotransplantation. *Z. Gesamte Exp. Med., 155*, 253–261.
21. Senge, T., Richter, K. D. and Lunglmayr, G. (1972): Vitality of human adenomatous prostatic tissue grafted into neonatal rats. *Invest. Urol., 10*, 115–119.
22. Faul, P., Klosterhalfen, H. und Schmidt, E. (1971): Erfahrungen mit der Feinnadelbiopsie (Saug- bzw. Aspirationsbiopsie nach Franzén) der Prostata. *Urologe, 10*, 120–126.

23. Franks, L. M. (1960): Estrogen-treated prostatic cancer. *Cancer (Philadelphia), 13,* 490–501.
24. Fergusson, J. D. (1972): The basis of endocrine therapy. In: *Endocrine Therapy in Malignant Disease,* pp. 237–246, Editor: B. Y. Stoll, Saunders, Philadelphia.
25. Huggins, C., Scott, W. W. and Hodges, C. V. (1941): Studies on prostatic cancer. III. The effects of fever, of desoxycorticosterone and of estrogen on clinical patients with metastatic carcinoma of the prostate. *J. Urol., 46,* 997–1006.
26. Kahle, P. I., Schenken, I. R. and Burns, E. L. (1943): Clinical and pathologic effects of diethylstilbestrol and diethylstilbestrol dipropionate on carcinoma of the prostate gland. *J. Urol., 50,* 711–732.
27. Ruppert, H. (1953): Zur Histopathologie der Hormonbehandlung beim Prostatakrebs. *Z. Urol., 46,* 443–456.
28. Dhom, G. (1979): Personal communication.
29. Thomas, J. A. and Manandhar, M. (1975): Effects of prolactin and/or testosterone on nucleic acid levels in prostate glands of normal and castrated rats. *J. Endocrinol., 65,* 149–150.
30. Johansson, R. (1976): Effect of some synandrogens and antiandrogens on the conversion of testosterone to dihydrotestosterone in the cultured rat ventral prostate. *Acta Endocrinol. (Copenhagen), 81,* 398–408.
31. Cowley, T. H., Brownsey, B. G., Harper, M. E., Peeling, W. B. and Griffiths, U. (1976): The effect of ACTH on plasma testosterone and androstenedione concentrations in patients with prostatic carcinoma. *Acta Endocrinol. (Copenhagen), 81,* 310–320.

Discussion

H. Becker (Hamburg, FRG): Did you look for metabolites of $3\alpha,17\beta$-androstanediol in the dog prostate?

F. Neumann: No, we did not.

N. Bruchovsky (Edmonton, Canada): Was there any specific reason for using 3α-androstanediol for inducing prostate hyperplasia?

F. Neumann: No, there was not. The only reason for using the androstanolone metabolite was the fact that the same compound has been used by Walsh and Wilson (*J. Clin. Invest., 57,* 1093 [1978]). As you know, these investigators were not able to induce prostate hyperplasia in dogs by using androstanolone in their first experiment, which was not in beagles.

I have learned in the meantime that they showed androstanolone to be as active as the diol in inducing prostate hyperplasia in beagle dogs. This, of course, makes sense and would have been expected because, as everybody knows, the diol can be transformed back to androstanolone, so both androgens should be identical with regard to their ability to induce prostate hyperplasia in dogs.

M. Krieg (Hamburg, FRG): In what kind of dogs did you induce benign prostatic hyperplasia?

F. Neumann: Adult beagles.

P. M. D. Robel (Bicêtre, France): In the castrated dog, does cyproterone acetate counteract hyperplasia induced by previous treatment with androstanediol?

F. Neumann: We have not completed this experiment up to now. There is one experiment still in progress in which we are following up this problem but it is known from experiments by Neri, Casmer, Zeman, Fielder and Tabachnick (*Endocrinology, 82,* 311 [1968]) and also from veterinary medicine (Schmidtke and Schmidtke, *Kleintier-Praxis, 13,* 146 [1968]) that spontaneously-occurring prostate hyperplasia in dogs can be cured within a few months by treatment with cyproterone acetate at a dose of 1 to 3 mg/kg/day, given orally or subcutaneously.

The role of testosterone metabolism in the mesenchymal induction of the rat prostate gland in vitro

D. R. Bard, I. Lasnitzki and T. Mizuno
Strangeways Research Laboratory, Cambridge, England, and Department of Zoology, Faculty of Science, University of Tokyo, Tokyo, Japan

Induction of the rat prostate gland

The differentiation of the male accessory sex organs, including the prostate gland, depends on the presence of testicular hormones, in particular testosterone. This has been demonstrated by Jost who suppressed the development of the male accessory sex organs in undifferentiated rabbit embryos by surgical castration [1, 2].

The prostate gland develops from its anlage, the urogenital sinus, as epithelial buds projecting into the surrounding mesenchyme, at approximately 19 to 20 days' gestation (Fig. 1). In their pioneering studies, Price and Pannabecker have shown that testosterone or foetal testes promote

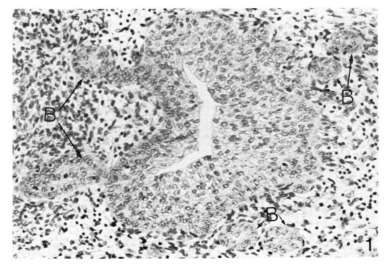

Fig. 1. Urogenital sinus from a 19.5 day rat embryo showing prostatic buds (B) which have penetrated the surrounding mesenchyme. (Haematoxylin-Eosin, ×.370).

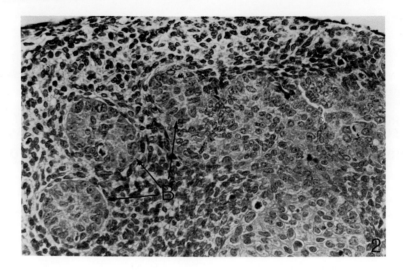

Fig. 2. Urogenital sinus from 16.5 day female rat embryo grown for 5 days with 1.5 µg/ml of testosterone showing development of prostatic buds (B). (Haematoxylin-Eosin, × 370).

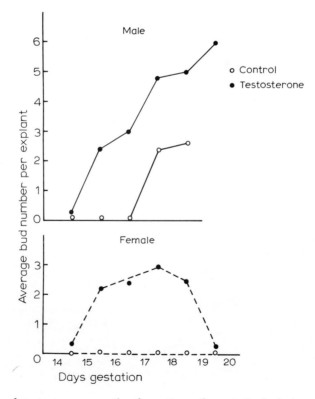

Fig. 3. Effect of testosterone on the formation of prostatic buds in male and female urogenital sinuses grown in organ culture and expressed as average bud number per explant.

differentiation of the gland in rat urogenital tracts grown *in vitro* [3, 4].
However, in their system prostatic buds also appeared in the absence of
testosterone.

This result raised some doubt as to the role of testosterone as an initiator
and it seemed possible that the induction of the gland is due to direct genetic
programming while the hormone supports its further growth and differentiation. The exact role of testosterone in this process has therefore been explored in rat urogenital sinuses grown in organ culture [5]. Sinuses obtained
from 14.5 to 19.5 day embryos were grown on agar clots [6] and exposed
to testosterone or androstanolone (dihydrotestosterone).

Addition of testosterone to the culture medium induced prostatic buds in
the 15.5 and 16.5 day male sinuses (Figs. 2 and 3) but not in the youngest
14.5 day sinus. The older male sinuses formed a small number of buds in the
absence of testosterone while exposure to the hormone increased their
number. Since rat testes begin to synthesize testosterone from an early foetal
stage [7, 8] the appearance of prostatic buds in control medium may be due
to exposure to endogenous testosterone before explantation.

Female sinuses never formed buds in androgen-free medium; testosterone
induced them in all except the youngest and the oldest sinus (Fig. 3).

Using 16.5 day male sinuses, the effect of testosterone was also examined
as a function of dose (Fig. 4); it was found that a concentration of 0.0015
μg/ml of medium was already highly effective in eliciting prostatic buds.

Androstanolone proved to be at least as active as testosterone and increased
the number of buds formed over that after testosterone treatment (Fig. 5).
In addition, the hormone elicited bud formation in the youngest (14.5 day)
sinuses of both sexes. The result suggests that their failure to respond to
testosterone is due to a lack of 5α-reductase and that the synthesis of the
enzyme may start between day 14 and 15 of foetal development.

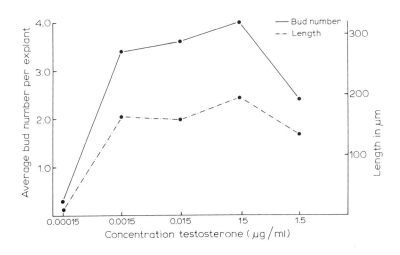

*Fig. 4. Effect of testosterone on prostatic bud formation on 16.5 day male urogenital
sinuses grown in organ culture as function of dose and expressed as average bud number
and length per explant.*

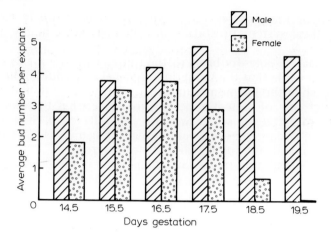

Fig. 5. Effect of androstanolone on the formation of prostatic buds in rat male and female urogenital sinuses grown in organ culture expressed as average bud number per explant.

Role of the mesenchyme

In organ culture the two main tissue components, epithelium and stroma, are preserved *in vitro*. In this system, foetal and postnatal prostate glands remain androgen-dependent and responsive [3–5, 9–11]. In contrast, mouse and human prostatic epithelium separated from its stroma did not respond to testosterone [12] or broke down [13]. Similarly, isolated rat urogenital epithelium was found to be no longer hormone-responsive [9]. If cultured in the presence of testosterone or androstanolone the cells failed to form prostatic buds and after a few days showed signs of degeneration (Fig. 6) and finally broke down. Since androstanolone was as ineffective as testosterone the breakdown of the epithelium could not be attributed to a loss of 5α-reductase.

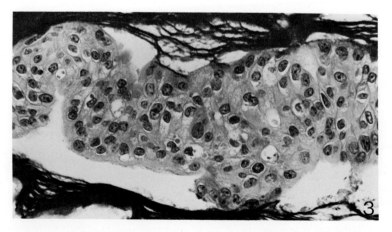

Fig. 6. Epithelium isolated from 16.5 day male urogenital sinus and grown protected by vitelline membrane for 5 days in presence of testosterone. The cells have lost their polarity and show cytoplasmic vacuolisation. (Haematoxylin-Eosin, × 450).

Experiments by Cunha involving cultivation of epithelial-mesenchymal recombinants followed by implantation into male hosts indicate a decisive role of the mesenchyme in the morphogenesis of the mouse prostate [14]. However, his final result may have been modified by the presence of other hormones in the host. This possible complication can be avoided by using an *in vitro* system throughout. The influence of the mesenchyme on the induction of the rat prostate has, therefore, been studied in recombinants of urogenital epithelium and mesenchyme with each other (Fig. 7) and with heterotypic epithelia and mesenchymes grown in organ culture [9].

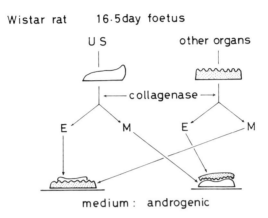

Fig. 7. *Arrangement of experiment to separate and recombine epithelium (E) and mesenchyme (M) from urogenital sinus (US) or other organs.*

Epithelium and mesenchyme from 16.5 day male or female rat foetuses were separated by treatment with collagenase and the completeness of the separation and viability of the two tissues confirmed by light microscopy. Urogenital epithelium was combined with urogenital mesenchyme or with mesenchymes derived from bladder, stomach or skin from foetuses at the same stage of development, grown in the presence of testosterone or androstanolone. In all cases the epithelium remained viable but formed prostatic buds only in association with urogenital mesenchyme. Conversely, epithelia from bladder, stomach or skin, when combined with urogenital mesenchyme, failed to develop prostatic buds.

These results pointed to a mutual specificity between sinus epithelium and sinus mesenchyme but it was not clear whether bud formation was due to hormone-primed epithelium or hormone-primed mesenchyme. This was explored in recombinants of androgen-pretreated and untreated urogenital epithelia and mesenchymes. The design of the experiment (Fig. 8) was based on the finding [5] that in the 16.5 day sinus a short exposure to testosterone followed by cultivation in androgen-free medium suffices to induce prostatic buds. Urogenital sinuses were exposed to testosterone or androstanolone for 24 hours and then separated by collagenase. Androgen-treated epithelium was combined with untreated mesenchyme, and untreated epithelium with androgen-treated mesenchyme and the recombinants grown for 4 days in hormone-free medium. The table shows that androgen-pretreated mesenchyme induces buds in most of the untreated epithelia (Fig. 9) while recombinants of pretreated epithelia with untreated mesenchyme were much less active: prostatic buds were either few in number and small or absent (Fig. 10).

The greater effectiveness of the androgen-treated mesenchyme suggested that it plays an active part in the induction of the gland and may be a target for androgens.

It is now thought that, as in the mature organ [15, 16], the induction and

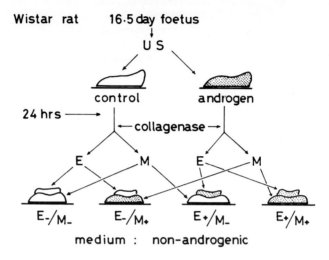

Fig. 8.   Arrangement of experiment to recombine androgen-treated and untreated urogenital epithelia and mesenchymes. + treated with androgens; − untreated.

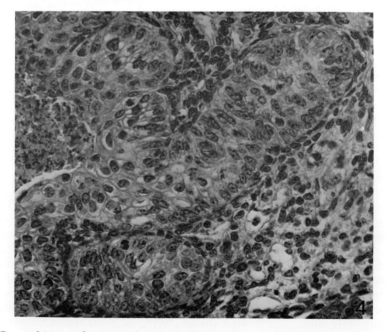

Fig. 9. Recombinant of untreated urogenital epithelium with testosterone-treated mesenchyme grown for 4 days without androgens. Note development of prostatic buds. (Haematoxylin-Eosin, × 370).

Table *Average bud number per explant and bud length in recombinants of untreated (−) and testosterone (T) – or androstanolone (DHT) – pretreated urogenital epithelium (E) and mesenchyme (M).*

Recombination		Bud formation	Average bud number	Bud length in μm
E_-	$/M_-$	0/14	0.0	0
E_-	$/M_T$	18/20	1.5 ± 0.16	169 ± 26
E_-	$/M_{DHT}$	9/11	1.4 ± 0.24	142 ± 36
E_T	$/M_-$	6/20	0.3 ± 0.12	18 ± 7
E_{DHT}	$/M_-$	7/11	0.7 ± 0.18	33 ± 9
E_T	$/M_T$	14/14	2.7 ± 0.26	143 ± 12

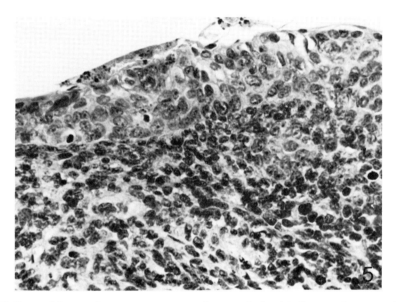

Fig. 10. *Recombinant of testosterone-treated urogenital epithelium and untreated mesenchyme grown for 4 days in androgen-free medium. Note absence of prostatic buds. (Haematoxylin-Eosin, × 370).*

differentiation of the foetal prostate by testosterone is mediated by its principal metabolite androstanolone [17]. The intact sinus converts testosterone to androstanolone [18] but it is not certain whether the conversion occurs in the epithelium or mesenchyme, or in both.

Metabolism of testosterone

The conversion of testosterone was measured by thin layer chromatography [19] in urogenital epithelia and mesenchyme from 17 day male and female sinuses separated by collagenase treatment and compared with that shown by the whole sinus [20]. The results were expressed as pM (= $M \times 10^{-12}$) per mg of deoxyribonucleic acid (DNA). The volume of the mesenchyme in the whole sinus greatly exceeded that of the epithelium and separated mesenchyme contained 13−15 times as much DNA as epithelium from the same number of sinuses.

Epithelium, mesenchyme and intact sinus from both sexes reduced testosterone to androstanolone and in epithelium this androgen was the principal metabolite. Although epithelium formed much more androstanolone than the mesenchyme or the intact sinus, most of it was released into medium and tissue levels were similar in all three types of explants (Fig. 11).

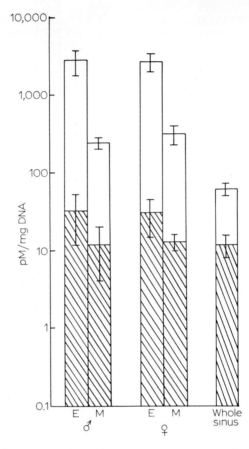

Fig. 11. Formation of androstanolone from testosterone in isolated male and female urogenital epithelia (E), mesenchyme (M) and whole sinus. Concentration in medium: □. Concentration in tissue: ▨.

The whole sinus and its separate components also formed $3\alpha,17\beta$-androstanediol, androstanedione and androsterone (Figs. 12–14). Thus, epithelium formed 80–100 times as much androstanedione as mesenchyme, but only half as much $3\alpha,17\beta$-androstanediol when the results are expressed as pM/mg DNA. If allowance is made for the different volumes of tissue in the whole sinus these ratios become 6 and 0.04 respectively. Androsterone, a relatively minor metabolite in both isolated epithelium and mesenchyme, was produced by the whole sinus in quantities almost equal to those of androstanolone and tissue levels (pM/mg DNA) were 8–10 times higher than in either component.

This last observation suggests that, in the whole sinus, the 3α- and 17β-hydroxysteroid dehydrogenases, located in the mesenchyme and epithelium

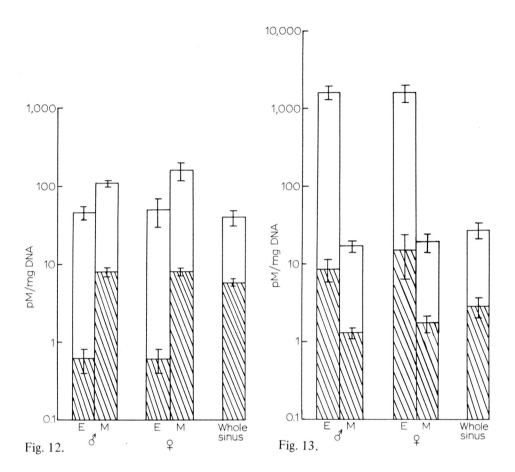

Fig. 12.   Fig. 13.

Fig. 12.   Formation of 3α,17β-androstanediol from testosterone in isolated male and female urogenital epithelia (E), mesenchyme (M) and whole sinus. Concentration in medium: □. Concentration in tissue: ▨.

Fig. 13.   Formation of androstanedione from testosterone in isolated male and female urogenital epithelia (E), mesenchyme (M) and whole sinus. Concentration in medium: □. Concentration in tissue: ▨.

respectively, act together to convert androstanolone to androsterone, the intermediates 3α,17β-androstanediol and androstanedione moving freely between the two tissues. It is tempting to speculate that androsterone, a potent androgen in its own right [16] may have a separate role, distinct from that of androstanolone in the induction of the rat prostate.

Summary and conclusions

Testosterone and androstanolone induce prostate glands *de novo* in rat urogenital sinuses grown in organ culture and the mesenchyme plays a decisive role in this process.

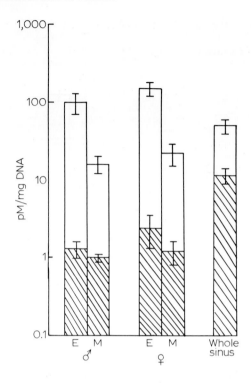

Fig. 14. Formation of androsterone from testosterone in isolated male and female uro-genital epithelia (E), mesenchyme (M) and whole sinus. Concentration in medium: ☐. Concentration in tissue: ▧.

Measurements of testosterone metabolism in isolated urogenital epi-thelium and mesenchyme show that both tissues convert testosterone to various metabolites, although in different proportions, and that the principal metabolite is androstanolone. The whole sinus also forms androsterone in similar quantities to androstanolone and it is possible that androsterone, in addition to androstanolone, is involved in the differentiation of the rat prostate gland.

Acknowledgments

We are indebted to the Ministry of Education, Science and Culture of Japan for a grant-in-aid for cancer research. Ilse Lasnitzki is a Leverhulme Emeritus Fellow.

References

1. Jost, A. (1953): Problems of foetal endocrinology: the gonadal and hypophyseal hormones. *Recent Prog. Horm. Res., 8,* 379.
2. Jost, A. (1968): Modalities in the action of androgens on the foetus. *Research on Steroids, 3,* 207.
3. Price, D. and Pannabecker, R. (1956): Organ culture studies of the foetal reproduc-tive tracts. *Ciba Foundation Colloquia on Aging, 2,* 3.
4. Price, D. and Pannabecker, R. (1959): Comparative responsiveness of homologous

sex ducts and accessory glands of foetal rats in culture. *Arch. Anat. Microsc. Morphol. Exp., 48*, 223.

5. Lasnitzki, I. and Mizuno, T. (1977): Induction of the rat prostate gland by androgens in organ culture. *J. Endocrinol., 74*, 47.
6. Wolff, E. and Haffen, K. (1952): Sur une méthode de culture d'organes embryonnaires *in vitro. Tex. Rep. Biol. Med., 10*, 463.
7. Noumura, T., Weisz, J. and Lloyd, C. W. (1966): *In vitro* conversion of 7⁻³ progesterone to androgens by the rat testis during the second half of foetal life. *Endocrinology, 78*, 245.
8. Warren, D. G., Haltmeyer, G. C. and Eik-Nes, K. B. (1973): Testosterone in foetal rat testis. *Biol. Reprod., 8*, 560.
9. Lasnitzki, I. and Mizuno, T. (1979): Role of the mesenchyme in the induction of the rat prostate gland in organ culture. *J. Endocrinol.*, in press.
10. Lasnitzki, I. (1976): The action of androgens on rat prostate glands in organ culture. In: *Organ Cultures in Biomedical Research*, p. 241. Editors: M. Balls and M. A. Monnickendam. Cambridge University Press, Cambridge.
11. Gittinger, J. W. and Lasnitzki, I. (1972): The effect of testosterone metabolites on the fine structure of the rat prostate gland in organ culture. *J. Endocrinol., 52*, 459.
12. Franks, L. M. and Barton, A. A. (1960): The effects of testosterone on the ultrastructure of the mouse prostate *in vivo* and in organ culture. *Exp. Cell Res., 19*, 35.
13. Franks, L. M., Riddle, P. N., Carbonell, A. W. and Gey, G. O. (1970): A comparative study of the ultrastructure and lack of growth capacity of adult human prostatic epithelium separated from its stroma. *J. Pathol., 100*, 113.
14. Cunha, G. R. (1976): Epithelial stromal interactions in development of the urogenital tract. *Int. Rev. Cytol., 47*, 137.
15. Bruchovsky, N. and Wilson, J. D. (1968): The conversion of testosterone to 5-androstan-17β-ol-3-one by rat prostate *in vivo* and *in vitro. J. Biol. Chem., 243*, 2012.
16. Baulieu, E. E., Lasnitzki, I. and Robel, P. (1968): Metabolism of testosterone and action of metabolites on prostate glands grown in organ culture. *Nature (London), 219*, 1155.
17. Wilson, J. D. and Siiteri, P. K. (1973): The role of steroid hormones in sexual differentiation. In: *Aspects in Fetal Endocrinology*, p. 1051. Editor: R. O. Scaw. Elsevier Publishing Company Inc., New York.
18. Wilson, J. D. and Lasnitzki, I. (1971): Dihydrotestosterone formation in fetal tissues of the rabbit and rat. *Endocrinology, 89*, 659.
19. Lasnitzki, I. and Franklin, H. R. (1972): The influence of serum on the uptake, conversion and action of testosterone in rat prostate glands in organ culture. *J. Endocrinol., 54*, 333.
20. Bard, D. R., Lasnitzki, I. and Mizuno, T. (1979): Metabolism of testosterone by isolated epithelium and mesenchyme of the rat urogenital sinus. *J. Endocrinol.*, in press.

Discussion

F. Neumann (West Berlin, Germany): Have you also tested other compounds like oestrogens and antiandrogens in your model? I think this is an ideal model to answer the question whether oestrogens have a direct effect on the prostate or not.

I. Lasnitzki: We have studied the effect of oestradiol and cyproterone acetate on the induction of the rat prostate and found that both compounds inhibit the formation of prostatic buds in the 16.5 day sinus but do not affect it in the older, 18.5 day sinus. The difference in response may be connected with the fact that the older sinuses have been exposed to endogenous testosterone before explantation.

F. H. Schröder (Rotterdam, The Netherlands): Did you check the purity of the separation of stroma and epithelium prior to recombination and how did you do this? Could impurity explain the presence of reduction in both fractions?

I. Lasnitzki: The completeness of the separation of epithelium and stroma was examined by light microscopy. We never found any tags of epithelium adhering to the mesenchyme or vice versa. In contrast to adult tissues, separation is usually easier in embryonic tissues, particularly in the urogenital sinus which consists of one discrete mass of epithelium surrounded by mesenchyme. Although 5α-reduction was present in both components the proportion of metabolites formed was different in epithelium and stroma.

F. Rommerts (Rotterdam, The Netherlands): Are the steroid concentrations of the various metabolites in medium and cells steady state concentrations or are they changing during the incubation period? This is important for correlation of cellular-steroid concentration and physiological effects.

I. Lasnitzki: In the tissue, the metabolites reach a steady state concentration after approximately 12 hours' incubation.

K.-D. Voigt (Hamburg, West Germany): You very nicely demonstrated the age dependency of bud formation in prostate. Does there also exist a dose dependency?

I. Lasnitzki: We have examined prostatic bud formation in the 16.5 day sinus as a function of testosterone concentration. The hormone induced an appreciable number of buds at a concentration of $5 \times 10^{-9}M$ and the optimum effect was seen after a concentration of $5 \times 10^{-7}M$.

K.-D. Voigt: You explained the insensitivity of this process, at the very early stage to testosterone, but not DHT, by a lack in 5α-reductase activity. Do you have clinical evidence for that assumption?

I. Lasnitzki: No.

Prostatic binding protein (PBP): an androgen-dependent protein secreted by rat ventral prostate

W. Heyns
Laboratory for Experimental Medicine, Rega Institute, Leuven, Belgium

The binding of androgens to the androgen receptor in rat ventral prostate has been the subject of numerous investigations [1]. A constant finding in these studies is the presence in this organ of a marked degree of non-receptor binding. It has been shown [2, 3] that this non-receptor binding is due to an abundant 'prostatic binding protein' (PBP) which has been purified and characterized [4]. This communication summarizes some of our results on the properties of this protein, its physiological significance and the mechanism of its regulation by androgens.

Steroid-binding properties

PBP binds a number of non-polar steroids with relatively low affinity [2, 3]. The strongest binding is observed for pregnenolone and androstenedione but other steroids such as testosterone and androstanolone also show significant binding. Because of the very high concentration of the protein this binding is not negligible in spite of its low affinity. Furthermore, binding increases markedly after moderate heating or after delipidation.

General properties [3, 4]

The native protein has an estimated molecular weight (mw) of 50,000 and a sedimentation coefficient in sucrose density gradients of 3.7 S. Under denaturing conditions (sodium dodecylsulphate (SDS), guanidine) the purified protein dissociates into 2 different subunits (F and S), which differ in size and amino acid composition. Reduction of disulphide bridges results in a further dissociation of each subunit into 2 components. Subunit F dissociates into component 1 (mw 8,000) and component 3 (mw 14,000), subunit S into component 2 (mw 10,500) and component 3.

Location of PBP

By measurement of its binding activity it could be shown [2, 3] that PBP is located primarily in the rat ventral prostate and that it is also secreted by this gland. This observation has been confirmed with a more sensitive immunological technique [5]. Using immunofluorescence the largest fraction of PBP is found at the apical border of the epithelial cells and within the acinar lumen. The detection of measurable amounts of this protein in prostatic fluid, rat semen and male rat urine also confirms that it is secreted by the prostate.

Concentration of PBP in prostatic cytosol as a function of age

PBP is present in low but detectable amounts in the prostates of 5-day old rats. From day 15 on its relative concentration increases gradually, reaching about 46% of the total cytosolic protein in adult rats [5].

Effect of castration and hormonal treatment

Castration results in a gradual but marked decrease in total PBP content and also of the relative concentration of PBP [5]. After 21 days the amount of PBP is only 0.5% of the control while its concentration has decreased to 3.9% of total protein. Administration of androgens to castrated rats, on the other hand, produces a marked increase in PBP content and relative concentration. This is not the case for estradiol, progesterone or cyproterone acetate. The latter steroid, however, counteracts stimulation by androgens.

In vitro synthesis of PBP by prostatic slices

After incubation of prostatic slices with ^{3}H-leucine, incorporation of the latter into PBP was measured by specific immunoprecipitation [6]. In prostates of intact adult rats 31.8% of the newly-formed peptides corresponded to PBP. This value went down to 6.9% 7 days after castration and returned to 22.9% after 4 days of treatment with testosterone. These data indicate that PBP synthesis occurs in the prostate and that this synthesis is regulated by androgens.

Translation of prostatic messenger ribonucleic acid (mRNA)

Addition of prostatic ribonucleic acid (RNA) to a cell-free translation system derived from wheat germ [7] or microinjection of prostatic RNA into Xenopus oocytes [8] results in both cases in the formation of peptides which are immunologically related to PBP. In Xenopus oocytes these peptides are identical to the components of native PBP but in wheat germ they have a slightly different size, probably indicating that precursor proteins are formed which need further processing. The mRNA activity of prostatic RNA decreases strongly after castration with a specific effect on the mRNA activity corresponding to PBP, which amounts to 29.7% of the total mRNA activity in intact rats and 4.9% in 6-day castrated rats. Conversely, androgen treatment results in a specific increase in mRNA activity. Consequently, androgens act on PBP levels through changes of its mRNA and thus, probably, by transcriptional regulation.

Discussion and conclusions

The rat ventral prostate contains and secretes large amounts of a protein which we have called PBP because of its steroid-binding properties. This protein, which has been purified and characterized, is probably responsible for the 'receptor' binding of pregnenolone [9] and for the 'α-protein' binding of androgens [10] observed in this organ. It is also likely that it is identical with prostatein, a major protein in rat ventral prostate, recently described [11].

The function of this protein is unknown and it is not sure that the steroid-binding properties are of functional importance. Indeed, the affinity for natural steroids is low, although it was reported at this meeting by Gustafsson *et al.* that there is very strong binding of the synthetic steroid derivative estramustine. The secretion of PBP in semen suggests that it plays a role in reproductive physiology. It is unknown at present whether similar proteins are present in the prostates of other species but our preliminary data on canine and human prostate are negative.

In spite of lack of a clear insight into its role, PBP has some interest for the study of the mechanism of action of androgens, for investigation of the action of which the rat ventral prostate constitutes a classical model system. Consequently, the presence of a major androgen-dependent protein in this organ forms an interesting end-point for such studies. In fact, the androgen-dependent changes in concentration and synthesis of PBP and of its mRNA are in good agreement with the observation of major changes in abundant populations of mRNA, described recently [12]. These data strongly suggest a transcriptional control mechanism, although other factors such as cell proliferation may also be involved.

Acknowledgments

The author thanks D. Bossyns, P. De Moor, M. Hertogen, J. Mous, B. Peeters, W. Rombauts and B. Van Damme for their contribution to these investigations. This investigation was supported by Grant 20168 of the Fund for Medical Scientific Investigation and by Grant OT/VI/34 of the Research Fund of the Catholic University of Leuven.

References

1. Mainwaring, W. I. P., Ed. (1977): *The Mechanism of Action of Androgens.* Springer Verlag, New York, Heidelberg, Berlin.
2. Heyns, W., Verhoeven, G. and De Moor, P. (1976): A comparative study of androgen binding in rat uterus and prostate. *J. Steroid Biochem., 7,* 987–991.
3. Heyns, W. and De Moor, P. (1977): Prostatic binding protein: a steroid-binding protein secreted by rat prostate. *Eur. J. Biochem., 78,* 221–230.
4. Heyns, W., Peeters, B., Mous, J., Rombauts, W. and De Moor, P. (1978): Purification and characterisation of prostatic binding protein and its subunits. *Eur. J. Biochem., 89,* 181–186.
5. Heyns, W., Van Damme, B. and De Moor, P. (1978): Secretion of prostatic binding protein. Influence of age and androgen. *Endocrinology, 103,* 1090–1095.
6. Heyns, W., Peeters, B., Mous, J., Rombauts, W. and De Moor, P. (1979): Androgen dependent synthesis of a prostatic binding protein by rat prostate. *J. Steroid Biochem., 11,* 209–213.
7. Heyns, W., Peeters, P. and Mous, J. (1977): Influence of androgens on the concentration of prostatic binding protein (PBP) and its mRNA in rat prostate. *Biochem. Biophys. Res. Commun., 77,* 1492–1499.
8. Mous, J., Peeters, B., Rombauts, W. and Heyns, W. (1977): Synthesis of rat prostatic binding protein in Xenopus oocytes and in wheat germ. *Biochem. Biophys. Res. Commun., 79,* 1111–1116.

9. Karsznia, R., Wyss, R. H., Leroy Heinrichs, W. M. and Herrmann, W. L. (1969):
Binding of pregnenolone and progesterone by prostatic 'receptor' proteins. *Endocrinology, 84,* 1238–1246.
10. Fang, A. and Liao, S. (1971): Androgen receptors. Steroid- and tissue-specific retention of 17β-hydroxy-5α-androstan-3-one protein by the cell nuclei of ventral prostate. *J. Biol. Chem., 246* 16–24.
11. Lea, O. A., Petrusz, P. and French, F. S. (1977); Isolation and characterization of prostatein, a major secretory protein of rat ventral prostate. *Fed. Proc., 36,* 780 (Abstract).
12. Parker, M. G. and Scrace, G. T. (1978): The androgenic regulation of abundant mRNA in rat ventral prostate. *Eur. J. Biochem., 85,* 399–406.

Discussion

N. Bruchovsky (Edmonton, Canada): In view of the observation by Dr. Robel that most of the intracellular androstanolone is found in the nucleus; do you think that PBP has any role in the retention of androstanolone by the cell?

W. Heyns: The retention of androstanolone occurs indeed mainly in the nuclei of the prostate whereas the largest amount of PBP is found extracellularly. For this reason it is unlikely that PBP plays a role in the intracellular retention of androstanolone although it may have an effect on the accumulation or retention of some steroids or steroid derivatives within the organ.

P. M. D. Robel (Bicêtre, France): How do you compare the subunits A and B of α-protein and the subunits of PBP?

W. Heyns: The F and S subunits described by us are observed during polyacrylamide gel electrophoresis in the presence of SDS which leads to dissociation of the protein. The A and B forms of Liao, on the other hand, are observed during polyacrylamide gel electrophoresis performed without SDS. They probably arise from spontaneous dissociation. From a comparison of both techniques it seems likely that the A form corresponds to the F subunit and the B form to the S subunit.

New aspects of androgen action in prostatic cells: stromal localization of 5α-reductase, nuclear abundance of androstanolone and binding of receptor to linker deoxyribonucleic acid

N. Bruchovsky, P. S. Rennie and R. P. Wilkin
Department of Medicine, University of Alberta, Edmonton, Canada

Introduction

Androstanolone is accumulated in the prostate by a complex process sustained by stromal-epithelial interactions, steroid-converting enzymes, binding reactions between androgen receptors and deoxyribonucleic acid (DNA) and possibly receptor-independent transport mechanisms within the cell. Fully integrated, this system yields a whole-tissue concentration of androstanolone of 130–210 ng (= g × 10^{-9})/100 g tissue in normal prostate [1, 2]. The resultant concentration in benign prostatic hyperplasia (BPH), however, is considerably higher at 400–1,300 ng/100 g tissue [1–5] while in carcinoma it falls at an intermediate level [3, 4, 6]. These differences are illustrated by the data in figure 1A. Concerning the excessive capacity of BPH to retain androstanolone, Bruchovsky and Lieskovsky [7] have suggested that this is due to an approximately 3-fold increase in the activity of 5α-reductase (Figure 1B). However, since the concentration of androstanolone in prostatic carcinoma is high (Figure 1A) relative to the activity of 5α-reductase (Figure 1B) it remains possible that the enzyme is not a major factor contributing to the accumulation of androstanolone.

In studying the pathogenesis of BPH, Cowan *et al.* [8] found that the greater part of the 5α-reductase activity in BPH tissue was localized in stroma. Their data, taken together with the results of Bruchovsky and Lieskovsky (Figure 1B; reference [7]), imply that BPH stroma is characterized by a raised level of 5α-reductase activity. The experiments described in our present report were designed to test this premise. In addition we examined two other aspects of the regulation of androgen uptake by the prostate, namely the relationship between the quantity of receptor and the steady-state concentration of androstanolone and the role of DNA in fostering the nuclear retention of androgen receptor.

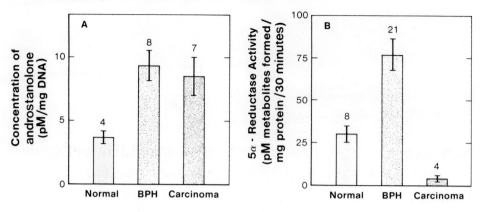

Fig. 1. Concentration of androstanolone and 5α-reductase activity in human prostate. Whole-tissue homogenates of prostatic tissue were analysed for (A) the concentration of androstanolone as determined by radioimmunoassay and (B) the activity of 5α-reductase. Data in B are modified from Bruchovsky and Lieskovsky [7].

Materials and methods

Tissue specimens

Normal prostates were obtained either at autopsy 2–15 hours after death or from brain-dead kidney donors. The age range of this group was 17–71 years. Hyperplastic prostates were obtained within 1 hour of suprapubic or retropubic extirpation. The age of the patients with BPH ranged from 53–90 years. Carcinomatous tissue was obtained at the time of radical prostatectomy. The age range of the cancer patients was 59–73 years. In each instance the diagnosis was confirmed by pathological examination. Studies on malignant tissue were confined to well-differentiated carcinoma.

At the time of operation or autopsy, the prostates were quickly chilled and brought on ice to the laboratory. The specimens were divided into smaller samples usually weighing 1–3 g and either processed immediately or stored in plastic jars at −80°C until analysed.

Homogenization of stroma and epithelium

Separation of prostate into stromal and epithelial fractions was accomplished by forcing finely minced tissue through a stainless steel wire screen (30 mesh, 0.55 mm grid) with a Teflon pestle. Fragments of epithelium were collected by intermittently percolating a total of 30 ml of 0.01 M TES buffer, pH 7.0 containing 0.5 mM mercaptoethanol and 0.05 M NaCl (incubation buffer) through the tissue pulp. Stroma retained by the screen was detached with forceps and transferred to a test tube containing a small amount of incubation buffer. It was then converted to a fine suspension using a Polytron homogenizer and diluted to a final volume of 30 ml. Lastly, this diluted suspension and the preparation of epithelium were homogenized manually in a Dounce apparatus with 25 strokes of a loosely fitting pestle A. The final homogenate was diluted with incubation buffer to bring the protein concentration to about 300 μg/ml.

The histological appearance of the stroma is shown in figure 2A and

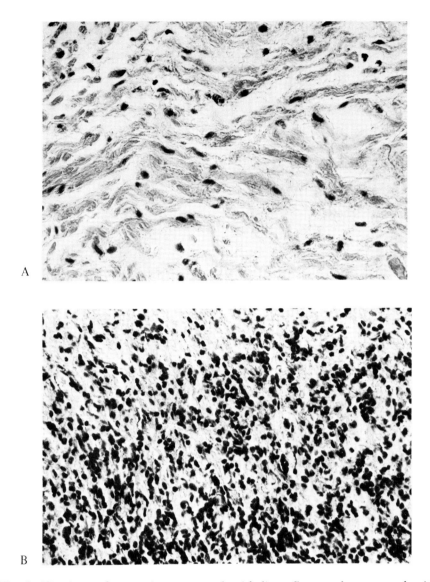

Fig. 2. Histology of prostatic stroma and epithelium. Separated stroma and epithelium were fixed in 4 % formaldehyde, stained with hematoxylin and eosin, and examined by light microscopy. Magnification × 220. A: stroma; B: epithelium.

that of the epithelium in figure 2B. Stroma consists of spindle-shaped fibromuscular cells and collagen while the epithelium is made up of sheets of densely packed cuboidal cells with round, darkly-staining nuclei. From a detailed microscopic analysis of such fractions from eight different prostates, it was established that the purity of the stroma was virtually 100% in all cases; in contrast, the purity of the epithelium ranged from 50–100% owing to contamination by stromal debris. About 40% of the whole-tissue DNA and protein was recovered in the stromal fraction (Table I).

Table I DNA and protein content of prostatic tissue.

Assay	Tissue		
	Normal	BPH	Carcinoma
DNA content			
a) total (mg/g tissue)	3.5 ± 0.5 (4)	2.6 ± 0.5 (6)	6.4 ± 0.9 (6)
b) recovered in stroma (%)	39.0 ± 8.3 (3)	51.7 ± 3.6 (6)	42.8 (2)
Protein content			
a) total (mg/g tissue)	110.6 ± 6.6 (5)	99.4 ± 6.4 (12)	104.3 ± 9.4 (6)
b) recovered in stroma (%)	41.5 ± 4.9 (3)	40.9 ± 2.1 (7)	41.2 (2)

Homogenates of whole tissue, stroma and epithelium were analysed for DNA and protein as described in the Materials and Methods section. The percentage of total DNA and protein in each fraction was then calculated. Values are presented as the mean ± SEM; the number of prostates examined is shown in parentheses.

Incubation conditions

Incubation mixture contained in a final volume of 2 ml the following components: 1.6 ml of the diluted homogenate, 50 nM-radioactive androgen and either an NADPH-generating system [7] for measuring 5α-reductase and $3\alpha(\beta)$-hydroxysteroid dehydrogenase (reductive) activities or 5×10^{-4}M NAD for measuring $3\alpha(\beta)$-hydroxysteroid (oxidative) activity. The samples were incubated at $37°$C in an oscillating water-bath for 30 minutes. At the end of incubation, 10 ml chloroform:methanol (2 : 1, v/v) were added to each sample. Steroids in the organic phase were identified by thin layer chromatography (TLC) and quantitated as described by Bruchovsky and Lieskovsky [7]. For each normal prostate two different sections of tissue were analysed to obtain a final mean velocity. Sampling of hyperplastic and carcinomatous prostatic tissue was limited to one section per gland.

Estimation of 5α-reductase activity was based on the percentage formation of androstanolone and $3\alpha(\beta)$-androstanediol from testosterone. $3\alpha(\beta)$-Hydroxysteroid dehydrogenase (reductive) activity was estimated from the percentage formation of $3\alpha(\beta)$-androstanediol from androstanolone. The oxidative activity of the dehydrogenase reaction was examined using 3α-androstanediol as substrate and estimating the percentage formation of androstanolone.

Purification of nuclei

Fragments of epithelium were collected essentially as described in the section on homogenization. However, the 0.01 M TES buffer, pH 7.0 (tris buffer was occasionally substituted), used for the recovery of nuclei contained 0.5 mM mercaptoethanol, 1.5 mM $CaCl_2$ and 0.25 M sucrose. The suspension, in a final volume of 30—40 ml of the above solution, was filtered through 2 layers of gauze and homogenized in a Dounce apparatus with 25 strokes of a loose-fitting pestle A followed by 10 strokes of a tight-fitting pestle B. Centrifugation of the filtrate at 800 g for 15 minutes yielded a crude nuclear pellet. This was suspended in 40 ml of an unbuffered aqueous solution, pH 6.5–7.0, containing 0.44 M sucrose, 0.2 mM neutral lead diacetate and 0.3% (v/v) triton N-101, and transferred to the Dounce apparatus. The pellet was dispersed with 10 strokes of pestle A and 10 strokes of pestle B. Centrifugation of the sample at 800 g for 15 minutes yielded a pellet of partially purified nuclei. The pellet was transferred to a Dounce apparatus and homogenized as before in a second unbuffered aqueous solution, pH 6.5–7.0, containing 0.44 M sucrose, 1 mM $MgCl_2$ and 0.3% (v/v) triton N-101. Nuclei were recovered by centrifugation at 800 g for 15 minutes, suspended in 0.01 M TES buffer, pH 7.0, containing 0.5 mM mercaptoethanol, 0.5 mM $CaCl_2$ (gradient buffer) and 0.88 M sucrose, and homogenized in the Dounce apparatus with 10 strokes of pestle A. The preparation of nuclei was layered over a discontinuous sucrose gradient consisting of 5 ml of 2.2 M sucrose and 5 ml of 1.8 M sucrose in gradient buffer. A final centrifugation of the sample at 53,000 g for 90 minutes in a Beckman-Spinco ultracentrifuge yielded a pellet of purified nuclei. The pellet was resuspended in 0.01 M TES buffer, pH 7.0, containing 0.5 mM mercaptoethanol; a small aliquot was stained with methylene blue and examined by light microscopy. As shown in Table II, the mean number of nuclei obtained was 4.3×10^7, 3.3×10^7 and 3.1×10^7 per g in normal, BPH and carcinomatous tissues respectively. Based on the theoretical number of nuclei per g of tissue the recovery was 13–24%. However, the theoretical number was calculated assuming that the nuclei were recovered from both stroma and epithelium, whereas in fact they were purified almost entirely from the epithelial portion of the tissue. Since the epithelium accounts for only about 60% of the whole-tissue content of DNA (Table I) the recovery of nuclei was probably in the vicinity of 22–40% of the total number.

Similar procedures were followed to obtain purified nuclei from rat ventral prostate. Detailed descriptions of the methods have been reported by Bruchovsky *et al.* [9] and, more recently, by Rennie [10]. The yield of nuclei averaged $9.8 \times 10^7 \pm 1.9 \times 10^7$ (mean ± standard error of mean (SEM), n = 15) per g of tissue using 250–300 g Wistar rats as the source of prostate.

Table II Recovery of prostatic nuclei.

Tissue	DNA content of whole tissue (mg DNA/g tissue)	DNA content of nucleus (pg DNA/ nucleus)	Theoretical nuclei/g tissue	Yield of nuclei/g tissue	Recovery of nuclei (%)
Normal	3.5 ± 0.5 (4)	13.7 ± 1.7 (5)	2.6×10^8	$4.3 \pm 0.5 \times 10^7$ (5)	17
BPH	2.5 ± 0.5 (6)	19.1 ± 1.5 (15)	1.4×10^8	$3.3 \pm 0.3 \times 10^7$ (23)	24
Carcinoma	6.4 ± 0.9 (6)	27.6 ± 2.7 (7)	2.4×10^8	$3.1 \pm 0.3 \times 10^7$ (10)	13

The DNA contents of homogenates of whole tissue and of known numbers of purified nuclei were measured as described in the Materials and Methods section. The theoretical number of nuclei/g of tissue was obtained by dividing the DNA content of whole tissue by the DNA content of the nucleus. The yield of nuclei is the actual count of purified nuclei. Recovery was calculated by dividing the theoretical number by the yield. Values are presented as the mean ± SEM; the number of prostates examined is shown in parentheses.

Extraction of nuclei

a) Using 0.6 M-NaCl

The fraction of purified nuclei was centrifuged at 800 g for 10 minutes and the pellet overlaid with 0.5 ml of 0.01 M TES buffer, pH 7.0, containing 0.5 mM mercaptoethanol and 0.05 M NaCl. The nuclei were then sonicated with 2 × 5 second pulses of a Bronwill Biosonik III sonicator at an intensity setting of 40. After addition of an equal volume of buffer containing 1.15 M NaCl, the resultant viscous solution was sonicated with 3 × 5 second pulses. Centrifugation of this solution at 18,000 g for 20 minutes yielded a supernatant fraction of solubilized chromatin.

b) Using micrococcal nuclease

About 1 × 10^8 purified nuclei were resuspended in 0.8 ml of 5 mM tris buffer, pH 8.0, containing 0.1 mM $CaCl_2$, and allowed to swell for 30 minutes. Disruption of the nuclei, accomplished with 3 × 5 second pulses of the sonicator, yielded a cloudy suspension of chromatin with an absorbance of 20–30 A_{260} units/ml. To 750 μl of such a suspension were added 200 μl of an aqueous solution containing 100 units of micrococcal nuclease. This mixture was then incubated at 20°C until 20% or more of the DNA was hydrolyzed into acid soluble products; usually a 30–40 minute interval was required. The enzyme reaction was stopped by the addition of 50 μl of 0.1 M EDTA bringing the final concentration of EDTA to 5 mM. Centrifugation of the sample in a Beckman Airfuge at 100,000 g for 40 minutes yielded a precipitate which was partially solubilized in 0.01 M TES buffer, pH 7.0, containing 0.5 mM mercaptoethanol and 0.6 M NaCl. After the suspension was centrifuged at 100,000 g for 10 minutes the supernatant was decanted and the pellet resuspended in buffer containing 1.2 M NaCl. The sample was again centrifuged at 100,000 g for 10 minutes; the supernatant was pooled with the one mentioned above to obtain the final nuclear extract.

Assay of nuclear receptor

About 0.5 ml of nuclear extract was incubated with 20 nM (1,2-^{3}H)-androstanolone or (17α-methyl-^{3}H)-metribolone at 4°C for 16–20 hours. Another 0.5 ml was treated similarly except that the sample also contained a 1,000-fold excess of non-radioactive androstanolone or metribolone. After incubation, both samples were analysed by gel-exclusion chromatography using a dual-column apparatus. This consisted of a column (0.5 cm × 15 cm) of Sephadex G-25 connected in series with a column (0.5 cm × 60 cm) of Sephadex G-100. The sample was introduced into a sample loop and subsequently pumped into the short column. It was then eluted in an upward direction with 0.01 M TES buffer, pH 7.0, containing 0.5 mM mercaptoethanol and 0.6 M NaCl at a flow rate of 2–3 ml/hour. Fractions of 0.5 ml were collected automatically and assayed for radioactivity. The amount of specific binding was calculated as the difference between total and non-specific binding in the receptor peak.

Isolation of chromatin

Nuclei were purified from rat ventral prostate and suspended in 10 ml of

0.01 M tris buffer, pH 7.0. After centrifugation at 20,000 g for 15 minutes the pellet was resuspended in 1 mM tris buffer, pH 7.0, and incubated at 0°C for 1 hour. Following this, the suspension was sonicated for 2 × 5 second intervals at an intensity setting of 40 and centrifuged at 20,000 g for 15 minutes to yield a pellet of chromatin. The pellet was resuspended in 2 ml of 0.01 M tris buffer, pH 7.0.

Labelling of chromatin with ^{3}H-androgen

Prostatic chromatin (1 ml of the above preparation) was incubated with 20 nM(1,2-^{3}H)-androstanolone while an equal part was incubated with both (1,2-^{3}H)-androstanolone and a 1,000-fold excess of non-radioactive androstanolone. Following incubation at 4°C for 18 hours the samples were diluted 10-fold with 0.01 M tris buffer, pH 7.0, and centrifuged at 20,000 g for 15 minutes. The pellet was resuspended in 5 mM tris buffer, pH 8.0, containing 0.1 mM CaCl$_2$, to a final concentration of 20 A$_{260}$ units/ml. An estimate of specific binding was obtained from the difference in the radioactivity between the sample without competing agent and the one with it.

Preparation of oligomeric nucleosomes

Labelled chromatin was warmed to 20°C for 4 minutes and digested at this temperature with micrococcal nuclease (5 units/A$_{260}$ unit) in 5 mM tris buffer, pH 8.0, containing 0.1 mM CaCl$_2$ for 1–60 minutes. The reaction was terminated by the addition of EDTA to a final concentration of 5 mM. An aliquot was mixed with an equal volume of a solution consisting of 0.8 M NaCl and 0.8 M HClO$_4$, incubated at 0°C for 30 minutes, and then centrifuged at 12,000 g for 3 minutes. The extent of digestion was calculated by dividing the amount of acid soluble DNA by the total amount of DNA in the sample. After 90 seconds of incubation, approximately 5% of the DNA was rendered acid soluble.

Separation of oligomeric nucleosomes

A 200 μl aliquot of the digested chromatin was layered on a linear density gradient (4.0 ml) containing 0.01 M tris buffer, pH 7.0, 5 mM EDTA and 7.6–76% (v/v) glycerol. The gradient was centrifuged at 130,000 g for 16 hours in a Beckman-Spinco ultracentrifuge. About 38 fractions were collected dropwise from the bottom of the centrifuge tube. After dilution to 1 ml with H$_2$O containing 5 mM EDTA, each of these was analysed for radioactivity and A$_{260}$.

Androgen-receptor complexes, not bound to chromatin, were separated on a linear density gradient containing 10 mM tris buffer, pH 7.0, 5 mM EDTA, and 5–20% (w/v) sucrose. The gradient was centrifuged at 246,000 g for 18 hours and fractions recovered as above.

Extraction and electrophoresis of DNA

DNA was extracted from the separated oligomeric nucleosomes by a modified Marmur technique [11, 12]. The appropriate fractions were mixed with 0.1 volumes of 5 M NaClO$_4$, 0.5 volumes chloroform:isoamylalcohol (24 : 1, v/v), and 0.5 volumes of phenol. These were shaken at 200 revolutions per minute (rpm) for 30 minutes on a mechanical rotator and then centrifuged at 2,500 g for 5 minutes. The aqueous layer was removed, dialysed at 4°C for 18 hours against three changes of 3 l of water and then lyophilized. The lyophilized material was dissolved in 10% (v/v) electrophoresis buffer consisting of 0.04 M tris, pH 7.8, 20 mM EDTA, 20 mM Na acetate and 10% (v/v) glycerol.

Samples (10–30 µl) containing 10 µg of DNA were electrophoresed on (by weight) 3% acrylamide (acrylamide:methylene bisacrylamide, 19 : 1): 0.5% agarose slab gels at 60 V for 4 hours. The gels were stained with 0.025% (w/v) Stains-all in 50% (v/v) formamide, destained in water, and scanned at 600 nm with a Gilford Model 250 spectrophotometer. The size of the DNA oligomers was determined by comparison with the electrophoretic mobility of PM2 DNA fragments after digestion with Hae III restriction endonuclease [13].

Radioimmunoassay

a) Extraction

Aliquots of whole-tissue, stromal and epithelial homogenates and samples of purified nuclei were diluted to 1 ml with H_2O. A small quantity (5,000 disintegrations per minute (dpm)) of (1,2-^{3}H)-androstanolone was added as an internal standard. Each sample was extracted with 4 ml of 10% (v/v) ethylacetate:hexane and the organic phase applied to a column (0.6 cm × 6.5 cm) of acid and solvent-washed Al_2O_3 [14]. Loading of the extract was completed by the application of 1.6 ml of 10% (v/v) ethylacetate:hexane. Androstanolone was then eluted with 0.45% (v/v) ethanol:hexane. Recovery of the internal standard was always 70–80%.

b) Assay

An aliquot of the eluate with androstanolone was transferred to a glass tube and dried in a vacuum oven at 45°C. After addition of 250 µl of dilute antiserum the solution was incubated firstly at 37°C for 1 hour and secondly at 20°C for 2 hours. An equal volume of saturated $(NH_4)_2SO_4$ was added and the precipitate removed by centrifugation; the supernatant was assayed for radioactivity and the androgen content was determined from a standard curve. Results were expressed in terms of pg (= g × 10^{-12})/ml, pmol (= mole × 10^{-12})/mg DNA and molecules/nucleus.

c) Antiserum and specificity

The antiserum was from rabbits immunized with an androstanolone-3-oxime-bovine serum albumin conjugate. Both testosterone and 5α-androstan-3β,17β-diol cross-reacted with the antiserum but, owing to the chromatographic purification of androstanolone, did not hinder the assay.

d) Sensitivity

The sensitivity as given by twice the standard deviation of replicate determinations on aqueous blanks (n = 9) was found to be 20 pg/ml.

e) Accuracy

Recovery experiments were performed to evaluate the accuracy of the assay by adding known amounts of androstanolone (100–800 pg/ml) to whole-tissue homogenates of ventral prostate from 24 hours castrated rats.

When the amount of steroid measured in the assay was correlated with the amount added, an r value of 0.99 was obtained.

f) Precision
   The within-assay and between-assay coefficients of variation were 5.0% (n = 5) and 9.7% (n = 3) respectively.

Other analytical procedures

Protein was measured by the method of Lowry *et al.* [15], using bovine serum albumin as the reference standard, or by the Bio-Rad Protein Assay, with bovine gamma globulin as standard. DNA was measured by the method of Burton [16] using calf thymus DNA as standard.
   Radioactivity was counted in a Beckman LS-250 liquid scintillation system using a diphenyloxazole/toluene solution which contained 6 g of diphenyloxazole, 75 ml of water and 126 g of Bio-solv BBS-3 per litre of toluene. The counting efficiency for ^3H was 35%.

Chemicals and reagents

Reagents used to prepare buffers and other solutions were purchased from Sigma Chemical Co., St. Louis, MO, USA. Micrococcal nuclease was also obtained from Sigma. Stains-all was supplied by Eastman Kodak, Rochester, NY, USA, and Bio-solv by Beckman Instruments, Fullerton, CA, USA. Steroids were obtained from Steraloids, Pawling, NY, USA. Chromatographic Al_2O_3 and the Bio-Rad Protein Assay were purchased from Bio-Rad Laboratories, Mississauga, ONT, Canada. The supplier of the androstanolone antiserum (DT 3–154) was Endocrine Sciences, Tarzana, CA, USA.
   (1,2-^3H)-Androstanolone (40 Ci/mM) and (17α-methyl-^3H)-metribolone (87 Ci/mM) were purchased from New England Nuclear, Boston, MA, USA. Purity was checked by TLC and the steroids were considered acceptable only if they were 95–100% pure.

Results

Stromal versus epithelial localization of 5α-reductase

The data in Table III indicate that the localization of 5α-reductase is predominantly in stroma irrespective of the normal or abnormal condition of the prostate. Moreover, the proportion of 5α-reductase activity associated with BPH stroma at 84.4 ± 2.3 percent (mean ± SEM) relative to the normal value of 71.2 ± 1.5 percent is significantly elevated (Student's t-test, $p < 0.05$). In contrast to the predominantly stromal distribution of 5α-reductase activity, the reductive and oxidative activities of 3$\alpha(\beta)$-hydroxysteroid dehydrogenase, are more evenly divided between stroma and epithelium.
   Data on the specific activities of the various enzymes in stroma and epithelium are presented in Table IV. As might be expected, the specific activity of 5α-reductase is uniformly higher in the stromal than in the epithelial fractions of all prostates examined. Comparing stromal fractions alone, it is clear that the mean specific activity of 5α-reductase in BPH stroma at 84.6 ± 13.1 pmol/mg protein/30 minutes is significantly greater than the corresponding

value in normal stroma, 31.6 ± 7.2 pmol/mg protein/30 minutes (Student's t-test, $p < 0.05$). This change accounts for the increased percentage of 5α-reductase activity in BPH stroma recorded in Table III. Stroma from carcinomatous prostate, on the other hand, is relatively poor in 5α-reductase activity.

Concentration of androstanolone in stroma and epithelium

To examine the effect of the high level of 5α-reductase activity in BPH stroma on the tissue distribution of androstanolone we measured the con-

Table III   Stromal versus epithelial localization of 5α-reductase and 3α(β)-hydroxysteroid dehydrogenase in human prostate.

Tissue	Percent of total enzyme activity in stroma		
	5α-Reductase	Dehydrogenase (r)	Dehydrogenase (o)
Normal	71.2 ± 1.5 (3)	35.5 ± 4.3 (3)	46.4 ± 5.6 (3)
BPH	84.4 ± 2.3 (9)	59.9 ± 6.1 (8)	71.5 ± 7.8 (8)
Carcinoma	71.0 (2)	36.6 (2)	49.9 (2)

Homogenates of stroma and epithelium were analysed for activity of 5α-reductase and 3α(β)-hydroxysteroid dehydrogenase (both oxidative (o) and reductive (r) pathways) as described in the text. Total enzyme activity was determined on the basis of the combined protein content of the stromal and epithelial fractions. The percentage of the total enzyme activity in each fraction was then calculated. Values are presented as the mean ± SEM; the number of prostates examined is shown in parentheses.

Table IV   5α-Reductase and 3α(β)-hydroxysteroid dehydrogenase activities in stroma and epithelium of human prostate.

Tissue	Enzyme activity (metabolites formed, pmol/mg protein/30 minutes)		
	5α-Reductase	Dehydrogenase (r)	Dehydrogenase (o)
Normal			
a) stroma	31.6 ± 7.2 (3)	15.0 ± 4.5 (3)	7.8 ± 1.3 (3)
b) epithelium	9.2 ± 3.0 (3)	19.7 ± 5.5 (3)	7.2 ± 2.5 (3)
BPH			
a) stroma	84.6 ± 13.1 (9)	20.9 ± 2.6 (8)	12.7 ± 1.7 (8)
b) epithelium	11.3 ± 1.9 (9)	11.7 ± 2.5 (9)	4.9 ± 2.1 (8)
Carcinoma			
a) stroma	12.4 (2)	13.2 (2)	8.4 (2)
b) epithelium	3.7 (2)	17.8 (2)	6.8 (2)

Homogenates of stroma and epithelium were analysed for activities of 5α-reductase and 3α(β)-hydroxysteroid dehydrogenase (both reductive (r) and oxidative (o)) pathways as described in the Materials and Methods section. The mean ± SEM for each set of results is shown for the number of experiments in parentheses.

centration of androstanolone in stroma and epithelium by radioimmuno-assay. The preliminary observations, recorded in Table V, suggest that BPH stroma and epithelium are both characterized by an above-normal level of androstanolone. The concentration appears to be highest in epithelium, giving a trend towards an elevated epithelial:stromal ratio of the concentrations of androstanolone in the separated fractions of BPH tissue. An elevated epithelial:stromal ratio of androstanolone concentration is also observed in one of the carcinomatous specimens.

Subcellular distribution and nuclear abundance of androstanolone

Since BPH tissue manifests an unusual propensity for accumulating andro-stanolone it was of interest to determine whether there is a specific location within the prostatic cell where this occurs. This was done by measuring the concentration of androstanolone in homogenates of whole tissue and in fractions consisting of purified nuclei and calculating the results with respect to DNA content of the samples. The difference between whole-tissue and nuclear concentrations gives the quantity of androstanolone in cytoplasm. From the data presented in Table VI it is clear that about 45% of andro-stanolone is held in the nucleus in normal and BPH tissues, compared with only an apparent 20% in carcinoma. In rat ventral prostate all androstano-lone is stored in the nucleus. Castration, while causing a marked reduction in concentration, does not change the relative distribution of this steroid.

The data in Table VI also show that the tendency for BPH tissue to ac-cumulate androstanolone is manifested to a similar degree in both cytoplas-mic and nuclear compartments. In contrast, the increase in concentration of androstanolone in carcinomatous tissue seems to be confined almost entirely to the cytoplasmic fraction.

Despite the differences in nuclear concentrations of androstanolone in human prostates, no significant variation is obvious in amounts of nuclear receptor. The finding that the concentration of receptor is 13–30 times lower than the concentration of androstanolone suggests that the nucleus of the prostatic cell is characterized by an abundance of free (non-receptor-bound) steroid. The concentration of nuclear receptor in rat ventral prostate, while almost 30 times greater than the concentration in human prostate, is nevertheless exceeded five-fold by the concentration of androstanolone.

Effect of DNA content on the nuclear concentration of androstanolone and androgen receptor

The data in Table VI suggest that there is no difference between concentra-tions of androstanolone in normal and carcinomatous nuclei and that nuclei from the three types of human prostate contain the same amount of recep-tor. However, when the data are adjusted to compensate for the varying amounts of DNA/nucleus (Table II) by normalizing on the basis of nuclear counts, a different perspective is obtained. Owing to the two-fold increase in the DNA content of carcinomatous nuclei, the concentrations of andro-stanolone and its receptor per nucleus are at least twice normal (Table VII). These observations strongly suggest that DNA exerts a positive influence on the nuclear retention of bound and unbound steroid.

Digestion of linker DNA and analysis of fragments

In view of the apparent direct relationship between the amounts of nuclear receptor and DNA we investigated the binding reaction between the two molecules in more detail as described by Rennie [10]. Extracts of nuclei from rat ventral prostate were digested with micrococcal nuclease to yield

Table V Concentration of androstanolone in stroma and epithelium.

Tissue	Concentration of androstanolone (pmol/mg DNA)		Ratio
	Stroma	Epithelium	E/S
Normal			
1	4.3	4.9	1.1
2	3.0	4.9	1.2
BPH			
1	5.4	7.1	1.3
2	11.8	20.0	1.7
3	6.4	9.1	1.4
4	6.0	9.0	1.5
Carcinoma			
1	5.6	5.1	0.9
2	5.9	15.0	2.5

The concentration of androstanolone was measured in separated stroma and epithelium by radioimmunoassay as described in the Materials and Methods section. Dividing the concentration in epithelium by that in stroma gives the E/S ratio.

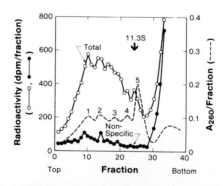

Fig. 3. Glycerol gradient separation of chromatin digests. Following digestion to 5% acid soluble with micrococcal nuclease, 200 µl of chromatin, labelled in vitro with 20 nM-[1,2-³H]-androstanolone and containing approximately 5 A₂₆₀ units, were applied to 7.6–76% (v/v) glycerol density gradients and centrifuged at 130,000 g for 16 hours. Fractions were collected from the bottom and analyzed for absorbance at 260 nm (broken line) and for radioactivity. The arrow indicates the position of the catalase sedimentation standard. Radioactivity recovered: (○) after incubation with isotope alone; (●) after incubation with isotope and a 1,000-fold excess of non-radioactive androstanolone. Modified from Rennie [10].

receptor-chromatin complexes of varying sizes; the complexes were separated on linear 7.6–76% (v/v) glycerol density gradients. After digestion of 5% of the DNA to acid soluble products most of the A_{260} and chromatin-bound radioactivity is recovered in fractions 1–28 of the gradient (Figure 3). Approximately 18% and 16% of the A_{260} and radioactivity respectively are associated with the pellet fraction (data not shown).

Within the gradient five A_{260} peaks are observed, the largest having a sedimentation value of about 11 S. Almost all of the specific binding is associated with the rapidly sedimenting components. Peak 1 is characterized by the highest mean value of dpm/A_{260} unit (5,826 ± 1,173; mean ± SEM, n = 4) which is 15%, 38%, 90% and 300% greater than the mean values for Peaks 2, 3, 4 and 5 respectively.

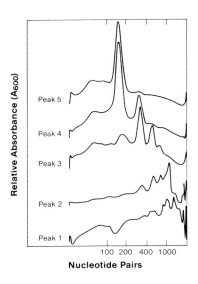

Fig. 4. Electrophoretic analysis of the DNA fragments recovered from glycerol gradient fractions. Fractions corresponding to the A_{260} peaks (numbers 1–5 in Figure 3) were recovered from six gradients, pooled, and the DNA in each peak extracted. Approximately 10 μg of DNA from each sample was applied to 3% acrylamide-0.5% agarose slab gels and electrophoresed at 60V for 4 hours. The gels were stained in Stains-all, destained in water, scanned at 600 nm and calibrated with PM2 DNA fragments. Modified from Rennie [10].

To determine the size of the DNA oligomers present in the A_{260} peaks, the appropriate fractions from six glycerol gradients were pooled and extracted. Aliquots containing 10 μg of the purified DNA were electrophoretically separated on 3% acrylamide-0.5% agarose slab gels. The gels were stained, scanned and calibrated with PM2 DNA fragments. The scans, reproduced in figure 4, indicate that some overlap of the DNA fragments occurs between adjacent A_{260} peaks and that the DNA fragments are integral multiples of a unit nucleosomal size [17] of 182 ± 3 (mean ± SEM, n = 6) base pairs. Peaks 1 and 2 contain large oligomeric forms of nucleosomes; Peak 3 is composed mainly of dimers and trimers with some monomers and tetramers; Peak 4 contains monomers and dimers; and Peak 5 contains principally monomers. Taken together these observations imply that fractions con-

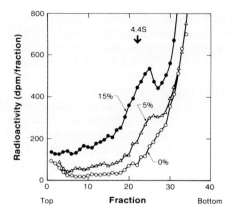

Fig. 5. Sucrose gradient analysis of nuclease digests. Chromatin samples, labelled in vitro with 20 nM [1,2-³H]-androstanolone and containing approximately four A_{260} units, were left undigested or underwent 5 or 15% digestion with micrococcal nuclease and centrifuged at 12,000 g for 10 minutes. The supernatant fractions (200 μl) were applied to 5–20% (w/v) sucrose density gradients and centrifuged at 246,000 g for 18 hours. Fractions were collected from the bottom and assayed for radioactivity. The arrow indicates the haemoglobin sedimentation standard. Modified from Rennie [10].

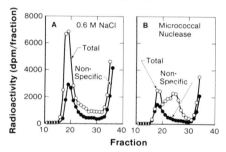

Fig. 6. Release of receptor from chromatin of normal human prostate by the action of micrococcal nuclease. Purified nuclei were either extracted with 0.6 M NaCl or disrupted and digested with micrococcal nuclease until 20% of the DNA was hydrolysed. In the latter procedure, the receptor-containing extract was prepared by solubilizing the precipitate formed during hydrolysis. The final extracts were incubated at 4°C for 16–20 hours in the presence of 20 nM [17α-methyl-³H]-metribolone. Non-specific binding was measured in duplicate samples. After incubation the extracts were analysed by Sephadex G25:G100 dual-column chromatography. Total (○) and non-specific (●) binding of radioactivity in nuclei treated with (A) 0.6 M NaCl; (B) micrococcal nuclease.

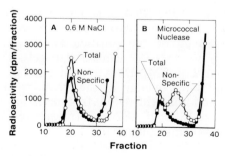

Fig. 7. Release of receptor from chromatin of BPH tissue by the action of micrococcal nuclease. Procedure as in legend to figure 6.

taining predominantly monomeric nucleosomes have low levels of labelled receptor, whereas fractions containing increasingly larger oligomeric nucleosomes have correspondingly higher levels of receptor.

Release of receptor from chromatin by the action of micrococcal nuclease

a) Chromatin from rat ventral prostate
   Micrococcal nuclease was used to digest preparations of labelled chromatin from rat ventral prostate. After varying amounts of hydrolysis, the nuclease-treated chromatin was analysed on 5–20% (w/v) sucrose density gradients to check for the presence of unbound nuclear receptors. As indicated by the results in figure 5, no peak corresponding to free receptors was observed in the undigested sample; after 5% digestion of DNA a small receptor peak appeared in the gradient. The peak is considerably augmented after 15% of the DNA is digested to acid soluble products. Thus the binding of androgen receptors to chromatin seems to depend on the region of DNA sensitive to nuclease attack.

b) Chromatin from human prostate
   Nuclear receptors are usually recovered from human prostatic nuclei in a free form if the nuclei are extracted with 0.6 M NaCl [18]. However, we have noted that this treatment is occasionally ineffective and that the receptor remains associated with chromatin. The failure to achieve the release of receptor with the use of salt is illustrated by the results in figures 6A and 7A. In the corresponding experiments on normal and BPH tissue respectively, purified nuclei were extracted with 0.6 M NaCl and the extracts incubated at 4°C for 16–20 hours in the presence of 20 nM(17α-methyl-^{3}H)-metribolone. Duplicate samples also contained 20 μM non-radioactive metribolone. Analysis of the labelled extracts by Sephadex G25:G100 dual-column chromatography indicated that the specific binding is limited to the void-volume fractions 15–25. However, if the purified nuclei are disrupted and treated with micrococcal nuclease until 20% of the DNA is hydrolysed to acid soluble products, the presence of free receptor is demonstrated as a peak of radioactivity in fractions 20–30 (Figures 6B and 7B). These findings reinforce the idea that there is a direct relationship between the amount of intact linker DNA and the amount of binding of receptor to chromatin. The relationship appears to hold for both rat and human prostates.

Discussion

Several processes contributing to the formation and retention of androstanolone by prostatic tissue have been studied. Concerning the function of different regions of the prostate, our results indicate that stroma is the primary site of conversion of testosterone to androstanolone in the human prostate owing to the prevalence in stroma of 5α-reductase. This finding is harmonious with the original conclusion of Cowan *et al.* [8] based on their experiments with BPH tissue. In the present report we show that 5α-reductase activity is largely confined to stroma in normal and carcinomatous prostates as well. We also demonstrate that the three-fold elevation of 5α-reductase activity previously observed in homogenates of whole BPH tissue [7] is mirrored by an increase of almost similar magnitude in the specific activity of the enzyme in BPH stroma. In analysing the degree of linear association between the variables of 5α-reductase activity and age, Bruchovsky and Lieskovsky [7] obtained a correlation coefficient that was consistent with a weakly positive relationship only; as a result they inferred that the rise in 5α-reductase activity is symptomatic of BPH and not exclusively of age. Allowing that age is indeed a negligible factor our present findings support the conclusion that BPH is characterized by an abnormally high level of stromal 5α-reductase activity.

In studying the post-formation disposal of androstanolone we observed that BPH stroma and epithelium are both characterized by an above normal level of androstanolone. Also the tendency for BPH to accumulate androstanolone appears to be equally pronounced in both the cytoplasm and the nucleus. A striking property of the nucleus is its ability to accumulate androstanolone well in excess of the quantity of receptor (Tables VI and VII); no exceptions to this rule are noticeable in any of the tissues examined. The simplest interpretation of this finding is that a large amount of androstanolone is transported into the nucleus by a non-receptor mediated process.

Despite the high nuclear concentration of androstanolone in BPH, the mean level of receptor, although elevated, is not significantly different from normal (Tables VI and VII). However, owing to a two-fold greater concentration of DNA, nuclei recovered from prostatic carcinoma are characterized by a proportional increase in the concentrations of both androstanolone and nuclear receptor (Table VII). It is possible, therefore, that the DNA content of the cell influences the nuclear concentration of these molecules.

The inferred relationship between the amount of nuclear receptor and DNA is supported by experimental proof that nuclear receptor is bound to linker DNA both in rat and human prostates. Three lines of evidence are

Table VI Subcellular distribution and nuclear abundance of androstanolone.

Tissue	Concentration (pmol/mg DNA)		Nuclear receptor
	Androstanolone		
	Whole tissue	Nucleus	
Human			
Normal	3.7 ± 0.5 (4)	1.5 ± 0.4 (5)	0.11 ± 0.02 (7)
BPH	9.3 ± 1.2 (8)	4.3 ± 0.7 (14)	0.14 ± 0.02 (17)
carcinoma	8.5 ± 1.5 (6)	1.7 ± 0.4 (7)	0.11 ± 0.01 (7)
Rat			
Normal	13.7 ± 0.6 (20)	18.2 ± 0.8 (5)	3.6 ± 0.7 (4)
Castrated	2.3 ± 0.3 (6)	2.0 ± 0.7 (4)	0.27 ± 0.05 (4)

The concentration of androstanolone in homogenates of whole tissue and in preparations of purified nuclei was measured by radioimmunoassay. Nuclear extracts were also analysed for the presence of androgen receptor by exchange labelling with [1,2-^{3}H]-androstanolone and [17α-methyl-^{3}H]-metribolone and Sephadex G25:G100 dual column chromatography, as described in the Materials and Methods section. Rats were castrated 24 hours before removal of prostate tissue. Results were normalized on the basis of the DNA content of the various fractions. The carcinomatous nucleus contains twice the normal amount of DNA. Values are presented as the mean ± SEM. The number of prostates examined is shown in parentheses.

Table VII Effect of DNA content on the nuclear concentration of androstanolone and androgen receptor in human prostate.

Tissue	Concentration (molecules/nucleus)	
	Androstanolone	Nuclear receptor
Normal	12,000 ± 3,000 (5)	900 ± 200 (7)
BPH	49,000 ± 8,000 (14)	1,600 ± 300 (17)
Carcinoma	29,000 ± 7,000 (7)	1,800 ± 200 (7)

The concentrations of androstanolone and nuclear receptor were normalized on a per nucleus basis to compensate for the greater amount of DNA/nucleus in carcinomatous cells (Table I). The number of molecules of receptor was estimated by assuming that one steroid molecule is equivalent to one receptor molecule. Values are presented as the mean ± SEM; the number of prostates examined is shown in parentheses.

presented. Firstly, more receptor is bound to large oligomeric nucleosomes than small ones (Figure 3); secondly, more receptor is released from chromatin as hydrolysis of DNA with micrococcal nuclease is allowed to proceed (Figure 5); thirdly, in cases where salt is ineffective, free receptor is generated in preparations of nuclei by the action of micrococcal nuclease (Figures 6 and 7).

The kinetics of androgen production and turnover are apparently quite different in BPH and carcinoma. While both tissues are characterized by a high concentration of androstanolone, stromal 5α-reductase activity is grossly elevated in BPH and abnormally low in carcinoma (Figure 1). Hence either 5α-reductase activity does not influence the accumulation of androstanolone, or this process is controlled by separate mechanisms in the two tissues.

Conclusions

1. The finding that 71.2 ± 1.5% (mean ± SEM), 84.4 ± 2.3% and 71.0% of the 5α-reductase activity in normal, BPH and carcinomatous prostates is recovered in separated stroma, confirms that 5α-reductase is a stromal enzyme.

2. Since the mean specific activity of 5α-reductase in BPH stroma at 84.6 ± 13.1 pmol/mg protein/30 minutes is grossly elevated relative to the values of 31.6 ± 7.2 and 12.4 pmol/mg protein/30 minutes in normal and carcinomatous stromal tissues, respectively, we conclude that BPH is characterized by an exceptionally high level of stromal 5α-reductase activity.

3. Possibly as a result of the stromal enzyme defect, BPH stroma and epithelium are both distinguished by an above-normal level of androstanolone.

4. The tendency for BPH tissue to accumulate androstanolone is manifested to a similar degree in both the cytoplasmic and nuclear compartments.

5. The observation that the concentration of nuclear receptor in human prostates is 13–30 times lower than the concentration of androstanolone suggests that the nucleus of the prostatic cell contains an abundance of free (non-receptor-bound) steroid.

6. Owing to a two-fold increase in the DNA of carcinomatous nuclei, the concentrations of androstanolone and its receptor per nucleus are at least

twice normal. This suggests that DNA exerts a positive influence on the nuclear retention of bound and unbound steroid.

7. The binding of androgen receptor to chromatin from both rat and human prostates seems to depend on the region of DNA sensitive to micrococcal nuclease. Thus we infer that nuclear receptor is bound to linker DNA.

Acknowledgments

Glenda Dennis provided valuable assistance in preparing this manuscript. Dr. T. K. Shnitka performed the histological and pathological examinations of the experimental tissues and gave generously of his time for this critical aspect of the study. Trudy Comeau was instrumental in supervising the performance of the various assays. The project was supported by grants from the Medical Research Council of Canada and the National Cancer Institute of Canada. One of us (P.S.R.) is a scholar of the latter.

References

1. Siiteri, P. K. and Wilson, J. E. (1970): Dihydrotestosterone in prostatic hypertrophy, 1: The formation and content of dihydrotestosterone in the hypertrophic prostate of man. *J. Clin. Invest., 49,* 1737–1745.
2. Geller, J., Albert, J., Lopez, D., Geller, S. and Niwayama, G. (1976): Comparison of androgen metabolites in benign prostatic hypertrophy (BPH) and normal prostate. *J. Clin. Endocrinol. Metab., 43,* 686–688.
3. Farnsworth, W. W. and Brown, J. R. (1976): Androgen of the human prostate. *Endocr. Res. Commun., 3,* 105–117.
4. Habib, F. K., Lee, S. R., Stitch, S. R. and Smith, P. H. (1976): Androgen levels in the plasma and prostatic tissues of patients with benign hypertrophy and carcinoma of the prostate. *J. Endocrinol., 71,* 99–107.
5. Krieg, M., Bartsch, W., Herzer, S., Becker, H. and Voigt, K. D. (1977): Quantification of androgen binding, androgen tissue levels, and sex hormone binding globulin in prostate, muscle and plasma of patients with benign prostatic hypertrophy. *Acta Endocrinol. (Copenhagen), 86,* 200–215.
6. Geller, J., Albert, J., Loza, D., Geller, S. and Stoltzing, W. (1978): DHT concentrations in human prostate cancer tissue. *J. Clin. Endocrinol. Metab., 46,* 440–444.
7. Bruchovsky, N. and Lieskovsky, G. (1979): Increased ratio of 5α-reductase:3α(β)-hydroxysteroid dehydrogenase activities in the hyperplastic human prostate. *J. Endocrinol., 80,* 289–301.
8. Cowan, R. A., Cowan, S. K., Grant, J. K. and Elder, H. Y. (1977): Biochemical investigations of separated epithelium and stroma from benign hyperplastic prostatic tissue. *J. Endocrinol., 74,* 111–120.
9. Bruchovsky, N., Rennie, P. S. and Vanson, A. (1975): Studies on the regulation of the concentration of androgens and androgen receptors in nuclei of prostatic cells. *Biochim. Biophys. Acta, 394,* 248–266.
10. Rennie, P. (1979): Binding of androgen receptor to prostatic chromatin requires intact linker DNA. *J. Biol. Chem., 254,* 3947–3957.
11. Marmur, J. (1961): A procedure for the isolation of deoxyribonucleic acid from micro-organisms. *J. Mol. Biol., 3,* 208–218.
12. Britten, R. J., Graham, D. E. and Neufeld, B. B. (1974): Analysis of repeating DNA sequences by reassociation. *Methods Enzymol., 29,* 363–418.
13. Kovacic, R. T. and Van Holde, K. E. (1977): Sedimentation of homogeneous double-strand DNA molecules. *Biochemistry, 16,* 1490–1498.
14. Furuyama, S., Mayes, P. and Nugent, C. A. (1970): A radioimmunoassay for plasma testosterone. *Steroids, 16,* 415–428.

15. Lowry, O. H., Rosebrough, N. J., Farr, A. L. and Randall, R. H. (1951): Protein measurement with the Folin phenol reagent. *J. Biol. Chem., 193,* 265–275.
16. Burton, K. (1956); a study of the conditions and mechanism of the diphenylamine reaction for the colorimetric estimation of deoxyribonucleic acid. *Biochem. J., 62,* 315–323.
17. Axel, R. (1976): The strucure of specific genes in chromatin. *Prog. Nucleic Acid Res. Mol. Biol., 19,* 355–371.
18. Lieskovsky, G. and Bruchovsky, N. (1979): Assay of nuclear androgen receptor in human prostate. *J. Urol., 121,* 54–58.

Discussion

P. Ekman (Stockholm, Sweden): How did you obtain your normal prostates?

N. Bruchovsky: At first we obtained the normal prostates at autopsy, the majority within 7 hours of death. Later our source was brain-dead kidney donors.

P. Ekman: The prostate may be subdivided into periurethral and peripheral lobes. BPH starts periurethrally while cancer starts peripherally. This is of importance when comparing results from 'normal', hyperplastic and cancerous prostates. From which part did you take your normal prostates?

N. Bruchovsky: No attempt was made to separate periurethral from peripheral zones when evaluating normal tissue. The data are from homogenates containing tissue from both zones. For comparative purposes the sampling of normal tissue need not be particularly zone-specific since the 5α-reductase activity is relatively low and invariant in all zones (N. Bruchovsky and G. Lieskovsky, *J. Endocrinol., 80,* 289, 1979).

R. Ghanadian (London, U.K.): You mentioned the value for androstanolone in BPH is over 9 pmol/mg DNA and for carcinomatous prostate about 8.0 pmol/mg. On the other hand you showed the level of 5α-reductase to be extremely low. I wonder how you reconcile these two findings. Your results on androstanolone in carcinomatous prostate are very high and do not agree with the data reported by Dr. Habib previously.

N. Bruchovsky: The puzzling discrepancy that you have alluded to between androstanolone levels and 5α-reductase activity in carcinoma of the prostate suggests to us that the retention of androstanolone by the prostate is not greatly influenced by the enzyme. Most investigators including Habib *et al.* (F. K. Habib, I. R. Lee, S. R. Stitch and P. H. Smith, *J. Endocrinol., 71,* 99, 1976) have found that the concentration of androstanolone in carcinomatous tissue is in the high normal range. Our mean value is well above normal but this might be explained by the fact that we have normalized our results on the basis of DNA content rather than dry or wet weight.

M. E. Harper (Cardiff, U.K.): How did you obtain your prostate samples? Were they from open prostatectomy (OP) or transurethral resection (TUR) samples? I feel very strongly that TUR specimens are of little use. We have measured various biochemical parameters in the same prostates obtained by different techniques, namely, prostatic cancer specimens obtained by cold punch and TUR and shown that the endogenous androgen content

is 5 to 10 times higher in the former. BPH samples obtained by open prostatectomy compared to TUR also have *n* 5 times greater concentrations. If
we turn to quite different fields, the polyamines, the content of these compounds and the enzymes involved in their synthesis is very much higher
in these OP to the TUR specimens (?). One could cite many more examples
such as platine activity in tissue culture, etc.

N. Bruchovsky: Samples were obtained at the time of open retropubic
prostatectomy. Immediately upon removal of the gland from the patient,
the hyperplastic nodules were dissected from the periurethral zone and
frozen at $-80°C$ within 15–20 minutes. No TUR specimens are included in
our study.

The use of heparin in extracting nuclei for estimation of nuclear androgen receptors in benign prostatic hyperplastic tissue by exchange procedures

J. A. Foekens, J. Bolt-de Vries*, J. C. Romijn* and E. Mulder
*Departments of Biochemistry (Division of Chemical Endocrinology) and
Urology, Medical Faculty, Erasmus University, Rotterdam, The Netherlands

Introduction

It is now generally accepted that steroid hormones mediate their effects in target tissues through binding to cytoplasmic receptor proteins. After translocation to the nucleus the steroid-receptor complex can initiate several biochemical processes [1]. The estimation of androgen receptor content in human tissues may be of importance in giving further insight into the development of benign prostatic hyperplasia (BPH) and the hormonal dependence of prostatic carcinoma, because the abnormalities are probably (in part) influenced by androgens. The measurement of cytoplasmic androgen receptor in prostatic tissues is complicated by the presence of a high proteolytic activity and the possibility of contamination with sex hormone binding globulin (SHBG) [2], which binds androstanolone (dihydrotestosterone, DHT) with high affinity. In addition, high levels of endogenous DHT have been measured in human prostatic tissue (5 ng (= g × 10^{-9})/g tissue) [3]. In spite of these difficulties the presence of cytoplasmic androgen receptor in prostatic tissues has been demonstrated [2, 4–17]. The levels reported varied between 0 and 80 fM (= M × 10^{-15})/mg protein, which is not surprising in the light of the differences in ligands, temperatures and separation techniques used. Because it can be expected from the high endogenous levels of DHT that most of the cytoplasmic receptor is translocated to the nucleus, it might be more meaningful to measure nuclear androgen receptor rather than cytoplasmic receptors. A rather wide variation in the contents of nuclear androgen receptors for BPH tissues has been found [11, 14, 15, 17, 18], probably due to differences in techniques used for tissue sampling, exchange conditions, homogenization procedures and the specific ligands used. We have attempted to overcome some of these technical difficulties and in this report we describe a rapid method for homogenization of prostate tissues and extraction of nuclear receptors with improved efficiency. The optimal conditions for exchange of unlabelled endogenous steroids with receptor-bound ^{3}H-DHT in heparin extracts of nuclear pellets were investigated. In addition a comparison was made between agar gel electrophoresis and protamine sulphate precipitation as methods for quantitative isolation of receptors.

Materials and methods

Tissue

Prostatic tissues were obtained from patients with BPH undergoing open prostatectomy. After surgery tissues were immediately placed on ice, divided into samples of $1-2$ g and stored at $-80°$C. Before processing the tissue was thawed on ice. Tissues were analyzed between 1 and 3 months after surgery.

Steroids

The following steroids were used: DHT, promegestone (R5020), metribolone (R1881), $(1,2,4,5,6,7-^3H)$-DHT (^{3}H-DHT) (specific activity 114 Ci/mM) and $(6,7-^3H)$-R1881 (^{3}H-R1881) (specific activity 58.2 Ci/mM).

^{3}H-R1881 and non-radioactive R1881 and R5020 were kindly supplied by Dr J. P. Raynaud, Roussel UCLAF, Paris, France. ^{3}H-DHT was purchased from the Radiochemical Centre, Amersham, England. Unlabelled DHT was obtained from Steraloids, Pawling, New York, U.S.A.

Preparation of nuclear extracts

Homogenization of tissue was carried out between two layers of stainless steel screens, after mincing the thawed tissue partly with scissors. During homogenization 0.5 g tissue was kept in 40 ml buffer A (50 mM trometamol (tris)-HC1, 2.5 mM KC1, 5 mM MgCl$_2$, pH 7.5), containing 0.55 M sucrose. After homogenization the suspension was divided into two equal parts and was layered on 25 ml buffer A, containing 0.88 M sucrose. Centrifugation was performed using an HB-4 rotor for 10 minutes at 3,500 revolutions per minute (rpm) in a Sorvall RC2B centrifuge.

The nuclear pellets were each resuspended in 1 ml buffer B (10 mM tris-HC1, 1.5 mM edetic acid (EDTA), 1.5 mM dithioerythritol, 0.05 M NaCl; pH 7.5) and were pooled.

The number of nuclei in 100 μl of the suspension were counted as described by Lieskovsky & Bruchovsky [18]. An average yield of 2×10^7 nuclei/0.5 g tissue was obtained. The remainder of the nuclear suspension (1,900 μl) was centrifuged for 10 minutes at 800 g and the nuclear pellet was extracted with a 2 mM phosphate buffer containing heparin at various concentrations for 1 hour without sonication. All procedures were performed at $0°$C.

Labelling of nuclear extracts

The nuclear extract was incubated for different periods of time and at different temperatures with $10-50$ nM ^{3}H-DHT or ^{3}H-R1881. In parallel experiments a $200-1,000$-fold excess of non-radioactive DHT, R1881 or R5020 was added.

Estimation of receptor levels

Samples were treated with a charcoal suspension (0.25% charcoal, 0.025% Dextran T-300 in buffer B). The charcoal treatment was performed for 10 minutes at 0°C followed by centrifugation for 10 minutes at 10,000 g. The supernatant fraction was analysed either with agar gel electrophoresis according to Wagner [19] or protamine sulphate precipitation according to Chamness et al. [20]. Agar gel electrophoresis was performed for 90 minutes at 130 mA. For the protamine sulphate precipitation assay, acid washed (12 × 75 mm) glass tubes were used. The tubes were incubated at 30°C for 15 minutes with 0.5 ml buffer B containing 0.1% bovine serum albumin and were then rinsed with 1 ml icecold buffer B. All subsequent procedures were carried out at 0°C. Protamine sulphate (Organon, Oss, The Netherlands) was diluted to 1–3 mg/ml in buffer C (10 mM tris-HCl; 1.5 mM EDTA; 1.5 mM dithioerythritol; 10% glycerol pH 7.5) and 250 μl was added to each tube. After treatment with charcoal, 50 μl of the nuclear extracts were added to 250 μl protamine sulphate solution, with 200 μl buffer C. The contents of the tubes were mixed using a Vortex and were subsequently left for 5–10 minutes at 0°C before centrifugation at 2,400 g for 15 minutes. The firmly coated precipitates were washed four times with 1 ml buffer C without further centrifugation. The pellets were dissolved in 0.5 ml toluene over 10 minutes at 60°C and counted for radioactivity.

Results

Extraction of the nuclear pellet

Nuclear pellets isolated after homogenization of BPH tissue between two stainless steel wire screens (Borel homogenizer) were extracted for 1 hour at 0°C either with 0.4 M KCl in buffer B or with a 2 mM phosphate buffer containing 1 mg/ml heparin. The nuclear extracts were labelled for 18 hours at 6°C with 10^{-8} M ^{3}H-DHT. In parallel experiments a 1,000-fold excess of non-radioactive DHT was added for measurement of aspecific binding. All samples were treated with charcoal for removal of non-specifically bound ^{3}H-DHT from the nuclear extracts and subsequently analysed by agar gel electrophoresis (Fig. 1).

Fig. 1A shows that the radioactive tracer stays at the application site during electrophoresis after 0.4 M KCl extraction, indicating an aggregated form of the receptor. After extraction of the nuclear pellet with a heparin-containing buffer (1 mg/ml), a change in electrophoretic mobility was demonstrated (Fig. 1B), which reflects deaggregation of the receptor proteins. Heparin extraction appeared to be about 30–50% more efficient than KCl extraction. In some experiments a residual peak also appeared at the application site on the agar gel after electrophoresis of heparin containing extracts. The amount of radioactivity present at the application site was also included in the amount of receptor-bound radioactivity estimated after agar gel electrophoresis of nuclear extract samples. This double peak partly consists of a peak at the application site and another peak having the same electrophoretic mobility as the peak presented in Fig. 1B.

The results in Fig. 2 illustrate the influence of the heparin concentration in the extraction buffer on the amount of extracted receptor. In the absence of heparin, 25% of the receptor molecules could be solubilized with phos-

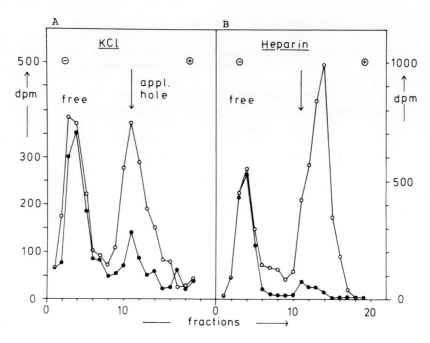

Fig. 1. *Agar gel electrophoretic patterns of labelled nuclear extracts of BPH tissue. Extraction of the nuclei with 0.4 M KCl (A) or with heparin (1 mg/ml) (B) was performed for 1 hour at 0°C, followed by centrifugation for 15 minutes at 100,000 g. Nuclear extracts were incubated for 18 hours at 6°C with 10^{-8} M ^{3}H-DHT (o——o) or with 10^{-8} M ^{3}H-DHT in the presence of a 1,000-fold excess of non-radioactive DHT (●——●). 'Free' = position of unbound steroid. 'Appl. hole' and arrow indicate position of sample at start of electrophoresis.*

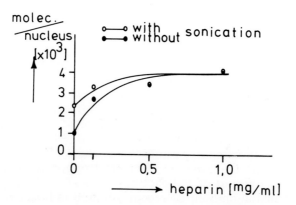

Fig. 2. *Effect of heparin concentration on number of extractable androgen receptor sites from nuclei of BPH tissue. Nuclear extracts were exchanged for 18 hour at 6°C with 10^{-8} M ^{3}H-DHT and specifically bound ^{3}H-DHT was determined by agar gel electrophoresis. ●——● Without sonication, o——o with sonication for 3 × 5 seconds and intermittent cooling with an MSE 100 W Ultrasonic Disintegrator. Sonication was performed at the beginning of the 1 hour extraction period (0°C).*

phate buffer without sonication. Sonication did not increase the maximal amount of receptors solubilized from the nuclear pellet with heparin solutions. Only at low heparin concentrations did there appear to be a positive effect of sonication on solubilization of receptor proteins. In further experiments a heparin concentration of 1 mg/ml was used without sonication. It appeared that extraction was almost complete after 1 hour at 0°C. As a standard procedure $1-2 \times 10^7$ nuclei were extracted with 1 ml extraction buffer for 1 hour at 0°C.

Labelling of nuclear extracts

The exchange of added radioactive steroid with endogenous receptor-bound steroid was studied at different temperatures up to 23°C for 18 hours with 10^{-8} M ^{3}H-DHT. From Fig. 3 it can be concluded that optimum exchange of added ^{3}H-DHT for endogenous-bound ligand could be achieved at ap-

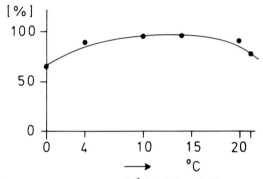

Fig. 3. Labelling of androgen receptors with ^{3}H-DHT at different temperatures. Samples were incubated for 18 hours with 10^{-8} M ^{3}H-DHT in the presence or absence of 2×10^{-6} M DHT and analysed by agar gel electrophoresis. Data are corrected for nonspecific binding and plotted as relative percentages of specifically bound steroid.

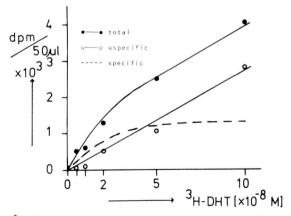

Fig. 4. Effect of ^{3}H-dihydrotestosterone concentration on labelling of androgen receptors for 18 hours at 10°C in nuclear extracts of BPH tissue. Values were obtained by the protamine sulphate precipitation technique. Data are plotted as total (●——●), aspecific (○——○) and specific binding (– – –). Aspecific binding was estimated by incubation of the nuclear extracts in the presence of a 200-fold excess of non-radioactive DHT. Specific binding was obtained by subtracting aspecific from total binding.

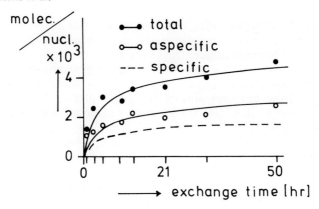

Fig. 5. *Labelling of androgen receptors in nuclear extracts of BPH tissue with 5×10^{-8} M*
^{3}H-DHT at 10°C for different periods. The amount of androgen receptors in the samples
was quantified by protamine sulphate precipitation. Data are plotted as total (●———●),
aspecific (○———○) and specific binding (– – –). Aspecific binding was estimated by in-
cubation of the nuclear extracts in the presence of a 200-fold excess of non-radioactive
DHT. Specific binding was obtained by subtracting aspecific from total binding.

proximately 10°C. In addition, the effect of variation in ^{3}H-DHT concentration during exchange under these conditions was studied (Fig. 4). A concentration of 5×10^{-8} M ^{3}H-DHT appeared to be optimal. This concentration was higher than the DHT concentration used for the experiments shown
in Fig. 3, therefore optimal exchange time was also studied in a series of experiments at 10°C with 5×10^{-8} M ^{3}H-DHT (Fig. 5). Maximal exchange
was reached after 20 hours and persisted up to at least 50 hours.

Comparison of protamine sulphate precipitation with agar gel electrophoresis

A comparison was made between the amounts of receptor-bound steroid
found with agar gel electrophoresis and with protamine sulphate precipitation. The results obtained for the estimation of optimal concentration for
exchange were measured by agar gel electrophoresis as well as protamine
sulphate precipitation. The results are listed in Table I. No difference was
found in the amount of detectable specifically bound steroid.

Table I *Agar gel electrophoresis and protamine sulphate precipitation of nuclear recep-*
tors from nuclear extracts labelled with different concentrations of ^{3}H-DHT (plus or
minus a 200-fold excess of non-radioactive DHT) for 18 hours at 10°C.

Concentration (nM) of labelled DHT		5	10	20	50	100
Agar gel electrophoresis	a	493	725	1,396	ND	4,041
	b	73	99	541	ND	2,669
Protamine sulphate precipitation	a	492	618	1,328	2,414	4,111
	b	63	90	517	1,115	2,880

a: disintegrations per minute (dpm) bound after incubation with ^{3}H-DHT.
b: dpm bound after incubation with ^{3}H-DHT and excess non-labelled DHT.
ND: not determined.

Absence of steroid-binding proteins other than DHT-receptors in the nuclear extracts

SHBG (sex hormone binding globulin) was not present in the nuclear extracts. SHBG migrates to the cathodic region during agar gel electrophoresis [19] and from Fig. 1 it can be concluded that no SHBG peak was present. SHBG is not precipitable with protamine sulphate [10] and the same amount of detectable specifically bound steroid was found with both agar gel electrophoresis and protamine sulphate precipitation (Table I). In experiments with the synthetic androgen metribolone as an exchange ligand no progesterone receptor could be demonstrated in the nuclear extracts (Table II). R5020 appeared to have lower competing capacity for ^{3}H-R1881 than for ^{3}H-DHT. In addition ^{3}H-R1881 binding was reduced much more with DHT than with R5020, indicating that R1881 was bound to androgen rather than to progesterone receptors.

Table II Competition of various steroids for nuclear androgen receptors from BPH tissue. Samples were quantified with the protamine sulphate precipitation technique after incubation of the nuclear extracts with 5×10^{-8} M ^{3}H-R1881 (A) or with 5×10^{-8} M ^{3}H-DHT (B) in the absence or presence of 10^{-5} M non-radioactive R1881, DHT and R5020 for 18 hours at $10°C$.

Competitor (10^{-5} M)	Molecules of labelled ligand per nucleus	Competition (%)
A) ^{3}H-R1881 binding		
none	3,719	0
R1881	0	100
DHT	0	100
R5020	2,814	24
B) ^{3}H-DHT binding		
none	4,249	0
R1881	0	100
DHT	0	100
R5020	2,016	53

Discussion

The results reported show that extraction of receptors from nuclear pellets of BPH tissue with a heparin-containing buffer offers several advantages over extraction with a KCl-containing buffer. Compared to KCl extraction the yield of solubilized receptor after heparin extraction was improved (30–50%). An additional advantage appeared to be the deaggregation of the receptor proteins. It had previously been shown that rat prostate nuclear androgen receptor could be deaggregated after storage at $-80°C$ by heparin [21]. The amount of nuclear receptor in BPH tissue estimated with the heparin extraction technique was of the same order of magnitude as the highest receptor levels reported in the literature [11, 14, 16–18].

The nuclear extract used in the present study contained negligible amounts of SHBG and cytoplasmic steroid receptors. Agar gel electrophoresis of the heparin-containing nuclear extracts did not give any evidence for steroid binding proteins with an electrophoretic mobility similar to SHBG.

In cytosol fractions obtained from BPH tissue the amount of SHBG was reported to be three times as high as the amount of cytoplasmic androgen receptor [9]. Progesterone binding protein appears to be present in BPH cytosol fractions [22, 23] but was not detected in the nuclear fractions as isolated in the present study.

The data presented show good agreement between nuclear androgen receptor content as estimated by either agar gel electrophoresis or protamine sulphate precipitation. We have recently also evaluated other techniques such as Sephadex LH-20 gel filtration, sucrose density gradient centrifugation and Sephadex G25–G150 gel filtration for the separation of androgen receptors from free steroid. The results of this comparison, which will be published elsewhere, showed that the techniques are comparable with respect to the amount of specifically bound ^{3}H-DHT.

In conclusion, we believe we have attained a further improvement in the measurement of nuclear androgen receptors in BPH tissue after storage at $-80°C$. The application of this procedure to the estimation of nuclear androgen receptor in prostatic carcinoma may be important in selecting the appropriate therapy for patients suffering from this disease. It is therefore our intention to adapt the method described for the estimation of androgen receptors in needle biopsies and small samples of carcinoma tissue.

Acknowledgments

We are grateful to Drs N. Bruchovsky, P. S. Rennie and H. J. van der Molen for discussions which led to the present studies.

References

1. Mainwaring, W. I. P. (1977): *The Mechanism of Action of Androgens,* Springer Verlag, Berlin.
2. Krieg, M., Grobe, I., Voigt, K. D., Altenähr, E. and Klosterhalfen, H. (1978): *Acta Endocrinol. (Copenhagen), 88,* 397.
3. Geller, J., Albert, J., Loza, G., Geller, S., Stoelzing, W. and de la Vega, D. (1978): *J. Clin. Endocrinol. Metab., 46,* 440.
4. Hansson, V., Tveter, K. J., Attramadal, A. and Torgersen, O. (1971): *Acta Endocrinol. (Copenhagen), 68,* 79.
5. Mainwaring, W. I. P. and Milroy, E. J. G. (1973): *J. Endocrinol. 57,* 371.
6. Davies, P. and Griffiths, K. (1975): *Mol. Cell. Endocrinol., 3,* 143.
7. Asselin, J., Labrie, F., Gourdeau, Y., Bonne, C. and Raynaud, J. P. (1976): *Steroids, 28,* 449.
8. Bonne, C. and Raynaud, J. P. (1976): *Steroids, 27,* 497.
9. Krieg, M., Bartsch, W., Herzer, S., Becker, H. and Voigt, K. D. (1977): *Acta Endocrinol. (Copenhagen), 86,* 200.
10. Menon, M., Tananis, C. E., McLoughlin, M. G., Lippman, M. E. and Walsh, P. C. (1977): *J. Urol., 117,* 309.
11. Mobbs, B. G., Johnson, I. E., Connolly, J. G. and Clark, A. F. (1978): *J. Steroid Biochem., 9,* 289.
12. Snochovsky, M., Pousette, Å., Ekman, P., Bression, D., Andersson, L., Högberg, B. and Gustafsson, J.-Å. (1977): *J. Clin Endocrinol. Metab., 45,* 920.
13. Ghanadian, R., Aug, G., Chaloner, P. J. and Chisholm, G. D. (1978): *J. Steroid Biochem., 9,* 325.
14. Menon, M., Tananis, C. E., Hicks, L. L., Hawkins, E. F., McLoughlin, M. G. and Walsh, P. C. (1978): *J. Clin. Invest., 61,* 150.
15. Shain, S. A. and Boesel, R. W. (1978): *Invest. Urol., 16,* 169.

16. Shain, S. A., Boesel, R. W., Lamm, D. L. and Radwin, H. M. (1978): *Steroids, 31,* 541.
17. Sirett, D. A. N. and Grant, J. K. (1978): *J. Endrocrinol., 77,* 101.
18. Lieskovsky, G. and Bruchovsky, N. (1979): *J. Urol., 121,* 54.
19. Wagner, R. K. (1978): *Acta Endocrinol., 88,* suppl. 218.
20. Chamness, G. C., Huff, K. and McGuire, W. L. (1975): *Steroids, 25,* 627.
21. Mulder, E., Foekens, J. A., Peters, M. J. and van der Molen, H. J. (1979): *Febs Lett., 97,* 260.
22. Cowan, R. A., Cowan, S. K. and Grant, J. K. (1976): *J. Endocrinol., 71,* 121.
23. Gustafsson, J.-Å., Ekman, P., Pousette, Å., Snochovsky, M. and Högberg, B. (1978): *Invest. Urol., 15,* 361.

Discussion

K.-D. Voigt (Hamburg, Federal Republic of Germany): Do you have any data on the purity of your nuclei?

J. A. Foekens: The nuclear pellet contained some residual endoplasmic reticulum fragments but the amount of SHBG and cytoplasmic steroid receptors was negligible.

Agar gel electrophoresis of the heparin-containing nuclear extracts did not give any evidence for steroid-binding proteins with an electrophoretic mobility similar to SHBG and progesterone binding protein was not detected in the nuclear fractions as isolated in the present study.

On the presence of a major protein, prostatic secretion protein or estramustine-binding protein, in the rat ventral prostate and in the human prostate

J.-Å. Gustafsson**, P. Björk*, K. Carlström‡, B. Forsgren*, T. Hökfelt***,
Å. Pousette** and B. Högberg*†
*AB Leo Research Laboratories, Helsingborg, Departments of **Chemistry
and Medical Nutrition, ***Histology, and †Pharmacology, Karolinska
Institute, and ‡Hormone Laboratory, Sabbatsberg Hospital, Stockholm,
Sweden

Introduction

This paper reports on the occurrence of a major protein secreted from rat ventral prostatic cells into the lumina of the ductuli. We detected this protein through its pronounced capacity to bind estramustine.

Estramustine phosphate (EP) is a nitrogen mustard derivative of estradiol phosphate in which the nitrogen mustard is attached to position 3 of the steroid via a carbamate link (Fig. 1). The drug was introduced in 1966 as a therapeutic agent for prostatic carcinoma. By now a number of reports have been published on the treatment of advanced prostatic carcinoma with EP (for references see [1]). The drug has mostly been used in patients previously orchiectomized and/or treated with oestrogens and with an advanced or relapsing carcinoma. Objective and/or subjective remissions including regression of the original tumour and soft tissue and skeletal metastases as well as relief of pain have been obtained in 20–50% of these cases.

When tested on experimental, transplanted tumours in rats and mice EP showed some tumour inhibitory effect suggestive of a weak cytostatic

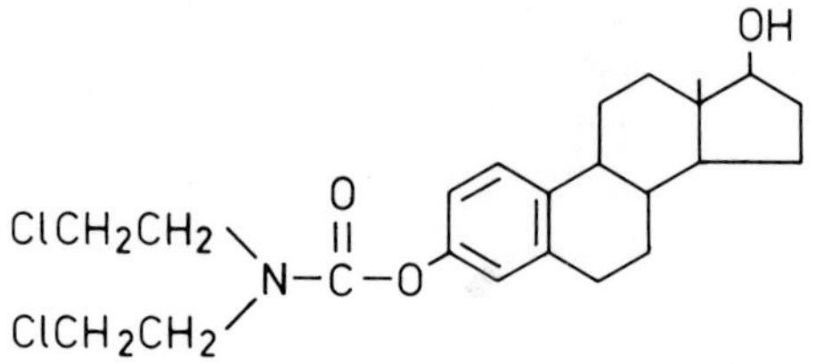

Fig. 1. Structural formula of estramustine.

action. Investigations using 7,12-dimethylbenz(a)anthracene(DMBA)-induced, hormone-dependent mammary tumours in the rat showed that the tumour inhibitory versus oestrogenic activity (measured as mouse uterus growth stimulation) was higher for EP than for estradiol [2]. Furthermore, EP had a growth inhibitory effect on DMBA-induced rat mammary tumours unaffected by initial treatment with estradiol [3]. Recently EP has also been shown to retard the growth of the hormone-sensitive, transplantable R-3327 rat prostatic adenocarcinoma (the Dunning tumour) [4].

When the effect of EP was studied in organ culture of rat ventral prostate thymidine incorporation experiments as well as histological analysis of the explants indicated that EP had a considerably stronger growth-inhibitory effect than estradiol [5].

When comparing the tissue distribution of radiolabelled EP, estradiol phosphate and estradiol, Plym Forshell and Nilsson found a selective uptake of radioactivity in the rat ventral prostate following intravenous administration of EP [6]. In extracts from the ventral prostate most of this selectively concentrated radioactivity could be accounted for as estramustine. Høisaeter confirmed the high uptake of estramustine in rat ventral prostate after a single intravenous dose of EP [7].

Materials and methods

Chemicals

[2,4,6,7-³H] Estramustine (80-107 Ci/mmol) was synthesized at AB Leo. The compound was purified before use to at least 99% purity by chromatography on Sephadex LH-20.

In addition to EP and estramustine, several unlabelled nitrogen mustard steroid derivatives synthesized at AB Leo were used in the ligand specificity studies. These compounds are summarized in Tables I-II. All reagents used were of analytical grade.

Preparation of cytosol

Wistar rats, 8–10 weeks old, were castrated 24 hours before removal of the ventral prostate. Pooled glands were homogenized in 3–10 volumes (v/w) of ice-cold 0.01 M tris-HCl, pH 7.2, 1 mM EDTA, 0.01 M KCl, 0.25 mM dithioerythritol and 10% (v/v) glycerol (TEKDG) buffer during 6 × 5 second periods with 55 second intervals using an Ultra-Turrax homogenizer. The homogenate was centrifuged for 1 hour at 105,000 g (Beckman L2-65B ultracentrifuge with an SW 56 or SW 27 rotor). The supernatant, the cytosol fraction, was used immediately or stored at −30°C. All preparation steps were carried out at 0–4°C. The protein concentrations of the cytosol preparations, determined according to Lowry *et al.* [8] using bovine serum albumin as a standard, were in the range 10–30 mg/ml.

Binding studies

The specificity and binding characteristics of the estramustine-binding protein were studied by incubation of duplicate samples (200 µl, 1.6 µg cytosol protein/ml TEKDG-buffer containing 0.1% gelatin) with 10 nM ³H-

Table I Relative binding affinity (RBA = excess of estramustine required for 50% inhibi-
tion/excess of competitor required for 50% inhibition) of various oestrogen nitrogen
mustard derivatives for the estramustine-binding protein in rat ventral prostate. For
compounds giving curves not parallel ($p < 0.05$) with that of estramustine (LS 275) RBA
was not calculated (n.c.). Under the conditions used the concentration of estramustine
required for 50% inhibition was 20 nM (2-fold excess). Saturation of the estramustine
binding sites was accomplished at approximately 100 nM estramustine.

Leo no.	R_1	R_2	R_3	RBA
LS 271	$= O$		H	1.16
LS 275	OH	H	H	1.00
LS 289	$O\overset{O}{\overset{\|}{C}}CH_3$	H	H	0.77
LS 299	$O\overset{O}{\overset{\|}{P}}(OH)_2$	H	H	0.002
LS 358	$O\overset{O}{\overset{\|}{C}}CH_2CH_3$	H	H	n.c.
LS 470	$O\overset{O}{\overset{\|}{C}}C(CH_3)_3$	H	H	n.c.
LS 453	$O\overset{O}{\overset{\|}{C}}N(CH_2CH_2Cl)_2$	H	H	n.c.
LS 675	OH	$C\equiv CH$	H	0.44
LS 1611	OH	H	OH	0.01
LS 2035	OH	H	$O\overset{O}{\overset{\|}{C}}CH_3$	0.02
LS 2179	H	OH	H	1.00

estramustine in the presence of various unlabelled steroids and steroid
derivatives in concentrations ranging from 1 nM to 45 μM. After 18 hours
at 15°C the samples were placed in ice water and 0.5 ml of ice-cold dex-
trancoated charcoal (DCC) suspension (1.5% (w/w) charcoal in 0.05 M tris-
HCl, pH 7.2, containing 1 mM EDTA, 0.1 mM dithioerythritol, 10% (v/v)
glycerol, 0.1% (w/v) gelatin, and 0.05% (w/v) Dextran T 70 (Pharmacia,
Uppsala)) added. After 20 minutes the charcoal was spun down and a
suitable volume of the supernatant analysed by scintillation counting for
protein-bound radioactivity. The result was expressed as percentage of

Table II Relative binding affinity (RBA) of some non-oestrogen nitrogen mustard deriva-tives and LS 298 for the estramustine-binding protein in rat ventral prostate. For further details, see legend to Figure 2.

$R = -\overset{\displaystyle O}{\overset{\displaystyle \|}{C}}-N-(CH_2CH_2Cl)_2$	Leo no.	RBA
	LS 275	1.00
	LS 452	0.23
	LS 524	0.16
	LS 451	0.007
	LS 298	n.c.

radioactivity bound in the absence of competitor. The linear log-logit trans-formation as described by Rodbard *et al.* [9] was used for calculation of 50% inhibition.

Results and discussion

Studies on the uptake and distribution of ³H-estramustine in vivo

Because of the rapid dephosphorylation of EP *in vivo* and the accumulation of estramustine as the main metabolite in the rat ventral prostate all studies were carried out using ³H-estramustine (specific radioactivity 80−110 Ci/nmol). Following administration of 0.5−5 µg ³H-estramustine/kg body weight to castrated rats the uptake and distribution of radioactivity in various tissues was studied using autoradiography and combustion analysis.

When administered intravenously ³H-estramustine was rapidly cleared from the blood [10]. As early as 5 minutes after injection higher levels of radioactivity were found in several tissues, e.g. liver, brain, salivary glands, and skeletal muscle than in blood. At this time radioactivity was also found in the epithelial cells of the ventral prostate gland and of the seminal vesicles. Fifteen minutes later the bile, intestinal contents, adrenal cortex, brown fat, liver, and pancreas, in decreasing order of magnitude, contained high levels of radioactivity. Among the sex accessory glands the preputial glands showed the highest accumulation of radioactivity. The ventral prostate gland also seemed to have an increased content of radioactivity, mainly confined to the epithelial cells. Four hours after injection the intestines and liver showed the highest amounts of radioactivity. Among the sex accessory glands the ventral prostate and seminal vesicles contained the highest concentrations of radioactivity. The radioactivity of the ventral prostate was also localized at this time point in the secretory contents of the lumina of the gland. In another experimental series, this observation was also made 2 hours following an intramuscular injection of ³H-estramustine. On the other hand, radioactivity from intramuscularly administered ³H-testosterone was found only in the epithelial cells and no radioactivity was detected in the lumina of the gland. Furthermore, combustion analyses [10, 11] showed that radioactivity from intramuscularly or intraperitoneally injected ³H-estramustine accumulated much more efficiently in the rat ventral prostate than from ³H-estradiol.

Combustion analyses also indicated that estramustine and its steroidal congener, estradiol, behave differently with respect to accumulation in several other tissues of the rat. Progressive accumulation of radioactivity from ³H-estramustine was particularly evident in the preputial, submaxillary and thyroid glands, in contrast to the rapid decrease in radioactivity from ³H-estradiol initially taken up by these organs.

In conclusion, the fate of estramustine and estradiol is quite different with regard both to uptake in various tissues and to distribution within the ventral prostate gland. The latter compound is confined to the prostatic epithelial cells, as is testosterone, while estramustine passes through the cells into the lumina and is most probably excreted together with prostatic secretory contents.

Binding of ³H-estramustine by rat ventral prostate cytosol

³H-Estramustine with high specific radioactivity was injected intraperitoneally into castrated male rats which were killed 2 hours following injection [11]. Cytosol (105,000 g supernatant) prepared from the ventral prostate gland was separated on a gel chromatography column (Ultrogel AcA-54) with a separation range of 6,000−70,000 daltons. A major peak of radioactivity

was eluted together with the main UV-absorbing peak at an elution volume corresponding to a molecular weight of 40,000–50,000. Thinlayer chromatographic analysis of the radioactive material easily extracted from the eluate organic solvent showed that it consisted mainly of estramustine.

The binding of estramustine by rat ventral prostate was further studied *in vitro* using cytosol preparations. ^{3}H-Estramustine was bound to macromolecules to a much higher extent than ^{3}H-estradiol or ^{3}H-androstanolone and this type of ^{3}H-estramustine binding was not present in plasma or cytosol preparations from liver or pancreas [12, 13]. Furthermore, gel filtration experiments indicated that estramustine was bound to a macromolecular species other than those binding estradiol or androstanolone.

Optimum *in vitro* binding of estramustine by rat ventral prostate cytosol occurred between pH 7 and 8.5 with a maximum at pH 7.8 [11]. The protein nature of the estramustine-binding species was indicated by its sensitivity to proteolytic enzymes and its inertness to deoxyribonuclease or ribonuclease treatment.

The estramustine-binding protein concentrated at pH 5 during isoelectric focusing in a sucrose gradient [13]. Sucrose density gradient centrifugation at low ionic strength indicated a sedimentation coefficient of the estramustine-protein complex of 3.7 S. Using this value and a Stokes radius of 2.9 nm (= m × 10^{-9}) (obtained by gel chromatography on a calibrated column) the molecular weight of the estramustine-binding protein was calculated [14] as 44,000 [13]. Using the linear relationship between the ratio of elution volume to void volume and the logarithm of the molecular weight [15], this parameter was determined as 48,000–50,000 [13, 17].

Ligand specificity of the estramustine-binding protein

Analysis of the binding characteristics of the estramustine-binding protein according to Scatchard [16] yielded an apparent K_d of 1–3 × 10^{-8} M (mean value 1.7 ± 0.3 (standard error (S.E.)) × 10^{-8} M, n = 7) (Fig. 2). In order to examine the ligand specificity of the estramustine-binding protein, various unlabelled steroids, steroid conjugates, and steroid nitrogen mustard derivatives in concentrations ranging from 1 nM (= M × 10^{-9}) to 45 μM were incubated together with 10 nM ^{3}H-estramustine in rat ventral prostate cytosol (Tables I-III). None of the steroids or steroid conjugates inhibited the binding of ^{3}H-estramustine by more than 35% even at 45 μM concentration (4,500-fold excess versus the tracer). The most efficient steroidal inhibitor at this concentration was progesterone (35% inhibition) followed by estrone (30%), pregnenolone (25%), androstenedione (20%), and dehydroepiandrosterone (10%). All other steroids or steroid conjugates tested decreased the binding of 10 nM ^{3}H-estramustine by less than 10% when added in 4,500-fold excess. On the other hand, most of the nitrogen mustard derivatives tested gave rise to displacement curves 'parallel' (p < 0.05) to the estramustine standard curve with concentrations for 50% inhibition ranging from 15–25 nM (estramustine) to 6–8 μM (EP), i.e. about 2-fold and 700-fold excess, respectively. The estrone nitrogen mustard LS 271 and the estradiol 3-N-derivative LS 2179 were as efficient competitors as estramustine. Substitution on the D-ring of the estradiol moiety diminished (LS 289, LS 358, LS 675) or virtually abolished (LS 2035, LS 1611, LS 299) the affinity of the ligand for the binding protein. The saturated compound LS 451 was a weak competitor whereas the dehydroepiandrosterone and 5-

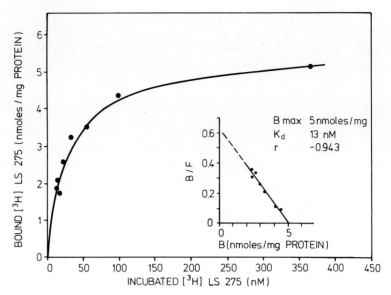

Fig. 2. Saturation and Scatchard analysis of estramustine-binding in cytosol from rat ventral prostate. Maximal specific binding capacity (B max) and apparent K_d were calculated after correction according to Chamness and McGuire [28].

Table III Effect of various steroids and steroid conjugates on the binding of ^{3}H-estramustine by rat ventral prostate cytosol. The table shows cytosol binding of 10 nM ^{3}H-extramustine in the presence of 45 μM competitor, i.e. a 4,500-fold excess, as a percentage of binding in absence of competitors. Estramustine gave 50% inhibition in 2-fold excess.

Competitor	Bound ^{3}H-estramustine (%)
No competitor	100
Progesterone	65
Estrone	70
Pregnenolone	75
Androstenedione	82
Dehydroepiandrosterone	90
Estradiol	92
Androstanolone	93
Testosterone	< 95
19-Nortestosterone	< 95
5α-Androstane-3β,17β-diol	< 95
Corticosterone	< 95
Hydrocortisone	< 95
Dexamethasone	< 95
Diethylstilboestrol	< 95
Ethinylestradiol	< 95
Estriol	< 95
Estrone sulphate	< 95
Estradiol, 3-sulphate	< 95
Estradiol, 3,17-disulphate	< 95
Estrone glucuronide	< 95
Estradiol, 17-glucuronide	< 95

androstene-3β,17β-diol nitrogen mustard derivatives (LS 452 and LS 524) retained substantial competitive capacity.

The maximal binding capacity of the estramustine-binding protein was calculated to be about 5 nmol/mg cytosol protein. Assuming that the protein binds one molecule of estramustine per molecule of protein and that the molecular weight of the protein is 45,000–50,000, it can be calculated that the estramustine-binding protein constitutes 20–25% of the total protein in cytosol from ventral prostate.

Purification of the estramustine-binding protein

In order to study the characteristics of the estramustine-binding protein further this macromolecule from rat ventral prostate was purified [17]. After labelling with ³H-estramustine cytosol was separated on a diethyl-aminoethyl (DEAE)-cellulose column. Radioactive fractions were pooled, concentrated, and filtered through a calibrated Sephadex G-100 Superfine column. The radioactive peak eluted at a position corresponding to a molecular weight of 48,000 was chromatographed on a column of Octyl-Sepharose. The final purification step consisted of polyacrylamide gel electrophoresis (PAGE) and yielded a homogeneous preparation of the estramustine-binding protein.

When analysed by PAGE in the presence of sodium dodecyl sulphate (SDS), the protein decomposed into two subunits with molecular weights of about 20,000 and 18,000, respectively. SDS-PAGE performed following reduction of disulphide bridges of the protein gave three protein bands with molecular weights of about 12,000, 11,000, and 8,000, respectively.

Amino acid analysis of purified estramustine-binding protein showed that

Table IV Amino acid composition of estramustine-binding protein.

Aminoacid	nmol amino acid per 100 nmol protein
Cysteic acid	3.57
Aspartic acid	9.78
Methionine	2.51
Threonine	5.93
Serine	6.31
Glutamic acid	15.97
Proline	3.63
Glycine	4.54
Alanine	4.71
Valine	8.62
Isoleucine	5.23
Leucine	8.91
Tyrosine	2.90
Phenylalanine	4.33
Glucosamine	1.96
Histidine	1.23
Lysine	6.82
Tryptophan	0.60
Arginine	2.46
Total	100.01

it contains about 6% of sulphur-containing amino acids and about 26% of acidic amino acids and indicated the presence of carbohydrate (Table IV).

Radioimmunoassay of the estramustine-binding protein

Antibodies against the purified estramustine-binding protein were produced in rabbits and used for radioimmunoassay of the protein in various tissues

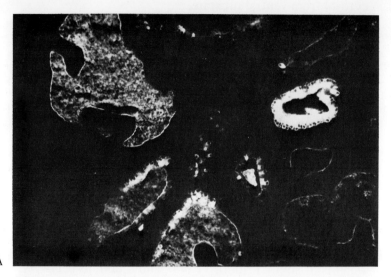

A

B

Fig. 3. Immunofluorescence micrographs of the rat ventral prostate gland. Sections of rat ventral prostate were incubated with rabbit antiserum to estramustine-binding protein (dilution 1:320) followed by fluoresceinisothiocyanate-conjugated sheep anti-rabbit antibodies. B represents a higher magnification of A. Several ductuli are seen. Immunoreactive epithelial cells are seen in several of them. Some exhibit fluorescence in the lumen and some both in the epithelial cells and in the lumen. In some ductuli profiles all epithelial cells are fluorescent.

of the rat [17]. In male rats estramustine-binding protein was present in high levels in the ventral prostate (about 18% of the total cytosol protein content) and in lower amounts in the lateral and dorsal lobes of the prostate (0.8 and 0.2% of total cytosol protein, respectively). In addition, estramustine-binding protein was found in much lower concentrations in several other tissues.

In female rats estramustine-binding protein was absent in most tissues and found only in low concentrations in the cerebral cortex, kidney, spleen, submaxillary gland, and pancreas.

Using the indirect immunofluorescence method of Coons [18], essentially as described elsewhere in detail [19], estramustine-binding protein-immunoreactive material was found in epithelial cells of many ductuli of the prostate gland (Fig. 3). Not all cells were positive in all ductuli, however, and some ductuli did not reveal any fluorescence as judged from examination of single sections. This fluorescence was not present in sections incubated with normal rabbit serum or with estramustine-binding protein-antiserum absorbed with estramustine-binding protein. A fluorescence of varying intensity could also be seen in the lumen of several ductuli. However, fluorescence was also seen sometimes in the lumen in controls, although with a markedly lower intensity.

Major steroid-binding proteins in rat ventral prostate

Several reports have been published on the binding of steroids to proteins in rat ventral prostate cytosol sedimenting between 3 S and 5 S and with molecular weights about 50,000. Liao and collaborators [20—22] reported on the presence of two androstanolone-binding proteins in rat ventral prostate cytosol. One protein ('β-protein') was the specific androgen receptor sedimenting at 7—9 S and binding androstanolone only. The second protein ('α-protein') sedimented at 3—3.5 S and bound a broader range of ligands including androstanolone, estradiol-17β and progesterone. The α-protein was claimed to interfere with the association of the androgen-receptor complex with the cell nuclei or chromatin. At the same time, Karsznia *et al.* described a protein in rat ventral prostate that sedimented at 3.5 S, had a molecular weight of 45,000—50,000 and that bound pregnenolone and progesterone [23]. This protein was not present in rat plasma or muscle.

In 1977, Lea *et al.* [24] described a protein, 'prostatein', which constituted a major part (20—30%) of the proteins in rat ventral prostate cytosol. Prostatein bound androstanolone with low affinity and high capacity and had an isoelectric point of 4.8 and a molecular weight of 46,000. Prostatein seemed to be a tetramer composed of two different subunits, with molecular weights of 9,000 and 14,000, respectively. It was localized in the lumen and epithelium of acinar glands as well as in semen. The production of prostatein by the rat ventral prostate was highly dependent on androgen stimulation, increasing with sexual maturation and decreasing more rapidly than total cytosol protein from day 3 after castration. Treatment with testosterone prevented the disappearance of prostatein following castration, and stimulated prostatein synthesis in the 6-day castrate.

Heyns *et al.* have recently reported on a steroid-binding non-receptor protein in rat ventral prostate cytosol [25, 26]. The protein — prostatic binding protein (PBP) — was precipitated with ammonium sulphate between 50 and 70% saturation, was eluted from Sephadex G-100 at a position corresponding to a molecular weight of 51,000 and sedimented at 3.7 S. The binding was not specific for particular steroids although pregnenolone and androstenedione seemed to be preferentially bound with a K_d value (for pregnenolone) in the range of 10^{-6} M. The amino acid composition of purified PBP was very similar to that of estramustine-binding protein [17, 27].

The similarities between the estramustine-binding protein, α-protein, prostatein and PBP are striking and it seems reasonable to assume that they may represent one and the same molecular species. Prostatein, PBP and estramustine-binding protein have all been reported to constitute 20% or more of the total protein content of cytosol from the ventral prostate of the rat. The quantitative predominance of this protein indicates that it has an important physiological function. The possibility cannot be excluded that it plays a role in the regulation of sperm activity as a steroid carrier. It is also possible that it may act inside the prostatic cell, perhaps in connection with androgen, as suggested by Liao for the α-protein. We would like to suggest that this major protein be called prostatic secretion protein (PSP).

Preliminary studies on the human prostate

Studies have recently been initiated to investigate the possible occurrence of estramustine-binding protein or a similar protein in human prostate tissue. Scatchard analysis of binding data obtained for estramustine in cytosol from a specimen of benign prostatic hyperplasia (BPH) indicated the existence of a high-affinity binding component (Fig. 4). Gel filtration on Ultrogel AcA-34 revealed an estramustine-binding macromolecule with a

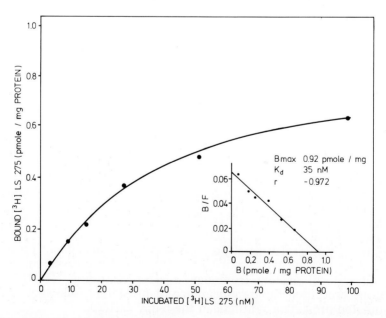

Fig. 4. Saturation and Scatchard analysis of estramustine binding in cytosol from a specimen of human BPH. Cytosol samples (200 μl, 2.5 mg cytosol protein/ml) were incubated at 15°C for 18 hours with 3 nM ³H-estramustine in the presence of varying amounts of unlabelled estramustine. For further details, see legend to Figure 2.

molecular weight in the range of 50,000. Following isoelectric focusing of a similar sample, radioactivity was concentrated at pH 5.

These data indicate that the human prostate contains an estramustine-binding protein with characteristics similar to the corresponding protein in rat prostate. Furthermore, radioimmunoassay of serial dilutions of cytosols from BPH tissues gave dose-response curves identical to the standard curve for rat estramustine-binding protein. It would therefore seem as if human prostate tissue contains a protein similar or identical to rat estramustine-binding protein.

The possible significance of the estramustine-binding macromolecule in the BPH tissue may as yet only be speculated upon. Its presence in human prostate tissue may provide an explanation for the efficiency of estramustine phosphate in the treatment of prostatic carcinoma: the estramustine-binding protein might concentrate estramustine from the blood and provide the tissue with a high concentration of the drug. Interindividual differences in prostatic content of estramustine-binding protein might be related to varying responses in prostatic cancer patients treated with estramustine phosphate.

Summary

The chemical and physical characteristics of a major protein in rat ventral prostate that interacts with estramustine, a nitrogen mustard derivative of estradiol and a metabolite of the anti-cancer drug estramustine phosphate, have been investigated. The binding of estramustine and related nitrogen mustard derivatives by this protein has been studied and the occurrence of the protein in tissues other than the rat ventral prostate has been examined.

The estramustine-protein complex was found to have a molecular weight of 45,000–50,000, a sedimentation coefficient of 3.5–4 S, a Stokes radius of about 3 nm, a frictional ratio of 1.2–1.3, and an isoelectric point at pH 5. The capacity of the protein to bind estramustine was about 5 nmol ligand per mg ventral prostate cytosol protein, and the complex had a K_d of about 20 nM.

The estramustine-binding protein constituted about 20% of the total rat ventral prostate cytosol protein content. Estramustine-binding protein was purified from rat ventral prostate cytosol using chromatography on DEAE-cellulose, Sephadex G-100 Superfine, Octyl-Sepharose CL-4B, and polyacrylamide gel electrophoresis. Amino acid analysis showed that the protein contains about 6% of sulphur-containing amino acids and about 26% of acidic amino acids, and that it contains glucosamine. The protein was found to consist of two subunits with molecular weights of about 20,000 and 18,000, respectively. Following reduction with β-mercaptoethanol the protein gave rise to three peptides with molecular weights of about 12,000, 11,000 and 8,000, respectively. The binding of estramustine by the protein *in vitro* occurred within a broad range from pH 7 to pH 8.5 with maximal binding at pH 7.8. The presence of the nitrogen mustard group at position 3 of the steroid moiety seemed to be essential for high-affinity binding, since none of the natural steroids tested inhibited the binding of ^{3}H-estramustine by more than 35%, even when added in 4,500-fold excess.

Tissue distribution of ^{3}H-estramustine and of the estramustine-binding protein was studied by use of autoradiography and radioimmunoassay, respectively. The ventral prostate gland showed the most efficient capacity to concentrate ^{3}H-estramustine and the highest concentration of the protein. The autoradiographic results indicate that the estramustine-binding protein is a secretory protein. It may be speculated that the protein is involved in regulation of the function of spermatozoa.

Preliminary results indicate that cytosol from specimens of BPH contain an estramustine-binding macromolecule similar or identical to estramustine-binding protein in rat ventral prostate. It is suggested that this protein may be of importance in the mechanism of action of estramustine phosphate in the treatment of prostatic carcinoma.

Acknowledgments

This study was in part supported by a grant from the Swedish Cancer Society.

References

1. Jönsson, G., Högberg, B. and Nilsson, T. (1977): Treatment of advanced prostatic carcinoma with estramustine phosphate (Estracyt^R). *Scand. J. Urol. Nephrol. 11*, 231.
2. Fredholm, B., Jensen, G., Lindskog, M. and Müntzing, J. (1974): Effects of estramustine phosphate (Estracyt) on growth of DMBA-induced mammary tumours in rats. *Acta Pharmacol. Toxicol., 35, Suppl. I*, 28.
3. Müntzing, J., Jensen, G. and Högberg, B. (1979): Pilot study on the growth inhibition by estramustine phosphate (Estracyt^R) of rat mammary tumours sensitive and insensitive to oestrogen. *Acta Pharmacol. Toxicol. 44, 1.*
4. Müntzing, J., Kirdani, R. Y., Saroff, J., Murphy, G. P. and Sandberg, A. A. (1977): Inhibitory effects of Estracyt on R-3327 rat prostatic carcinoma. *Urology, 10, 439.*
5. Høisaeter, P. A. (1975): Incorporation of ^{3}H-thymidine into rat ventral prostate in organ culture. Influence of hormone-cytostatic complexes. *Invest. Urol., 12, 479.*
6. Plym Forshell, G. and Nilsson, H. (1974): The distribution of radioactivity after administration of labelled estramustine phosphate (Estracyt^R), estradiol-17β-phosphate and estradiol to rats. *Acta Pharmacol. Toxicol., 35, Suppl. I*, 28.
7. Høisaeter, P. A. (1976): Studies on the conversion of oestradiol linked to a cytostatic agent (Estracyt^R) in various rat tissues. *Acta Endocrinol. (Copenhagen), 82, 661.*
8. Lowry, O. H., Rosebrough, N. J., Farr, A. L. and Randall, R. J. (1951): Protein measurement with the Folin phenol reagent. *J. Biol. Chem., 193, 265.*
9. Rodbard, D., Rayford, P. L., Cooper, J. A. and Ross, G. T. (1968): Statistical quality control of radioimmunoassays. *J. Clin. Endocrinol. Metab., 28, 1412.*
10. Appelgren, L.-E., Forsgren, B., Gustafsson, J.-Å., Pousette, Å. and Högberg, B. (1978): Autoradiographic studies of ^{3}H-estramustine in the rat ventral prostate. *Acta Pharmacol. Toxicol., 43, 368.*
11. Forsgren, B., Gustafsson, J.-Å., Pousette, Å. and Högberg, B. (1979): Binding characteristics of a major protein in rat ventral prostate cytosol that interacts with estramustine, a nitrogen mustard derivative of estradiol-17β. *Cancer Res.*, submitted for publication.
12. Forsgren, B. and Högberg, B. (1977): Binding of a nitrogen mustard derivative of estradiol to rat ventral prostate gland and cytosol. In: *Research on Steroids, Transactions of the Seventh Meeting of the International Study Group for Steroid Hormones, Rome 1975*, Vol. VII, p. 431. Editors: A. Vermeulen, P. Jungblut, A. Klopper, L. Lerner and F. Sciarra. North-Holland Publishing Co., Amsterdam.
13. Forsgren, B., Högberg, B., Gustafsson, J.-Å. and Pousette, Å (1978): Binding of estramustine, a nitrogen mustard derivative of estradiol-17β, in cytosol from rat ventral prostate. *Acta Pharm. Suecica, 15, 23.*
14. Siegel, L. M. and Monty, K. J. (1966): Determination of molecular weights and

frictional ratios of proteins in impure systems by use of gel filtration and density gradient centrifugation. Application to crude preparations of sulfite and hydroxyl-amine reductase. *Biochim. Biophys. Acta, 112,* 346.

15. Determann, H. and Michel, W. (1966): The correlation between molecular weight and elution behaviour in the gel chromatography of proteins. *J. Chromatogr., 25,* 303.

16. Scatchard, G. (1949): The attractions of proteins for small molecules and ions. *Ann. N.Y. Acad. Sci., 51,* 660.

17. Forsgren, B., Björk, P., Carlström, K., Gustafsson, J.-Å., Pousette, Å. and Högberg, B. (1979): Purification and distribution of a major protein in the rat prostate that binds estramustine, a nitrogen mustard derivative of estradiol-17β. *Proc. Natl. Acad. Sci. U.S.A., 76,* 3149.

18. Coons, A. H. (1958): Fluorescent antibody methods. In: *General Cytochemic Methods,* p. 399. Editor: J. F. Danielli. Academic Press, New York.

19. Hökfelt, T., Fuxe, K., Goldstein, M. and Joh, T. H. (1973): Immunohistochemical localization of three catecholamine synthesizing enzymes: Aspects of methodology. *Histochemistry, 33,* 231.

20. Fang, S., Anderson, K. M. and Liao, S. (1969): Receptor proteins for androgens. On the role of specific proteins in selective retention of 17β-hydroxy-5α-androstan-3-one by rat ventral prostate *in vivo* and *in vitro. J. Biol. Chem., 244,* 6584.

21. Fang, S. and Liao, S. (1971): Androgen receptors. Steroid- and tissue-specific retention of a 17β-hydroxy-5α-androstan-3-one-protein complex by the cell nuclei of ventral prostate. *J. Biol. Chem., 246,* 16.

22. Liao, S., Tymoczko, J. L., Liang, T., Anderson, K. M. and Fang, S. (1971): Androgen receptors: 17β-Hydroxy-5α-androstan-3-one and the translocation of a cytoplasmic protein to cell nuclei in prostate. In: *Advances in Biosciences,* Vol. 7, p. 155 (*Schering Workshop on Steroid Hormone Receptors, Berlin 1970*). Editor: G. Raspé. Pergamon Press, Oxford.

23. Karsznia, R., Wyss, R. H., LeRoy Heinrichs, Wm. and Hermann, W. L. (1969): Binding of pregnenolone and progesterone by prostatic 'receptor' proteins. *Endocrinology, 84,* 1238.

24. Lea, O. A., Petrusz, P. and French, F. S. (1977): Prostatein: A dihydrotestosterone binding protein secreted by the rat ventral prostate. *Proceedings of the 59th Annual Meeting of the Endocrine Society, Chicago 1977,* p. 165.

25. Heyns, W. and De Moor, P. (1977): Prostatic binding protein. A steroid-binding protein secreted by rat prostate. *Eur. J. Biochem., 78,* 221.

26. Heyns, W., Verhoeven, G. and De Moor, P. (1976): A comparative study of androgen binding in rat uterus and prostate. *J. Steroid Biochem., 7,* 987.

27. Heyns, W., Peeters, B., Mous, J., Rombauts, W. and De Moor, P. (1978): Purification and characterisation of prostatic binding protein and its subunits. *Eur. J. Biochem., 89,* 181.

28. Chamness, G. C. and McGuire, W. L. (1975): Scatchard plots: Common errors in correction and interpretation. *Steroids, 26,* 538.

Discussion

J.-P. Raynaud (Romainville, France): Have you any idea of the effect of long-term treatment (i.e., toxicology) of estramustine phosphate on biological parameters and do you know which tissues concentrate this compound?

J.-Å. Gustafsson: Estramustine, the dephosphorylated metabolite of estra-mustine phosphate, seems to be well tolerated during long-term treatment of patients with advanced prostatic carcinoma who fail to respond to conventional endocrine therapy. The effects of estramustine phosphate on biological parameters are those of an oestrogen, with decreased plasma levels of testosterone, follicle-stimulating hormone and luteinizing hormone and increased levels of hydrocortisone, transcortin, and prolactin. The oestrogenic side-effects, however, are small, as reflected by the lower incidence of gynecomastia and other feminizing side-effects registered.

The cytotoxic activity of estramustine phosphate is weaker than that of conventional alkylating agents. Though active against experimental animal tumours (rat DMBA-induced mammary tumour and hepatoma AH130), estramustine phosphate has a weak general cytostatic effect and causes little or no marrow depression at conventional therapeutic dosage. It has no immunosuppressant effect.

The concentration of the estramustine-binding protein measured in cytosol preparations from various tissues is shown in the following Table.

Table

Tissue	*Male rat* ng/mg of total cytosol protein	*Female rat* ng/mg of total cytosol protein
Epiphysis	—	—
Pituitary gland	63	—
Cerebral cortex	28	99
Submaxillary gland	278	6
Thyroid gland	48	—
Lung	—	—
Liver	—	—
Pancreas	167	167
Adrenal gland	210	—
Kidney	—	4
Spleen	—	3
Uterus		—
Ovary		—
Oviduct		—
Vagina		—
Ventral prostate	177,000	
Lateral prostate	8,350	
Dorsal prostate	1,817	
Seminal vesicle	394	
Coagulating gland	503	
Epididymis	50	
Testis	—	
Preputial gland	184	—
Skeletal muscle	—	—

J.-P. Raynaud: What do you think is the biological significance of the estramustine-binding protein?

J.-Å. Gustafsson: The quantitative predominance of this protein indicates that it has an important physiological function. It cannot be excluded that it plays a role in regulation of sperm activity, possibly as a steroid carrier. It is also possible that it may act inside the prostatic cell, perhaps in connection with androgen action, as suggested by Liao for the α-protein.

J.-P. Raynaud: Can you give a short survey of the biological profile of estramustine?

J.-Å. Gustafsson: The mode of action of estramustine phosphate is complex and has not been completely elucidated. The general effects in animals and patients treated with the drug are those of an oestrogen, as judged from its antigonadotropic and anti-androgenic properties, including atrophy of the testes and accessory sex organs, antagonism of testosterone-induced growth of the ventral prostate in castrated rats, reduction in serum testosterone levels, decrease of 5α-reductase activity of the prostate and of the prostatic acid phosphatase activity, changes in lipid and carbohydrate metabolism as well as decreased β-glucuronidase activity. However, the oestrogenic activity of estramustine phosphate is weak compared to that of estradiol and experiments in both animals and patients have shown that estramustine phosphate has a considerably stronger cell growth inhibitory effect than estradiol.

F. Rommerts (Rotterdam, The Netherlands): In one of your slides you showed fluorescence dependent on the presence of the binding protein. I noticed that not all of the cells were stained. Could this be an indication that the prostate cells have cycling activities?

J.-Å. Gustafsson: Yes, this is certainly possible. In several cases only the cells were stained, in other cases only the secretion fluid was stained. This may indicate a synchronized discharge of extramustine-binding protein in some ductuli, a process that may be cyclic or occur irregularly.

Binding, metabolism and tissue level of androgens in human prostatic carcinoma, benign prostatic hyperplasia and normal prostate

M. Krieg, W. Bartsch and K. D. Voigt
Department of Clinical Chemistry, 2nd Medical Clinic, University of Hamburg, Hamburg, Federal Republic of Germany

Introduction

We have compared binding, *in vitro* metabolism and endogenous tissue concentration of androgens in 14 prostatic carcinomas (CA), 14 benign prostatic hyperplasias (BPH) and 7 normal prostates (NPR). In this paper we would like to summarize results which have been published elsewhere [1–3]. The reader will find details concerning the experimental procedures in these original papers. Furthermore, particularly in one publication [3] our results are critically discussed in the light of findings reported by other research groups. The present publication also contains as yet unpublished data on *in vitro* metabolism of testosterone (T) in separated epithelium and stroma from BPH and NPR.

Results

Binding studies

Using tritiated 5α-dihydrotestosterone (DHT) receptor- and sex hormone-binding globulin (SHBG)-bound radioactivity was found in the 14 CA cytosols analysed. In 2 of the 14 BPH cytosols receptor-bound radioactivity could not be demonstrated. In the 7 NPR cytosols receptor-binding of radioactivity was never assayable. When calculating the assayable cytosol receptor and SHBG concentrations in CA and BPH from the amount of tritiated DHT displaced by an excess of unlabelled DHT, it was found (Table I) that CA cytosol had significantly ($p < 0.04$) higher assayable receptor concentrations than BPH. This holds true also for SHBG ($p < 0.01$). Dividing CA samples into a group consisting exclusively of adenocarcinoma and a group consisting predominantly of a cribriform and/or poorly-differentiated tumour pattern, in the latter group significantly ($p < 0.05$) higher amounts of assayable receptor sites (mean: 37.8 fmol/mg protein;

number of samples (n) = 8) are present than in adenocarcinoma (mean: 21.7 fmol/mg protein; n = 6). No significant difference exists on comparing both groups with respect to SHBG.

Metabolic studies

Table II summarizes the main metabolites found after incubation of CA, BPH and NPR homogenates with either tritiated T, DHT, or 5α-androstane-3α,17β-diol (3α-Diol). Four points seem remarkable: 1. In CA, significantly more of the added T remained unmetabolized than in BPH and NPR and formation of DHT plus 5α-androstane-3α,17β-diol + 5α-androstane-3β, 17β-diol (Diol) was approximately 15% lower. However, the amount of

Table I Assayable receptor and SHBG concentrations (fmol/mg protein) in the 100,000 g cytosol of CA, BPH and NPR.

	Number of samples	Receptor concentration		SHBG concentration	
		Mean	Range	Mean	Range
CA	14	30.9[1]	6.0–93.5	93.2[2]	35.7–225
BPH	14	12.3	0–37.8	39.9	18.1–84.7
NPR	7	not assayable		not determined	

[1] Significantly different from BPH ($p < 0.04$).
[2] Significantly different from BPH ($p < 0.01$).

Table II Main metabolites (mean ± standard deviation (sd)) obtained by thin layer chromatography of homogenate of CA, BPH and NPR found after incubation of homogenate, diluted 1:2 with buffer, with tritiated T, DHT and 3α-Diol for 30 minutes at 37°C in the presence of $NADPH_2$ (for T and DHT) or NADP (for 3α-Diol).

Metabolites found (pmol)		Tritiated steroids (pmol) added per g homogenate					
		T (15.4 ± 2.4)		DHT (16.8 ± 2.5)		3α-DIOL (23.2 ± 1.6)	
CA	T	5.1 ± 2.8[1]	(10)	<0.5	(5)	<0.5	(4)
	DHT	6.6 ± 3.2	(10)	13 ± 2.5[3]	(5)	1.8 ± 0.2	(4)
	DIOL	3.3 ± 2.4[2]	(10)	3.9 ± 2.1[2]	(5)	20 ± 0.6	(4)
BPH	T	0.8 ± 0.5	(16)	<0.5	(16)	<0.5	(6)
	DHT	5.5 ± 1.7	(16)	6.8 ± 1.9	(16)	1.2 ± 0.4	(6)
	DIOL	6.2 ± 2.7	(16)	7.3 ± 3.0	(16)	21 ± 1.3	(6)
NPR	T	1.2 ± 0.8	(7)	<0.5	(7)	<0.5	(2)
	DHT	4.3 ± 1.7	(7)	5.5 ± 2.7	(7)	<0.5	(2)
	DIOL	7.3 ± 2.5	(7)	10.5 ± 3.6	(7)	22.6 ± 1.8	(2)

[1] Significantly different from BPH and NPR ($p < 0.01$).
[2] Significantly different from BPII and NPR ($p < 0.05$).
[3] Significantly different from BPH and NPR ($p < 0.001$).

Table III Main metabolites (mean ± sd) obtained by thin layer chromatography of homogenate of human BPH and NPR diluted 1:2 with buffer and incubated with tritiated T or DHT for 30 minutes at 37°C without NADPH supplementation.

Metabolites found (pmol)		Tritiated steroids (pmol) added per g homogenate			
		T (15.4 ± 2.4)		DHT (16.8 ± 2.5)	
BPH	T	8.1 ± 3.9[1]	(15)		
	DHT + DIOL	5.5 ± 2.8[2]	(15)		
NPR	T	13.0 ± 1.2	(6)		
	DHT + DIOL	1.5 ± 0.3	(6)		
BPH	DHT			12.3 ± 2.7	(15)
	DIOL			0.7 ± 0.6	(15)
NPR	DHT			12.8 ± 1.7	(6)
	DIOL			0.5 ± 0.2	(6)

[1] Significantly different from NPR ($p < 0.002$).
[2] Significantly different from NPR ($p < 0.001$).

Table IV Relative metabolic activities found in CA, BPH and NPR after incubation of organ homogenates with tritiated T or DHT for 30 minutes at 37°C in the presence of 30 µmol NADPH/g homogenate.

	T		5α-Reduction		DHT	
	5α-Reduction		3α (β)-Reduction		DIOL	
CA	0.62 ± 0.42[1]	(10)	3.1 ± 1.8	(5)	4.3 ± 2.4[2]	(5)
BPH	0.07 ± 0.04	(16)	2.0 ± 1.4	(16)	1.4 ± 1.4	(16)
NPR	0.10 ± 0.08	(7)	1.2 ± 0.4[3]	(7)	0.7 ± 0.5	(7)

5α-Reduction = DHT + DIOL found after T-incubation.
3α (β)-Reduction = DIOL found after DHT-incubation.
DHT/DIOL = ratio of DHT and DIOL found after DHT-incubation.
[1] Significantly different from BPH and NPR ($p < 0.01$).
[2] Significantly different from BPH and NPR ($p < 0.02$).
[3] Significantly different from BPH and CA ($p < 0.05$).

Table V Main metabolites (mean ± sd) obtained by thin layer chromatography of epithelium and stroma fraction of BPH and NPR incubated with tritiated T for 30 minutes at 37°C in the presence of NADPH. The concentration of added T was 1 pmol per mg protein of the epithelium and stroma fractions.

Metabolites found (pmol × 10/mg protein)	BPH (10)		NPR (1)	
	Epithelium	Stroma	Epithelium	Stroma
T	7.4 ± 2.3	2.0 ± 1.8	0.9	2.6
DHT	1.2 ± 0.6	3.2 ± 1.1	2.2	2.2
DIOL	0.9 ± 0.4	2.9 ± 2.0	6.5	4.3

Numbers in brackets = number of experiments.

DHT formed was as high as in BPH or NPR. 2. In CA, significantly more of the added DHT remained unmetabolized than in BPH or NPR and formation of Diol was significantly lower. 3. For all three tissues, there was very little conversion of added 3α-Diol to DHT. 4. Comparing BPH and NPR, the latter converted much more of the added DHT to Diol, although the difference is slightly above the 5% confidence limits.

A further difference between BPH and NPR was found when androgen metabolism was studied in the homogenates without NADPH supplementation (Table III). While in BPH even without cofactor supplementation a significant amount of DHT plus Diol was found, in NPR the high conversion of T to DHT plus Diol recorded in Table II stops nearly completely without cofactor supplementation. If DHT was added as substrate differences between BPH and NPR were not found.

In Table IV the metabolic data are compiled according to relative metabolic activities. Besides the significantly higher ratios in CA compared with BPH and NPR, which confirm the significant differences in metabolism mentioned above, it seems remarkable that the ratio 5α-reduction to 3α(β)-reduction is significantly lower in NPR than in BPH and CA.

In a first attempt to analyse T metabolism in BPH and NPR after separating the tissue into epithelium and stroma according to Cowan *et al.* [4], we found (Table V) that in BPH most of the 5α-reductase activity is located in the stroma, while, in the one NPR so far investigated, the epithelium seems to be more active in terms of 5α-reductase activity.

Endogenous androgen tissue levels

Table VI summarizes the endogenous androgen concentrations found in CA, BPH and NPR homogenates. The following differences are statistically significant: 1. The high T concentration in CA compared with BPH and NPR. 2. The low DHT concentration in NPR compared with CA and BPH. 3. The low 3α-Diol concentration in BPH compared with CA and NPR.

Table VI   Endogenous levels (ng/g tissue; mean ± sd) of T, DHT and 3α-DIOL in homogenate of human CA, BPH and NPR, measured by radioimmunoassay.

	Endogenous androgen level		
	CA	BPH	NPR
T	1.2 ± 0.8^1 (7)	0.3 ± 0.1 (11)	0.2 ± 0.1 (7)
DHT	3.9 ± 0.3 (3)	4.5 ± 1.4 (14)	1.6 ± 1.0^2 (6)
3α-DIOL	1.6 ± 0.8^3 (7)	0.6 ± 0.7 (14)	1.7 ± 0.3^3 (3)

[1] Significantly different from BPH and NPR ($p < 0.002$).
[2] Significantly different from CA and BPH ($p < 0.05$).
[3] Significantly different from BPH ($p < 0.05$).

Concluding remarks

After finishing the manuscript for this Amsterdam meeting two points prompted us to re-examine morphologically and biochemically what we name 'epithelium and stroma fraction': 1. The absence of significant 5α-reductase activity in the epithelium of the BPH, which is in complete contradiction to basic knowledge of androgen metabolism in epithelial cells of rat and dog prostate. 2. The striking difference between BPH and NPR in T metabolism of the epithelium fraction.

Without going into details, which will be published later, the re-examination revealed that the epithelium fraction of BPH consists predominantly of nuclei of epithelial cells freed of their surrounding cytoplasm. On the other hand, the epithelium fraction of NPR showed predominantly intact epithelial cells. Furthermore, compared to the whole organ homogenate, acid phosphatase activity in the epithelium was unexpectedly low.

After modifying the method of tissue processing, we now obtain predominantly intact cells in the epithelium of BPH also and, in concomitance, find a much higher conversion of T in this fraction. Concerning the stroma of BPH, androgen metabolism remained high, indicating that high 5α-reductase activity is still located in the stroma. From these very preliminary data, which have to be substantiated by a larger series, it may be deduced that epithelium from BPH is far more active in metabolizing T than shown in Table V.

Nevertheless, from the results presented, the following may be concluded:

1. The NPR seems to be protected against excessive accumulation of T and DHT due to the shift of androgen metabolism towards Diol not, in general, bound with high affinity to the cytosolic androgen receptors.

2. Compared to NPR, androgen metabolism in CA and BPH is shifted significantly towards T and DHT, both of which have a high affinity for cytosolic androgen receptors.

It is tempting to speculate that this acquired error in androgen metabolism could play an important role in the development and hormone responsiveness of BPH and PCA.

Acknowledgments

This work was supported by the Deutsche Forschungsgemeinschaft (DFG), Sonderforschungsbereich 34 'Endokrinologie'.

References

1. Krieg, M., Bartsch, W., Herzer, S., Becker, H. and Voigt, K. D. (1977): Quantification of androgen binding, androgen tissue levels, and sex hormone-binding globulin in prostate, muscle and plasma of patients with benign prostatic hypertrophy. *Acta endocrinol. (Copenhagen), 86,* 200.
2. Krieg, M., Grobe, I., Voigt, K. D., Altenähr, E. and Klosterhalfen, H. (1978): Human prostatic carcinoma: Significant differences in its androgen binding and metabolism compared to human benign prostatic hypertrophy. *Acta endocrinol. (Copenhagen), 88,* 397.
3. Krieg, M., Bartsch, W., Janssen, W. and Voigt, K. D. (1979): A comparative study of binding, metabolism and endogenous levels of androgens in normal, hyperplastic and carcinomatous human prostate. *J. Steroid Biochem., 11,* 615.
4. Cowan, R. A., Cowan, S. K., Grant, J. K. and Elder, H. Y. (1977): Biochemical investigations of separated epithelium and stroma from benign prostatic tissue. *J. Endocrinol., 74,* 111.

Discussion

P. Ekman (Stockholm, Sweden): The prostate may be subdivided into periurethral and peripheral lobes. BPH starts periurethrally while cancer starts peripherally. This is of importance when comparing results from 'normal', hyperplastic and cancerous prostates. From which part did you take your normal prostates?

M. Krieg: The 'whole' normal prostate was processed. Only in one case have we divided the normal prostate into a periurethral and peripheral part and we could not find striking differences in androgen metabolism and tissue concentrations.

P. Ekman: How did you obtain your normal prostates?

M. Krieg: The seven normal prostates were obtained from the Institute of Forensic Medicine. The men were in the age range 19–43 years (mean: 33) and the time span between death of the men and tissue processing was up to 6 hours. The absence of any pathological alteration was verified by histological examination.

R. Ghanadian (London, UK): I found your DHT level in tissues with CA to be very high, compared to NPR, or even relatively high compared to BPH. Do you have any comment on this?

I have also a comment on the metabolism of T in CA. Our studies suggest that the conversion of T to androstenedione occurs in all carcinomatous tissues. This cannot be demonstrated in BPH tissues.

M. Krieg: Our DHT levels in CA tissue are nearly identical to those reported very recently by Geller *et al. (Cancer Res., 38,* 4349, 1978). Furthermore, our DHT levels in BPH and NPR are nearly identical to those reported very recently by Meikle *et al. (J. Clin. Endocrinol. Metab., 47,* 909, 1978). On the other hand we know that compared to BPH relatively low DHT levels were found in CA by Geller *et al. (J. Clin. Endocrinol. Metab., 46,* 440, 1978) and Habib *et al. (J. Endocr., 71,* 99, 1976), while Farnsworth and Brown *(Endocr. Res. Comm., 3,* 105, 1976) reported just the opposite. Therefore, it seems too early to make definite statements concerning DHT levels in CA until further research groups have published their results.

R. Ghanadian: Were all the patients with carcinoma of the prostate untreated?

M. Krieg: Yes.

F. K. Habib (Edinburgh, UK): Your demonstration of high levels of DHT in the malignant tissue is a rather interesting observation, particularly in view of the low 5α-reductase activity. Could these levels be accounted for in terms of a high reversible 3α(β)-hydroxysteroid dehydrogenase or is it perhaps due to a change of emphasis in the binding properties of the malignant prostate?

M. Krieg: Concerning the 3α(β)-hydroxysteroid dehydrogenase activity, we found that very low back-conversion of 3α-Diol to DHT takes place in the human prostate, particularly if compared with respective data on the rat prostate. From our data we concluded that the drastically decreased conversion of DHT to Diol leads to a relatively higher 5α-reductase than 3α(β)-hydroxysteroid dehydrogenase activity in CA, thus shifting the androgen metabolites to T as well as DHT.

Changes in the binding properties of the malignant prostate could additionally favour the accumulation of DHT in CA. However, the latter point is, so far, speculative.

M. E. Harper (Cardiff, UK): How did you obtain your prostate samples? Were they from open prostatectomy (OP) or transurethral resection (TUR) samples? I feel very strongly that TUR specimens are of little use. We have measured various biochemical parameters in the same prostates obtained by different techniques and prostatic cancer specimens obtained by cold punch and TUR show that the endogenous androgen content is 5 to 10 times higher in the former. BPH samples obtained by OP compared to TUR also have a 5 times greater concentration. If we turn to quite a different field, the polyamines, the content of these compounds and the enzymes involved in their synthesis is very much higher in OP than in TUR specimens. One could cite many more examples such as platine activity in tissue culture, etc.

M. Krieg: CA samples were obtained during the course of open perineal cryosurgery. BPH samples were obtained during OP.

Concerning TUR specimens, we have also bad experiences. So far, in no case could a receptor protein be demonstrated.

F. Rommerts (Rotterdam, The Netherlands): The enzyme activities you measured in homogenates were *potential* activities. Within the cell the enzyme activities depend on cofactor availability and enzyme can even be latent. The *actual* intracellular enzyme activities may therefore be different from your data. This is important when you try to explain the different amounts of androgens in prostate tissue.

M. Krieg: You are right in saying that we have measured 'potential' enzyme activities. What actually takes place intracellularly is more or less unknown. On the other hand it seems remarkable that, despite experimental limitations, our predictions of endogenous tissue concentrations of androgens deduced from the *in vitro* metabolic data are fulfilled with only one exception, thus indicating that the *in vitro* metabolism might reflect, at least partly, the *in vivo* situation.

J. C. Romijn (Rotterdam, The Netherlands): How did you separate epithelium and stroma of the prostatic tissue? How did you check for the purity of the tissue fractions? Were the metabolism studies with separated fractions performed with 'intact' fractions or with homogenates made of it? Did you add cofactors?

M. Krieg: 1. We have separated the tissue according to the method of Cowan *et al.* (*J. Endocr.*, *74*, 111, 1977).

2. The purity of the fractions was checked by measuring the concentrations of acid phosphatase and hydroxyproline. So far, epithelium as well as stroma were contaminated by each other in the range of 5–10%. Further-

more, the fractions were checked by light microscopy.

3. The metabolism was studied in fractions which were not homogenized. However, concerning the epithelium, the recovery of intact cells was very low.

4. The metabolism was studied in the presence of a high excess of NADPH.

Receptor proteins for androgens in benign prostatic hypertrophy and carcinoma of the prostate

R. Ghanadian and G. Auf
Prostate Research Laboratory, Department of Surgery, Royal Postgraduate Medical School and Institute of Urology, University of London, London, United Kingdom

Introduction

Hormone therapy of prostatic carcinoma is based on the role of testicular hormones in the growth and development of the tumour. The response to this treatment is variable and unpredictable [1]. Failure of endocrine treatment can be attributed to the lack of a reliable index for prediction of responders and non-responders. The predictive role of steroid receptors in the assessment of responsiveness of most breast tumour cases to hormonal manipulation is now well-established. It has been reported that patients whose breast tumours contain either modest or negligible amounts of oestrogen receptors have very little chance of benefiting from adrenalectomy, hypophysectomy or other forms of hormone manipulation. However, most patients whose cancer tumours contain substantial receptor levels will respond objectively to endocrine therapy [2]. The significance of the measurement of oestrogen receptors in the nuclei of breast tumour cells has also been emphasised [3]. The references cited indicate the role of both cytoplasmic and nuclear receptors in predicting response to endocrine treatment in breast cancer patients.

Progress in the development of techniques required for the quantitative measurement of steroid receptors in the human prostate has lagged behind that for mammary tumours. The nature and characteristic features of prostatic tumours have been the main reasons for the failure of most of the early attempts to measure cytoplasmic receptors in this tissue.

The high level of endogenous androgens [4] bound to most of the androgen receptors in the human prostate accounts for the limited number of remaining binding sites available and, often, for failure to detect them.

Another important problem is the strong enzymic activity of this tissue which results in metabolism of testosterone to androstanolone (DHT) and androstanediols [5]. Other problems include the presence of a high level of sex hormone-binding globulin (SHBG) which exhibits a high affinity for DHT [6], whilst the existence of two different types of cells, epithelial and fibromuscular, and their uneven distribution can seriously affect the interpretation of results [7].

During the last decade these problems have been tackled by several research groups. Their efforts have resulted in the development of a number of techniques which have overcome some of the above-mentioned difficulties involved in the assay of androgen receptors in prostate tissue [8–11]. In this study we report on a technique developed in our laboratory for the measurement of cytoplasmic and nuclear androgen receptors in the human prostate and present data on 15 patients with benign hypertrophy (BPH) and 54 patients with carcinoma of the prostate (CA). However, the data for receptor assay have not been correlated with the clinical progress of the patients for this report.

Materials and methods

Steroids

DHT, progesterone (P), oestradiol (E), and cortisol (17-hydroxycorticosterone, C) were purchased from Sigma Chemicals. Metribolone (R1881) was a gift from Roussel Uclaf. The following radioactive steroids were also used: 1,2-^{3}H-DHT (^{3}H-DHT), 60 Ci/mM, 1,2,6,7-^{3}H-P (^{3}H-P), 87 Ci/mM (purchased from the Radiochemical Centre, Amersham) and 6,7,-^{3}H-R1881 (^{3}H-R1881), 55.5 Ci/mM (kindly given by Roussel Uclaf). Stock solutions of 50 pM (= M × 10^{-12})/ml ^{3}H-P and ^{3}H-DHT in methanol and of 50 pM/ml ^{3}H-R1881 in toluene: methanol, 9:1 were prepared and stored at −20°C.

Buffers

Trometamol (tris)-edetic acid (EDTA) buffer containing 20 mM tris and 1.5 mM EDTA with 2 mM mercaptoethanol (pH 7.4) was used as the standard buffer. For tissue homogenization procedures and preparation of dextran-coated charcoal 250 mM sucrose were added to the standard buffer. Dextran-coated charcoal was prepared in two concentrations, for stripping endogenous steroids (5% charcoal and 0.5% dextran T 70 (Pharmacia)) and for removal of free from bound tritiated steroids (1.25% charcoal and 0.625% dextran T 70).

Patients

Prostatic tissues were obtained from 54 patients with CA and 15 patients with BPH. Patients with CA were classified into 3 groups:
1) Untreated: These patients received no treatment for their disease prior to operation.
2) Treated: These patients received a variety of treatments for varying periods of time prior to surgery. They underwent operation due to onset of urological complications.
3) Unclassified: Carcinoma had been established by histological examination in all tissues investigated in this group. However, at this stage case histories have not been followed-up.

Tissues

BPH and CA tissues were obtained by transurethral resection (TUR). Burned tissue was removed from the surface of the chips and the residue cleansed of contaminating fluids prior to freezing in liquid nitrogen. Tissues were stored at $-40°C$ before being assayed.

Receptor assays were performed for all prostatic tumours without prior knowledge of the clinical status of the patients. At the present time clinical data on the patients has not been finalized and hence no attempt has yet been made to correlate clinical response of the patients with the level of androgen receptors in tissue.

Preparation of cytosol and nuclear extracts

Prostatic tumours were sliced and pulverized in a microdismembrator (Braun Melsungen) for two cycles, each lasting 30 seconds, with a cooling period of 1 minute in liquid nitrogen. The powdered tissue was transferred into 3 volumes of ice-cold buffer and the mixture gently homogenized with a motor-driven Teflon pestle to yield an even homogenate. Tissue homogenates were transferred to precooled 10 ml centrifuge tubes and spun at 600 g for 10 minutes at $4°C$ to yield a supernatant fraction and a crude nuclear pellet. Cytosol fractions were obtained by centrifuging the resultant supernatant fractions at 105,000 g for 1 hour at $2°C$. Crude nuclear pellets were suspended in 10 volumes of ice-cold buffer and filtered through a double layer of nylon gauze (Nybolt T25). The filtrates were then centrifuged at 800 g for 10 minutes at $4°C$. The resulting nuclear pellets were further washed with 2×5 ml buffer. Finally, the nuclear pellets were disrupted by resuspending them in sucrose buffer containing 0.4 M KCl (1:3 w/v) for 30 minutes at $4°C$. Nuclear extracts were then prepared by centrifuging the disrupted nuclear suspension at 20,000 g for 30 minutes at $2°C$.

Removal of free endogenous hormones

Aliquots of cytosol and nuclear extracts were incubated with dextran-coated charcoal (10:1 v/v) for 10 minutes at $4°C$. At the end of the incubation period the steroid bound to charcoal was precipitated by centrifugation at 3,700 g for 20 minutes at $4°C$. This procedure yields cytoplasmic and nuclear fractions stripped of endogenous hormones.

Specificity studies

The specificity of binding of ^{3}H-R1881 to cytoplasmic androgen receptor was examined at both $0°C$ and $15°C$. The experiments were carried out by the incubation of either the 105,000 g cytoplasmic fraction directly or the protamine sulphate-precipitated receptors.

Specificity studies at $0°C$: Aliquots (100 μl) of cytosol were incubated with 5 nM (= M $\times$ 10^{-9}) ^{3}H-R1881 or ^{3}H-P in the presence or absence of increasing concentrations of radio-inert R1881, DHT and P for 16–20 hours. In parallel experiments, C (10^{-7} M) was included in the media to inhibit the binding of ^{3}H-P to C-binding globulin (CBG). All experimental procedures were performed as previously described [10]. The specificity of the nuclear receptors was similarly examined by incubating the nuclear extracts with ³H-R1881 in the presence or absence of a 100-fold excess of radio-inert competitor.

In another series of experiments the binding of ³H-R1881, ³H-DHT and ³H-P to cytoplasmic androgen receptors was investigated using protamine sulphate-precipitated receptors. In this procedure aliquots (100 μl) of cytosol were equilibrated with an equal volume of protamine sulphate solution (1 mg/ml). The resultant precipitates were incubated with 5 nM ³H-R1881, ³H-DHT or ³H-P in the presence or absence of 100-fold excess R1881, DHT or P, as described elsewhere [12]. The results were expressed as the percentage inhibition of total specific binding, following correction for background count rate.

Specificity studies at 15°C: Aliquots (100 μl) of cytosol were incubated in triplicate with 30 nM ³H-R1881 in the presence or absence of increasing concentrations of radio-inert R1881, DHT, P or E (30 nM – 600 nM) for 20 hours at 15°C. Bound steroid was separated from free by incubation with 50 μl dextran-coated charcoal for 10 minutes at 0–4°C and subsequent centrifugation at 1,000 g for 15 minutes. Bound radioactivity was determined in 100 μl of the resulting supernatant.

The results were plotted as excess molar concentration of competitor versus 1/Y (where $Y = \dfrac{\text{counts per minute (cpm) in presence of competitor}}{\text{cpm in absence of competitor}}$).

Corrections for non-specific binding were applied by subtracting the cpm obtained in the presence of 100-fold excess R1881 from all other values.

The conditions applying to direct specificity studies in the cytosol at 15°C prohibit the use of ³H-DHT as the radioligand, mainly due to the presence of SHBG. For this reason, we modified the protamine sulphate-precipitation technique in such a manner as to enable us to use ³H-DHT as the radioligand. This made it possible to compare the results with ³H-R1881 with those with ³H-DHT-labelled receptors at 15°C.

In this procedure, cytosol was equilibrated with protamine sulphate (1 mg/ml, 1:1 v/v) and the resulting precipitate collected by centrifugation at 800 g. The precipitate was then washed three times with buffer and reconstituted in 0.6 M KCl prepared in sucrose buffer. It was found that the addition of 0.6 M KCl solubilizes the receptor protein from the protamine precipitate. Following this procedure, aliquots (100 μl) of KCl-solubilized fraction were incubated with 30 nM ³H-DHT in the presence or absence of 30–6,000 nM radio-inert competitor at 15°C for 20 hours.

Measurement of cytoplasmic receptors

The procedure for assay of cytosol receptors and the analysis of the results have been reported elsewhere [10].

Measurement of nuclear receptors

The procedures adopted for assay of nuclear receptors and for calculation of results are basically similar to those for cytoplasmic receptors [10]. Following preparation of the nuclear extract and removal of unbound endogenous steroids as previously described, aliquots (100 μl) were incubated with increasing amounts of ³H-R1881 in the presence or absence of a 100-fold excess of radio-inert R1881 at 15°C for 20–24 hours. Separation of free from bound steroid was achieved by treatment with dextran-coated charcoal.

Results

Specificity of binding of R1881 to cytoplasmic receptors

The specificity of binding of R1881 to cytoplasmic androgen receptor proteins was examined under various conditions. Table I shows that, under 0–4°C incubation conditions, R1881 was the most potent competitor for the binding of ^{3}H-R1881, followed by P (85%) and then DHT (58%). In order to determine whether binding of ^{3}H-R1881 was to an androgen- or to a progesterone-binding component, a similar experiment was carried out using ^{3}H-P as the binding ligand. The results show that the main competitor in this case was P (60%) with R1881 (10%) and DHT (20%) displaying very little competition. Inclusion of 10^{-7} M C in the incubation media abolished the competing ability of P for ^{3}H-P-binding, whereas it had no effect on the binding of ^{3}H-R1881. The specificity of binding of ^{3}H-R1881 was also assessed and compared with binding of ^{3}H-DHT and ^{3}H-P to cytoplasmic receptors precipitated by protamine sulphate. Protamine sulphate precipitates were incubated with either ^{3}H-R1881, ^{3}H-P or ^{3}H-DHT at 0–4°C for 16 hours. The results (Table II) show that R1881, P and DHT are all strong competitors for the binding of ^{3}H-R1881 and ^{3}H-DHT. However, ^{3}H-P displayed negligible binding to precipitated cytoplasmic receptor proteins (cf. Table I).

The specificity of R1881 binding to androgen receptors was also examined at 15°C. The relative competition indices of R1881, DHT, P and E as

Table I Specificity of binding of ^{3}H-R1881 and ^{3}H-P to androgen receptors at 0°–4°C in the cytosol of human BPH.

Competitors (100-fold excess)	% Inhibition of specific binding			
	^{3}H-R1881	^{3}H-P	^{3}H-R1881 (plus 10^{-7} M C)	^{3}H-P
R1881	100	10	100	0
P	85	60	88	0
DHT	58	20	60	0

Table II Specificity of binding of ^{3}H-R1881, ^{3}H-DHT and ^{3}H-P to protamine sulphate-precipitated receptors at 0–4°C in the cytosol of human BPH.

Competitors (100-fold excess)	% Inhibition of specific binding		
	^{3}H-R1881	^{3}H-DHT	^{3}H-P
R1881	100	87	16
P	90	71	11
DHT	86	100	10

inhibitors of ³H-R1881 binding were found to be 100%, 40%, 4% and 3%, respectively (Fig. 1). The shift in the binding specificity of cytoplasmic androgen receptor proteins with increase in incubation temperature was also observed when ³H-DHT was used as the radioligand. Results are shown in Fig. 2. In this case, the relative competition indices of R1881, DHT, P and E as competitors to ³H-DHT binding were 100%, 33%, 3% and 1%, respectively.

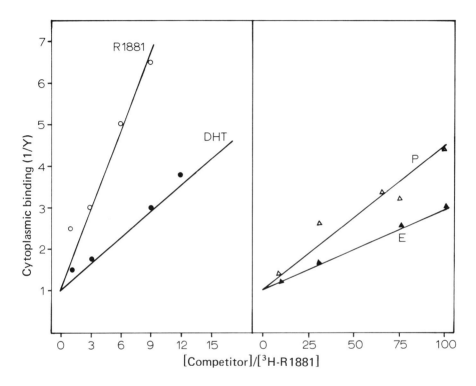

Fig. 1. Competition to cytoplasmic R1881-binding in human BPH by R1881, DHT, P and E. The experiment was carried out by incubation of cytosol with ³H-R1881 in the absence or presence of different amounts of radio-inert competitors at 15°C for 24 hours. ³H-R1881 bound to cytosol was analysed as described in materials and methods. From the relative competition plot, the slopes were calculated, and the relative competition index obtained.

Specificity of R1881 binding to nuclear receptors

The apparent steroid specificity of human prostate nuclear androgen receptors was evaluated following incubation of nuclear extracts with ³H-R1881 at 0–4°C for 20–24 hours. The data indicate that the type of crossreactivity previously observed in the cytoplasm at 0–4°C differs from that found in the nuclei. Under similar experimental conditions, the crossreactivity of P with the binding of R1881 to cytoplasmic receptors was 85%, whereas in the nuclei it was found to be only moderate (50%). Table III shows that both R1881 and DHT are the major competitors for ³H-R1881 binding.

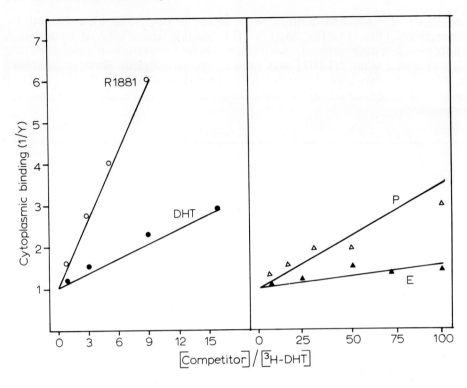

Fig. 2. *Competition to DHT-binding in KCl extract of protamine sulphate-precipitated cytoplasmic receptors in human BPH by R1881, DHT, P and E. The experiment was performed by incubation of KCl extract of precipitated receptors with ³H-DHT in the absence or presence of different amounts of radio-inert competitors at 15°C for 24 hours. ³H-DHT bound to receptors was analysed as described in materials and methods. From the relative competition plot, the slopes were calculated, and the relative competition index obtained.*

Table III *Specificity of ³H-R1881 binding to nuclear androgen receptors.*

Competitor (100-fold excess)	% Inhibition
R1881	100
DHT	81
P	50

Optimal conditions for nuclear receptor assay

Further studies were carried out to determine optimal conditions for nuclear androgen receptor binding to ³H-R1881. The results showed that maximum exchange occurred at 15°C following 20–24 hours incubation. Moreover, at this temperature, nuclear androgen receptor binding remained constant for a further incubation period of up to 10 hours (Fig. 3).

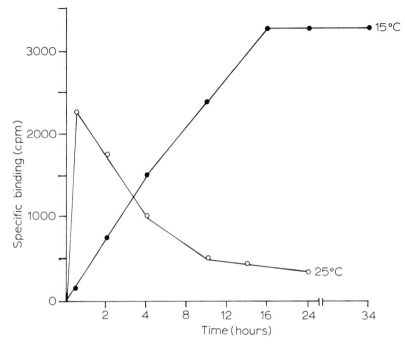

Fig. 3. Optimal temperature and incubation period for maximum labelling of the nuclear androgen receptor. Aliquots (100 µl) of nuclear extract were incubated with 30 nM ^{3}H-R1881 in the presence or absence of 100-fold excess of radio-inert R1881 at either 15°C or 25°C. Specific binding was calculated by subtracting the amount of radio-activity bound in the presence of competitor from that obtained in the absence of competitor.

Cytoplasmic and nuclear androgen receptor levels in BPH and CA

Having established the assay procedure, concentrations of the cytoplasmic and nuclear androgen receptors were measured in 15 benign hypertrophied and 54 carcinomatous prostates. The results are shown in Table IV.

Patients with carcinomatous prostates were divided into 3 groups: 16 untreated, 10 treated and 28 unclassified. Details of each group are given in the Materials and Methods section.

The results show that a considerable degree of variation in receptor levels exists for both BPH and CA tissues. There is also some degree of overlapping in receptor levels between BPH and the different types of CA tissues. These differences are illustrated in Figs 4, 5, 6, and 7. The results demonstrate that the concentration of total receptors in BPH is 20–30 times greater than that of free sites. A similar relationship can also be observed in patients with CA. However, it appears that hormonal manipulation of the tumour may alter this relationship. The mean ± standard error of the mean (sem) for free sites in untreated CA was $5.8 ± 1$ fM ($= M × 10^{-15}$)/mg protein. The corresponding value for treated patients was $14.3 ± 4.3$. This represents a significant difference between the two groups ($p < 0.05$). On the other hand, observed levels of bound receptor decreased following hormonal manipulation of the tumour, values being $84.9 ± 19.5$ and $58 ± 16.7$ fM/mg protein for untreated and treated CA, respectively ($0.05 < p < 0.1$).

Table IV Cytoplasmic and nuclear androgen receptor levels in BPH and CA.

Tissue	Cytoplasmic		Nuclear	
	free	total	bound	total
BPH	3.6 ± 0.5 (1.2–9.6)	110.0 ± 14.7 (35–222)	106.0 ± 14.7 (33.8–213)	236.0 ± 33.6 (96–510)
Untreated CA	5.8 ± 1.0 (0–17)	90.7 ± 19.5 (22–288)	84.9 ± 19.5 (21–282)	367.0 ± 123.0 (44–1,123)
Treated CA	14.3 ± 4.3 (1.5–53)	72.9 ± 20.5 (23–333)	58.0 ± 16.7 (3–180)	232.0 ± 30.6 (25–566)
Unclassified CA	10.4 ± 1.76 (1–29)	178.0 ± 23.3 (13–427)	168.4 ± 22.7 (7–417)	455.2 ± 94.16 (20–1,888)

Values are means ± sem expressed as fM/mg protein. Figures in brackets denote the range for each group. See also Figs 4, 5, 6, 7.

Attempts were made to measure the concentration of free receptors in nuclei. However, it was found that the level of free receptors was below the sensitivity of the method (> 1 fM/mg protein). The concentration of total nuclear androgen receptor was found to be 2–4 times higher than the total receptors in the cytosol (Table IV).

Discussion

In the present study, cytoplasmic and nuclear androgen receptors were measured by an exchange assay using the synthetic radioligand ^{3}H-R1881. The choice of a method for the measurement of androgen receptors in the human prostate is influenced by a variety of complicating factors which set limitations on the type of technique used. Any method, therefore, which contemplates the quantitative measurement of androgen receptors must take into account the complexity of human prostatic tissue, its high level of enzymic activity, the presence of several steroid-binding proteins, including SHBG, and the high level of endogenous steroids which interfere with receptor binding to the radioligand marker.

One of the earlier techniques used for the measurement of cytoplasmic androgen receptors in the prostate involved the *in vitro* incubation of tissue with ^{3}H-DHT and the subsequent separation of bound from free steroid by dextran-coated charcoal [13]. This method overestimates the receptor concentration due to its inability to separate ^{3}H-DHT binding to androgen receptors from that binding to SHBG. Further inaccuracies also result because of metabolism of DHT to androstanediols.

The introduction of agar gel electrophoresis, with its ability to separate androgen receptors from SHBG, offered a good prospect for androgen receptor measurements [8]. However, the conditions used for labelling the androgen receptors with ^{3}H-DHT necessitate the use of a low-temperature incubation (0–4°C) to avoid metabolism of DHT. This, in turn, only allows measurement of the available (unoccupied) binding receptor sites.

The use of glycerol gradient centrifugation for the isolation of 8S androgen receptors and the subsequent measurement of bound DHT by radioimmunoassay has also been reported [9]. Although this method has been applied for the measurement of both free and bound receptors in the human prostate, our experience, as well as that of others, suggests that the isolation of 8S androgen receptors is not always successful [14]. Furthermore, some authors originally even reported absence of androgen receptors in BPH tissue [15]. Apart from the tediousness of this technique for routine applications, some degree of inaccuracy in the estimation of total binding sites can result from dissociation of DHT from its receptor during long-term centrifugation.

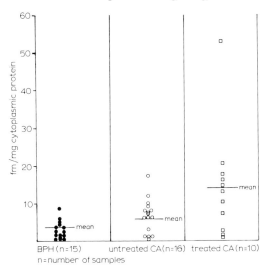

Fig. 4. Comparison between the levels of free cytoplasmic androgen receptors in prostatic tissues obtained from patients with BPH and CA.

Precipitation of androgen receptors by protamine sulphate and their subsequent labelling with ^{3}H-DHT has also been applied to the cytosol of human prostatic tissue [11] and to androgen receptors in breast cancer [16]. Apart from separating androgen receptors from SHBG this technique has the advantage of inactivating the enzymic system responsible for the conversion of DHT to 5α-androstanediols [17] and therefore allows application of exchange conditions for maximum labelling of the receptor. In our experience, however, this method underestimates the concentration of total receptor population due to losses during the receptor precipitation step. A modification of this technique for measuring unoccupied binding sites has also been reported [18]. In this procedure androgen receptors are labelled with ^{3}H-DHT and subsequently precipitated by protamine sulphate. Again, due to receptor losses which result during the precipitation step, this procedure does not offer any advantages.

The synthetic radioligand ^{3}H-R1881 has been used for measurement of androgen receptors [19, 20]. This compound possesses a high affinity for androgen receptors, does not undergo metabolism under exchange conditions and does not bind to SHBG. Several laboratories have examined the specificity of this compound [10, 21–23]. These laboratories found that P strongly cross-reacts with binding of R1881 during 0–4°C incubations with BPH cytosol. Moreover, R1881 was found to bind P-receptors in rat endometrium [21]. This, together with the ability of R5020 (17,21-dimeth-

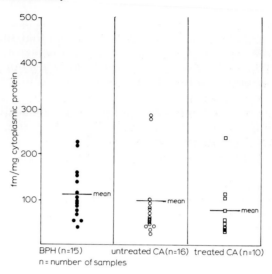

Fig. 5. *Comparison between the levels of total cytoplasmic androgen receptors in prostatic tissues obtained from patients with BPH and CA.*

yl-19-norpregna-4,9-diene-3,20-dione) to bind to specific proteins in BPH cytosol, led some of these investigators to suggest the presence of a P-binding component in the cytosol of human prostate and that use of R1881 may thereby lead to overestimation of the number of androgen-binding sites [24].

In the present investigation a comprehensive study was carried out to examine the binding specificity of R1881 to cytoplasmic androgen receptors. The results suggest that, at $0-4°C$, P competes strongly with binding of R1881. However, due to the fact that progestogens are strong competitors for binding of androgen receptors [25], this experiment was repeated using ^3H-P as the binding ligand. In this case both R1881 and DHT displayed little competition to binding of ^3H-P whereas radio-inert P was a strong competitor. The effect of 10^{-7} M C in these experiments was to abolish the ability of P to compete for binding of ^3H-P, whereas it did not alter the effects on ^3H-R1881 binding. In another series of experiments, the abilities of R1881, DHT and P to compete for binding of ^3H-R1881, ^3H-DHT and ^3H-P at $0-4°C$ were investigated following precipitation of cytoplasmic receptors by protamine sulphate. This study supported our previous findings in that, while R1881 and DHT bound the same specific site, specific binding for progesterone was not demonstrated. We therefore concluded that, under these experimental conditions, R1881 binds to androgen receptors in the human prostate.

Further support for this conclusion was obtained when the specificity of R1881 binding to cytoplasmic androgen receptors was examined at $15°C$. Under these experimental conditions the ability of P to inhibit specific binding of R1881 to cytoplasmic androgen receptor was less than that observed at $0-4°C$, whereas the competing ability of DHT increased. Identical results were obtained when the effect of these competitors on specific binding of ^3H-DHT to KCl-solubilized protamine sulphate-precipitated cytoplasmic androgen receptors was examined. Alteration in specificity behaviour of androgen receptors with temperature changes has also been reported in dog [26] and human prostates [27, 28].

An explanation for the changes in specificity with elevation in temperature may be sought in studies on glucocorticoid receptors of mouse thymocytes [29]. The workers concerned observed that, under 4°C incubation conditions, both dexamethasone and corticosterone were equipotent in competing for binding of ^{3}H-dexamethasone to cytoplasmic glucocorticoid receptors in suspensions of mouse thymocytes. When the incubation temperature was raised to 37°C, corticosterone became a less effective competitor than dexamethasone. On the basis of these results, the authors predicted the presence of a receptor transconformation system as described by Feldman *et al.* [30]. Dexamethasone stabilizes the receptor at raised temperatures whereas corticosterone does not, allowing differences in competition patterns and between dissociation rates of steroid-receptor complexes. A similar model of receptor transconformation can also be envisaged for cytoplasmic androgen receptors. Such a model would require the presence of at least two allosteric forms of androgen receptors, each with different specificity. The first, allosteric form of the receptors, representing unoccupied binding sites ('inactive form') would be stable at 0–4°C and transformed to the second 'active form' at 15°C. The 'inactive' receptor form would be less specific than the 'active' and transformation of 'inactive' receptors to 'active' forms at raised temperatures could therefore explain the differences in specificity of R1881 binding observed between 4°C and 15°C.

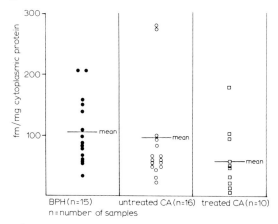

Fig. 6. Comparison between the levels of bound cytoplasmic androgen receptors in prostatic tissues obtained from patients with BPH and CA.

The specificity of binding of R1881 was also examined with nuclear androgen receptors following their extraction from partially purified nuclear preparations with 0.4 M KCl. The results suggest that the cross-reactivity of P towards R1881 binding is lower in nuclear extracts than in cytosol. Moreover, DHT was found to be a stronger competitor for R1881 binding in nuclear extract than in cytosol. Similar findings have been reported by others [23, 27, 31]. These findings suggest that R1881 binds to an androgen receptor protein in the nuclear extract. From our specificity data it can be concluded that R1881 is a suitable radioligand for androgen receptor assay in both cytosol and nuclei of human prostatic tissue.

Our results demonstrate wide variations in the level of androgen receptors in cytosol and nuclei in BPH and CA tissues. A distinct finding was that, in all cases, the level of bound receptors in nuclei was significantly higher than that in cytosol. It appears from our data that virtually all binding sites in nuclei are occupied by endogenous hormone. In contrast, the cytosol fraction contained both free and bound receptors. The level of bound receptors was 20—30 times higher than that of free receptors. This would suggest that techniques for the quantitative measurement of cytoplasmic receptors that employ short-term incubations at 0—4°C are not suitable.

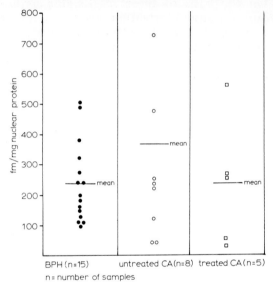

Fig. 7. Comparison between the level of total nuclear androgen receptors in prostatic tissues obtained from patients with BPH and CA.

There was a wide range of values for cytoplasmic and nuclear androgen receptors in treated and untreated CA tissues. This probably reflects differences in the hormonal status of each tissue, which in turn, may be related to response to hormonal manipulation. In the present investigation we have not correlated our receptor results with clinical response in patients. This correlation can only be made when the patients encompassed within this investigation have undergone an appropriate period of treatment. An interesting finding in this study was the raised level of free cytoplasmic receptors observed in treated patients. A similar finding has also been reported by others [18]. The increase in free receptor concentrations could be due to suppression of circulating androgens brought about by hormonal manipulation. This decline may in turn decrease prostatic androgen levels and thereby reduce the amount of endogenous hormone available for binding to cytoplasmic androgen receptors. The overall net effect would be an increase in free receptor concentration accompanied by a decrease in bound receptor level.

Summary

A method is described for the measurement of cytoplasmic and nuclear androgen receptors in prostatic tissues obtained from patients with benign prostatic hypertrophy (BPH) or carcinoma of the prostate (CA). The synthetic androgen, metribolone (R1881), was used either under exchange conditions (15°C for 16 hours) for the assay of total binding sites or at 0–4°C for 1 hour to measure available (free) sites. Specificity patterns of the binding of R1881 to cytoplasmic androgen receptors at these temperatures were examined. The ability of androstanolone (DHT) and progesterone (P) to compete with binding of R1881 to androgen receptors was found to vary between the different temperatures. However, this data confirms the suitability of this radioligand for androgen receptor assay in the human prostate. Androgen receptors were measured in the cytosol and nuclear extracts of 15 BPH and 54 CA tissues. Patients with CA had either received treatment for their disease prior to operation or were untreated. In the study described the response of patients to endocrine manipulation was nct correlated with the level of androgen receptors.

Acknowledgements

The authors are most grateful to the Cancer Research Campaign for financial support. Special thanks are also to Mr E. P. N. O'Donoghue, Mr G. Williams, Mr B. Richards and Mr M. R. C. Robinson for providing us with prostatic tissue, to the staff of the Prostate Research Laboratory for their co-operation in this investigation and to Mrs Lynette Sofras and Mrs Anne Ingram for their secretarial assistance.

References

1. Grayhack, J. T. and Wendel, E. F. (1974): Hormone dependent carcinoma of the prostate. In: *Male Accessory Sex Organs.* Chapter 17, p. 425. Editor: D. Brands. Academic Press, New York.
2. Jensen, E. V. (1977): Oestrogen receptors in human cancers. *J. Am. Med. Assoc., 238,* 59.
3. McGuire, W. L., Zava, D. I., Horwitz, K. B., Carola, R. L. and Chamness, G. C. (1978): Receptors and Breast Cancer. *J. Steroid Biochem., 9,* 461.
4. Sitteri, P. K. and Wilson, J. D. (1970): Dihydrotestosterone in prostatic hyperplasia. 1. The formation and content of dihydrotestosterone in the hypertrophic prostate of man. *J. Clin. Invest., 49,* 1737.
5. Ghanadian, R. (1976): Endocrine control of the prostate: mechanism of action of androgens. In: *Scientific Foundation of Urology,* Vol. II, Chapter 18, p. 138. Editors: D. I. Williams and G. D. Chisholm. Heinemann, London.
6. Cowan, R. A., Cowan, S. K. and Grant, J. K. (1975): The specificity of 5α-dihydrotestosterone binding in human prostate cytosol preparation. *Biochem. Soc. Trans., 3,* 537.
7. Cowan, R. A., Cowan, S. K., Giles, C. A. and Grant, J. K. (1976): Prostatic distribution of sex hormone-binding globulin and cortisol-binding globulin in benign hyperplasia. *J. Endocrinol., 71,* 121.
8. Wagner, R. K., Schulze, K. H. and Jungblut, P. W. (1975): Oestrogen and androgen receptors in human prostate and prostatic tumour tissue. *Acta Endocrinol. suppl., 193,* 52.
9. Rosen, V., Jung, I., Baulieu, E. E. and Robel, P. (1975): Androgen binding proteins in human benign prostatic hypertrophy. *J. Clin. Endocrinol. Metab., 41,* 761.
10. Ghanadian, R., Auf, G., Chaloner, P. J. and Chisholm, G. D. (1978): The use of methyltrienolone in the measurement of the free and bound cytoplasmic receptors for dihydrotestosterone in benign hypertrophied human prostate. *J. Steroid Biochem., 9,* 325.

11. Menon, M., Tananis, C. E., McLaughlin, M. G., Lippman, M. E. and Walsh, P. C. (1977): The measurement of androgen receptors in human prostatic tissue utilising sucrose density centrifugation and a protamine precipitation assay. *J. Urol., 117,* 309.

12. Ghanadian, R., Auf, G., Chisholm, G. D. and O'Donoghue, E. P. N. (1978): Receptor proteins for androgens in prostatic disease. *Br. J. Urol., 50,* 567.

13. Mobbs, B. G., Johnson, I. E. and Connolly, J. G. (1975): *In vitro* assay of androgen binding by human prostate. *J. Steroid Biochem., 6,* 453.

14. Mainwaring, W. I. P. and Milroy, E. J. (1973): Characterisation of a specific androgen receptor in the human prostate gland. *J. Endocrinol., 57,* 371.

15. Steins, P., Krieg, M., Hollmann, H. J. and Voigt, K. D. (1974): *In vitro* studies of testosterone and 5α-dihydrotestosterone binding in benign prostatic hypertrophy. *Acta Endocrinol. (Copenhagen), 75,* 773.

16. Lippman, M. and Huff, K. (1976): A demonstration of androgen and oestrogen receptors in a human breast cancer using protamine sulphate assay. *Cancer, 38,* 868.

17. Davies, P., Thomas, O. and Griffiths, K. (1977): Measurement of free and occupied cytoplasmic and nuclear androgen receptor sites in rat ventral prostate gland. *J. Endocrinol., 74,* 393.

18. Mobbs, B. G., Johnson, I. E., Connolly, J. G. and Clark, A. F. (1978): Androgen receptor assay in human benign and malignant prostatic tumour cytosol using protamine sulphate precipitation. *J. Steroid Biochem., 9,* 289.

19. Bonne, C. and Raynaud, J. P. (1975): Methyltrienolone, a specific ligand for the cellular androgen receptors. *Steroids, 26,* 227.

20. Bonne, C. and Raynaud, J. P. (1976): Assay of androgen binding sites by exchange with methyltrienolone (R1881). *Steroids, 27,* 497.

21. Asselin, J., Fernand, L., Gourdeau, Y., Bonne, C. and Raynaud, J. P. (1976): Binding of ³H-methyltrienolone (R1881) in rat prostate and human benign prostatic hypertrophy (BPH). *Steroids, 28,* 449.

22. Cowan, R. A., Cowan, S. K. and Grant, J. K. (1977): Binding of methyltrienolone (R1881) to a progesterone receptor-like component of human prostate cytosol. *J. Endrocrinol., 74,* 281.

23. Menon, M., Tananis, C. E., Hicks, L. L., Hawkins, E. F., McLaughlin, M. G. and Walsh, P. C. (1978): Characterisation of the binding of a potent synthetic androgen, methyltrienolone, to human tissues. *J. Clin. Invest., 61,* 150.

24. Gustafsson, J. Å., Ekman, P., Pousette, Å., Snochowsky, M. and Högberg, B. (1978): Demonstration of a progestin receptor in human benign prostatic hyperplasia and prostatic carcinoma. *Invest. Urol., 15,* 361.

25. Horwitz, K. B., Costlow, M. E. and McGuire, W. L. (1975): A human breast cancer cell-line with oestrogen, androgen, progesterone and glucocorticoid receptors. *Steroids, 26,* 785.

26. Boesel, R. W., Klipper, R. W. and Shain, S. A. (1977): Identification of limited capacity androgen binding components in nuclear and cytoplasmic fractions of canine prostate. *Endocr. Res. Commun., 4,* 71.

27. Shains, S. A., Boesel, R. W., Lamm, D. L. and Radwin, H. H. (1978): Characterisation of unoccupied (R) and occupied (R.A.) androgen binding components of the hyperplastic human prostate. *Steroids, 31,* 541.

28. Shain, S. A. and Boesel, R. W. (1978): Human prostate steroid hormone receptor quantitation: current methodology and possible utility as a clinical discriminant in carcinoma. *Invest. Urol., 16,* 169.

29. Duval, D. and Simon, J. (1977): Temperature dependent changes and specificity of glucocorticoid receptors in mouse thymocytes. In: *Multiple Molecular forms of Steroid Hormone Receptors, p. 229.* Editor: M. K. Agarwal. Elsevier/North-Holland Biomedical Press, Amsterdam.

30. Feldman, D., Funder, J. W. and Edelman, I. S. (1972): Subcellular Mechanisms in the action of adrenal steroids. *Am. J. Med., 53,* 545.

31. Sirett, D. A. M. and Grant, J. K. (1978): Androgen binding in cytosol and nuclei of human hyperplastic tissue. *J. Endocrinol., 77,* 101.

Discussion

P. Ekman (Stockholm, Sweden): How did you achieve material enough consisting of prostatic carcinoma to permit nuclear receptor studies? Electroresected specimens cannot be used due to protein denaturation. How carefully did you check that the specimens were not contaminated with normal or hyperplastic tissue?

R. Ghanadian: As I described before, the prostatic materials in this study were provided by TUR. The TUR chips were carefully cleaned and burned material removed. Samples from each chip were taken for histology which, in turn, would determine the percentage of the normal tissue and tumour. Biopsy materials provide very little tissue for receptor assay, especially if nuclear receptor is to be assayed. One has to be careful in using TUR materials. If the chips are large enough they can be used, but if the chips are small then the risk of denaturation is great. In our laboratory we only select large chips for receptor assay.

F. K. Habib (Edinburgh, United Kingdom): Perhaps you could tell us something about the type of carcinoma tissues you used in your receptor studies. Were they poorly or highly differentiated specimens?

R. Ghanadian: Samples have been taken for histology from each TUR chip. We hope that we will be able to relate our receptor data to the type of tumour. At this stage, however, we have not received a full report on the clinical and histological examination of each case and therefore I am not able to give you full answer.

M. Pavone-Macaluso (Palermo, Italy): Can metribolone be clinically employed as an antiandrogen?

R. Ghanadian: Metribolone is a strong androgen and is meant to be used only for laboratory purposes. Perhaps Dr. Raynaud could make more comments on this.

P. M. D. Robel (Bicêtre, France): Was the nuclear receptor assay made on nuclear extracts. It is difficult to compare RN and R receptors on a per mg protein basis. Have you made comparisons on a per cell basis?

R. Ghanadian: Yes. The receptor assay was carried out on the nuclear extracts. We have also measured the DNA content of the nuclei, and could express the results either as fM/mg DNA or fM/cell. This comparison will be made when we correlate the receptor results with clinical progress of the patients.

Androgen metabolism in fibroblasts from human benign prostatic hyperplasia, prostatic carcinoma and nongenital skin

H. U. Schweikert, H. J. Hein and F. H. Schröder
Department of Internal Medicine, Medical University-Polyclinic, University of Bonn, Bonn, Federal Republic of Germany, and Department of Urology, Erasmus University, Rotterdam, The Netherlands

The two major circulating androgens in man, testosterone and androstenedione, can serve as precursors or prohormones for two types of cellular hormone, each of which exerts unique actions within cells. On the one hand, the 4,5 double bond can be 5α-reduced to a variety of 5α-androstanes, principally androstanolone, which is thought to mediate many of the hormonal actions within androgen target organs. On the other hand, the A-ring of the circulating androgens can be aromatized in the peripheral tissue of both sexes to form oestrogen (Fig. 1). Thus the net effect of circulating testosterone represents the sum total of the actions of testosterone itself and these two types of metabolites.

Since oestrogen can antagonize some actions of testosterone [1, 2] and in some instances acts in concert with androgens to influence physiological processes [3, 4] it is clear that androgen action can only be understood if the regulation of both of these pathways in peripheral tissue is understood.

The present study was undertaken to examine both pathways. The metabolism of testosterone in fibroblasts from benign prostatic hyperplasia (BPH), prostatic carcinoma and nongenital skin was first examined. The possible conversion of androgen to oestrogen in fibroblasts derived from various prostatic sources as well as genital and nongenital skin was then investigated. Cultured fibroblasts were chosen for these experiments for the following reasons:

1. Several aspects of androgen physiology could be investigated in fibroblasts cultured from human skin [5–8].

2. In contrast to tissue specimens cultured fibroblasts offer the advantage that the hormonal milieu can be precisely controlled.

3. Fibroblast cell strains can be developed from a variety of prostatic sources.

4. Since fibroblasts are thought to develop from the stromal part of tissue and an increase in stroma is a common feature in BPH, studies to examine

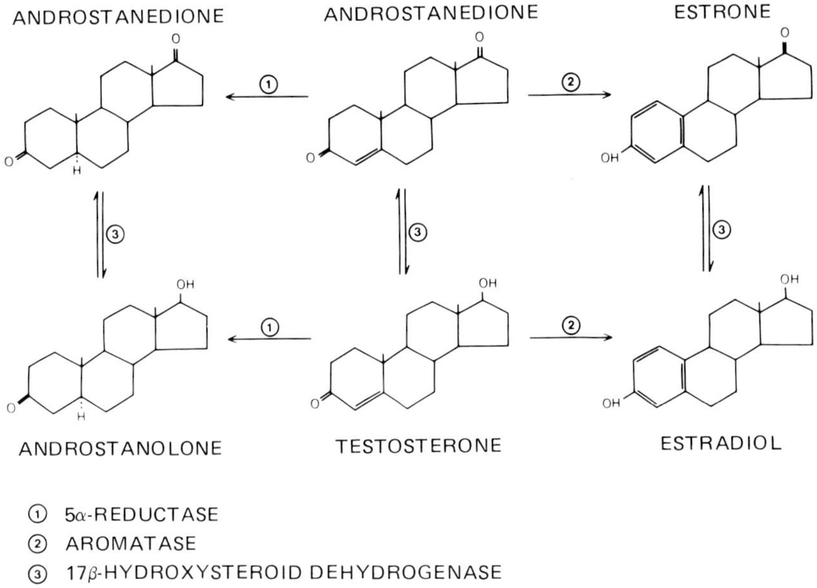

ANDROSTANEDIONE   ANDROSTANEDIONE   ESTRONE

ANDROSTANOLONE   TESTOSTERONE   ESTRADIOL

① 5α-REDUCTASE
② AROMATASE
③ 17β-HYDROXYSTEROID DEHYDROGENASE

Fig. 1. Principal metabolites formed from testosterone and androstenedione by peripheral tissues.

androgen metabolism in fibroblasts might prove to be of value in elucidating this common disorder.

The fibroblasts used were grown in Eagle's minimum essential medium containing 10% charcoal-treated foetal calf serum so that the media were essentially free of steroids. The incubation was performed when cells were in the semilogarithmic growth phase. The fibroblast strains used for these investigations were derived from prostates and from explants of genital and nongenital skin from normal males and from one individual with the 46, XX male syndrome. The prostates were obtained at open prostatectomy except for one which was obtained from a kidney donor with the consent of next of kin. The clinical diagnoses of all prostates were confirmed by histological examination of the corresponding tissue used for cell culture.

The methods utilized to develop fibroblasts from tissue, for incubation of fibroblasts with tritiated steroids and for steroid analysis have been described elsewhere [7–11]. In brief, for the determination of the androgen metabolites of testosterone, the cells were incubated with 25 nm (= M × 10^{-9}) [1,2,6,7-^{3}H]-testosterone. The cells were scraped off the dishes after incubation and the steroids extracted into chloroform. For purification the steroids were subjected to one or two successive thin-layer chromatography procedures. The identities of the metabolites recovered as well as of the unmetabolized substrate were finally confirmed by recrystallization either to constant specific activity or to constant ^{3}H/^{14}C ratio.

When fibroblasts grown from prostatic adenoma, prostatic carcinoma and nongenital skin were incubated with testosterone for periods of time ranging from 30 minutes to 24 hours, characteristic differences in their pattern of metabolism were found.

Results representative of this type of experiment are shown in figure 2. As can be seen, testosterone was much more rapidly metabolized by fibro-

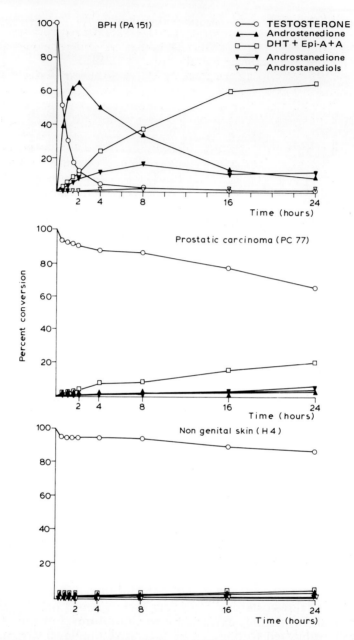

Fig. 2. Time course of the metabolism of [1,2,6,7-³H]-testosterone in different fibroblast cell strains derived from benign prostatic adenoma (upper panel), prostatic carcinoma (middle) and nongenital skin (lower panel). Cell growth, incubation and steroid analysis are as described in the text. □——□: *Sum of androstanolone (DHT), epiandrosterone (Epi-A) and androsterone (A).* ▽——▽: *Sum of androstane-3α,17β-diol and androstane-3β,17β-diol. (From [17].)*

blasts from BPH. About 90% of the substrate had disappeared after 2 hours. A peak of androstenedione after 2 hours suggests high activity of 17β-hydroxysteroid dehydrogenase. After 24 hours the androsterones and androstanolone are the predominant metabolites.

In contrast, fibroblasts grown from prostatic carcinoma metabolized testosterone to a much lower degree. Even after 24 hours incubation 70% of the substrate still remained unmetabolized. Metabolism was lowest in fibroblasts derived from nongenital skin, where 90% of the testosterone was still unmetabolized after 24 hours.

The relation between the concentration of substrate testosterone and rate of formation of 5α-androstanes was next studied in fibroblasts grown from BPH. The half-maximum rate of 5α-androstane formation was found to be 0.2 μM, a value similar to the one reported for fibroblasts derived from genital skin [12].

The time course of appearance of the various metabolites following incubation of 3 different cell strains grown from each of 3 different prostates with BPH, 3 carcinomas of the prostate and 2 cell strains originating from nongenital skin was then studied. The activity of 5α-reductase was determined from the sum of all 5α-reduced steroids formed. 5α-reductase was about 2–4 times more active in fibroblasts from BPH (8.9 pM (= M $\times$ 10^{-12})/mg protein/hour incubation) than in the corresponding cells from carcinoma (2.1 pM/mg protein/hour incubation). The formation of 5α-androstanes in fibroblasts from nongenital skin was on average between 10–20 times lower than in fibroblasts from BPH.

Thus we were able to show that fibroblasts with regard to androgen metabolism from prostatic tissue resemble, in many respects, whole tissue specimens, e.g. as with whole tissue slices fibroblasts derived from BPH metabolize testosterone to a much higher extent than cells grown from prostatic carcinoma [13, 14].

Comparing fibroblasts grown from these types of tumours it is also evident that activity of 5α-reductase was considerably higher in fibroblasts from BPH tissue than in fibroblasts cultured from prostatic carcinoma.

The rates of metabolism in fibroblasts from prostatic carcinoma are, furthermore, considerably higher than in skin fibroblasts from nongenital sites. This might suggest, as has been shown for skin fibroblasts, that the rate of metabolism in fibroblasts grown from different sources is a function of the original tissue [5, 6] and that fibroblasts grown from the human prostate retain this differentiative function of the original tissue for at least 15 passages.

The aromatization of androgen in cultured human fibroblasts from various prostatic sources, from nongenital skin and from genital skin (foreskin) was next examined under standardized conditions. The methods utilized for the routine assay of oestrogen formation have been described previously [8, 9, 16]. Radioactive androstenedione rather than testosterone was used routinely as substrate because of a more favourable rate of conversion. Briefly, the cells were routinely incubated with 50 nM [1,2,6,7-^{3}H]-androstenedione. Carbon-14-labelled estrone was then added as internal standard and the cells and media were extracted with chloroform. For purification of estrone the first step was chromatography on a small scale version of a celite column. The eluate containing ^{14}C-estrone was then subjected to four successive thin layer chromatography steps and recrystallization to constant ^{3}H/^{14}C ratio.

Having shown that fibroblasts grown from human prostates indeed aromatize androstenedione to estrone, attempts have been made to standardize te incubation procedure.

The time course of the appearance of estrone showed that its formation in fibroblasts cultured from prostate was linear with time from 2 to at least 16 hours (Fig. 3). The half maximum rate of estrone formation was observed both in fibroblasts derived from BPH and from prostatic carcinoma at a substrate concentration of about 0.1 μM, a value similar to that reported for human placental microsomes.

The results of a comparative study of aromatase activity in a total of 15 cell strains obtained from 11 subjects are illustrated in figure 4. Estrone formation in fibroblasts from BPH varied from 3.0 to 11.6 pM/100 mg protein/hour, values clearly higher than those from fibroblasts cultured from prostatic carcinoma, where estrone formation ranged from 0.8 to 2.0 pM/ 100 mg protein/hour. Estrone formation in fibroblasts from prostatic carcinoma was only slightly higher than that observed with fibroblasts from foreskin where estrone formation amounted to between 0.4 and 2.3 pM/100 mg protein/hour.

Finally, estrone formation in fibroblasts from nongenital skin sites was, in every instance, considerably lower than in fibroblasts grown from prostates. In 3 out of 4 nongenital skin strain values obtained for estrone formation were, in fact, less than twice the amount of the blank and therefore considered to be zero.

The finding of high estrone formation in fibroblasts from BPH as compared to that of carcinoma may be of importance in the elucidation of the cause of BPH since recent studies indicate that oestrogen may be causally linked to its development [4, 15].

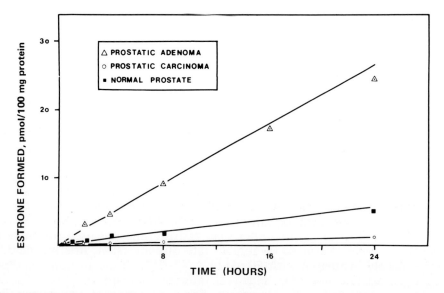

Fig. 3. Time course of estrone formation by fibroblast monolayers. Cells grown from a benign hyperplastic prostate, a prostatic carcinoma and a normal prostate were incubated with 10 ml Eagle's minimum medium containing 50 nM [1,2,6,7-³H]-androstenedione. At the indicated times the cells of each line were harvested and the amount of [³H]-estrone determined.

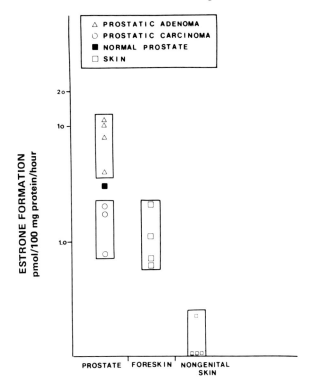

Fig. 4. Estrone formation from [1,2,6,7-³H]-androstenedione in 15 fibroblast strains derived from 11 individuals. The cells were cultured from prostates and nongenital skin sites such as the abdominal wall and the deltoid region of the arm. The cells were incubated with medium containing 50 nM [1,2,6,7-³H]-androstenedione. [³H]-estrone formed after 4 hours' incubation was determined. (From [16].)

Acknowledgments

The authors are grateful to Mrs. Petra Grünsfelder and Ms. Eva Wiebelhaus for providing excellent technical assistance during these studies. This investigation was supported by grants Schw 168/2–4 from the Deutsche Forschungsgemeinschaft.

References

1. Federman, D. D., Robbins, J. and Rall, J. E. (1958): Effects of methyl testosterone on thyroid function, thyroxine metabolism and thyroxine-binding protein. *J. Clin. Invest., 37*, 1024.
2. De Moor, P., Steeno, O., Heyns, W. and Van Baelen, H. (1969): The steroid binding β-globulin in plasma: Pathophysiological data. *Ann. Endocrinol., 30*, 233.
3. Baum, M. J. and Vreeburg, J. T. M. (1973): Copulation in castrated male rats following combined treatment with estradiol and dihydrotestosterone. *Science, 182*, 283.
4. Walsh, P. C. and Wilson, J. D. (1976): The induction of prostatic hypertrophy in the dog with androstanediol. *J. Clin. Invest., 57*, 1093.
5. Mulay, S., Finkelberg, R., Pinksy, L. and Solomon, S. (1972): Metabolism of 4-¹⁴C-testosterone by serially subcultured human skin fibroblasts. *J. Clin. Endocrinol. Metab., 34*, 133.

6. Wilson, J. D. (1975): Dihydrotestosterone formation in cultured human fibroblasts. Comparison of cells from normal subjects and patients with familial incomplete male pseudohermaphroditism, type 2. *J. Biol. Chem., 250,* 3498.
7. Griffin, J. E., Punyashthiti, K. and Wilson, J. D. (1976): Dihydrotestosterone binding by cultured human fibroblasts. *J. Clin. Invest., 57,* 1342.
8. Schweikert, H. U., Milewich, L. and Wilson, J. D. (1976): Aromatization of androstenedione by cultured human fibroblasts. *J. Clin. Endocrinol. Metab., 43,* 785.
9. Schweikert, H. U., Milewich, L. and Wilson, J. D. (1975): Aromatization of androstenedione by isolated human hairs. *J. Clin. Endocrinol. Metab., 40,* 413.
10. Milewich, L. and Schweikert, H. U. (1978): Synthesis of carbon-14-labelled C_{19}-steroids. *J. Label. Compounds Radiopharm., 14,* 427.
11. Schweikert, H. U., Hein, H. J. and Schröder, F. H.: Testosterone metabolism of fibroblasts grown from prostatic carcinoma, benign prostatic hyperplasia and nongenital skin. Submitted for publication.
12. Moore, R. J., Griffin, J. E. and Wilson, J. D. (1975): Diminished 5α-reductase activity in extracts of fibroblasts cultured from patients with familial incomplete male pseudohermaphroditism, type 2. *J. Biol. Chem., 250,* 7168.
13. Djøseland, O., Tveter, K. L., Attramadal, A., Hansson, V., Haugen, H. N. and Mathisen, W. (1977): Metabolism of testosterone in the human prostate and seminal vesicles. *Scand. J. Urol. Nephrol., 11,* 1.
14. Krieg, M., Grobe, I., Voigt, K. D., Altenähr, E. and Klosterhalfen, H. (1978): Human prostatic carcinoma: Significant differences in its androgen binding and metabolism compared to the human benign prostatic hypertrophy. *Acta Endocrinol. (Copenhagen), 88,* 397.
15. Seppelt, U. (1978): Correlation among prostate stroma, plasma estrogen levels and urinary estrogen excretion in patients with benign prostatic hypertrophy. *J. Clin. Endocrinol. Metab., 47,* 1230.
16. Schweikert, H. U. (1979): Conversion of androstenedione to estrone in human fibroblasts cultured from prostate, genital and nongenital skin. *Horm. Metab. Res., 11,* 589.
17. Schröder, F. H., Oishi, K. and Schweikert, H. U. (1978): The application of cell culture techniques to human prostatic carcinoma. Union International Contre le Cancer. Workshop on Prostatic Cancer, Geneva, Oct. 23–26 (in press).

Discussion

I. Lasnitzki (Cambridge, U.K.): Were the cell lines derived from the skin fibroblasts still androgen-dependent and did you grow them in the presence of androgens?

H. U. Schweikert: We did not investigate whether the fibroblasts used in our study were still androgen dependent.

The cell strains used were established in Eagle's minimum essential medium (EMM) containing 10% foetal calf serum (FCS). FCS contains considerable amounts of both androgens and oestrogens. For metabolic studies the cells were seeded at day 0 in EMM supplemented with 10% FCS. On days 3 and 6 the medium was replaced with fresh growth medium made up like the starting medium except that 10% charcoal-extracted FCS which was essentially free of hormones was used instead of ordinary FCS. On day 7 the medium was removed and the cells were incubated in EMM containing the radioactive androgen.

M. Pavone-Macaluso (Palermo, Italy): Is there any information on the presence of receptors or of enzymes involved in steroid metabolism in muscle cells in prostatic stroma?

H. U. Schweikert: To my knowledge there is still no information available as to the presence of receptors or enzymes in muscle cells isolated from prostatic sources. Recent studies, however, in separated stromal cells and separated epithelial cells obtained from BPH tissue (see the papers of Dr. Bruchovsky and Dr. Romijn at this workshop) might indicate a different quantitative pattern of metabolism in these two prostatic cell types.

Androgen metabolism and androgen receptors in separated epithelium and stroma of the human prostate

J. C. Romijn*, K. Oishi*, J. Bolt-de Vries*, H. U. Schweikert**, E. Mulder*** and F. H. Schröder*
* Department of Urology and *** Department of Biochemistry (Division of Chemical Endocrinology), Erasmus University, Rotterdam, The Netherlands; and **Medical Polyclinic of the University of Bonn, Bonn, Federal Republic of Germany

Introduction

In the human prostate different types of cells, which can be divided roughly into epithelial and stromal cells, are present in varying amounts. So far, little is known about the properties of the specific cell types with respect to their role in the functioning of the normal prostate or in the aetiology of prostatic diseases. It was shown by Cunha and co-workers, that the stroma is necessary for the induction of epithelial morphogenesis [1]. Franks et al. [2] have shown that separated epithelium is dependent on stroma for its maintenance in tissue culture. These results, which suggest that there is a specific stromal-epithelial interaction, have stimulated us to study the properties of the individual cell types after separation. As steroid hormones presumably play an important role in the regulation of growth and function of the human prostate, the study of steroid metabolism and steroid hormone receptors in separated fractions may lead to a better understanding of the interactions between stroma and epithelium. A separation technique, by which the epithelium of human prostatic tissue can be separated from the stroma and to a large extent purified, has been described recently by Oishi et al. [3]. In this paper we will present some studies on the metabolism of testosterone in the tissue fractions separated by this procedure and on the assay of androgen receptor in purified epithelial cells.

Materials and methods

Tissue

Prostatic tissue was obtained after radical prostatectomy. The tissue was put immediately in ice-cold saline under sterile conditions and processed in the laboratory without delay. In these studies tissues from hyperplastic prostates

(BPH) as well as carcinomatous tissue have been used. All specimens were examined histologically.

Separation of prostatic epithelium from stromal tissue

The procedure for the separation of epithelium and stroma of human hyperplastic prostates has been described in detail by Oishi *et al.* [3]. The basis of this method, which is essentially the same as that of the procedure described by Franks and co-workers [2], is detachment of the epithelium from prostatic tissue by the application of mechanical pressure. In brief, after decapsulation and washing the tissue is minced as finely as possible by scissors in a Petri dish. The small pieces of tissue are then squeezed gently between a glass surface and the bottom of the Petri dish. At this stage as a result of the cutting and squeezing a mixture is obtained of single epithelial and stromal cells (usually, also some erythrocytes), large sheets of epithelial cells and the remaining pieces of tissue, depleted in epithelium. From this mixture the epithelial cells are isolated in the form of epithelial sheets by means of differential sedimentation. The larger particles are allowed to sediment (first 5 minutes, unit gravity). The supernatant is sucked off. The epithelial sheets sediment from this during the next 30 minutes. This step is repeated once more to increase purity. To improve recovery the larger tissue pieces and the smaller particles sedimented along with them are resuspended and resedimented. This sedimentation procedure is performed 5–10 times with successive changes of culture medium. In the later steps, where the quantity of blood cells and stromal cells is very low, the cells are collected from the supernatant by centrifugation instead of sedimentation (3 minutes, 100 g).

For counting purposes, part of the suspension is subsequently incubated with edetic acid (EDTA) in calcium- and magnesium-free phosphate-buffered saline (PBS) for 10 minutes. After this period the suspension contains mainly single epithelial cells, the number of which can be counted with a haemocytometer.

For the studies on the stroma we used the pieces of tissue remaining after the squeezing procedure. These pieces are finely cut with a mechanical tissue chopper, treated with EDTA and filtered over nylon gauze (100 μ). The tissue mince retained on the filter appears to be largely devoid of epithelial elements. It will be referred to as 'stromal tissue'. In some experiments we have prepared a single cell suspension from this tissue after overnight incubation with 0.1% pronase at 37°C. This cell suspension will be referred to as 'stromal cells'.

Steroid metabolism studies

Metabolism of testosterone by prostatic fractions was studied by measurement of the conversion of tritium-labelled testosterone (1,2,6,7-³H-testosterone, 85 Ci/mM, New England Nuclear) added to the incubation medium at a concentration of 5×10^{-8} M. The quantity of cells or tissue was chosen such that it contained 2–3 mg of protein, corresponding, for example, to 10–12 million epithelial cells. Cells or tissue were suspended in Eagle's minimal essential medium (MEM) supplemented with 10% charcoal-extracted foetal calf serum (FCS). The final volume of the incubation mixture was 1.0 ml. The effect of cofactors such as nadide phosphate, reduced form

(NADPH) after addition to the incubation medium at different concentrations has also been studied. Further incubation conditions and procedures for analysis of the steroid metabolites were essentially the same as those used by Schweikert *et al.* [4] in their studies of testosterone metabolism in prostatic fibroblasts. In brief, the cells (or tissue) were incubated in 1 ml of a medium containing 50 nM radio-labelled testosterone at 37°C in a humidified incubator gassed with O_2/CO_2. After incubation for 30 minutes to 20 hours metabolism was stopped by addition of chloroform. After extraction of the steroid metabolites into the chloroform an aliquot of the organic phase washed out twice with water and subsequently dried over anhydrous magnesium sulphate was concentrated and spotted on silica gel thin-layer plates (Polygram Sil G-Hy, Macherey and Nagel, W-Germany) after addition of a carrier mixture containing 20 μg each of androstanedione, androstenedione, dihydrotestosterone, testosterone and androstanediol. The plates are developed in the solvent system dichloromethane – ethyl acetate – methanol (85:15:2; v/v/v/). After visualization all bands are cut out directly into counting vials and the radioactivity counted in an Isocap 300 liquid scintillation spectrometer.

Since dihydrotestosterone and androsterone do not well separate from each other in the system described above, we use for the analysis of these steroids a second thin-layer chromatography (after their acetylation in pyridine-acetic anhydride, 1:1) on aluminium oxide plates (Merck F 254, type E) (80:20, v/v). We have not attempted to separate the epimers of androstanediol.

Steroid receptor estimations

The assay used for (total) androgen receptor in isolated epithelial cells is similar to the procedure developed recently for the assay of the nuclear receptor in BPH-tissue [5]. By this procedure the receptor complex is extracted from the cells with a 2 mM phosphate buffer containing 0.1% heparin (HEP-buffer). It appeared that sonication of the cells (4 times 5 sec in a MSE sonificator at 20 kHz) is essential in order to obtain a complete extraction of the receptor complex; omission of this step always resulted in a considerably lower amount (about 60% lower) of detectable receptor sites.

The cell extract is incubated for 18 hours at 10°C with 50 nM ^{3}H-dihydrotestosterone (1,2,4,5,6,7-^{3}H-DHT, 114 Ci/mmol, Radiochemical Centre, Amersham); in parallel experiments a 1000-fold excess of non-radioactive dihydrotestosterone is added. After incubation the extracts are analyzed either by agar gel electrophoresis or by protamine sulphate precipitation as described by Foekens *et al.* [5].

This procedure can be performed with 10 to 20 million purified epithelial cells.

Other procedures

Protein amounts were determined by the method of Lowry *et al.* [6]. Deoxyribonucleic acid (DNA) was measured according to Giles and Myers [7]. Hydroxyproline was determined by means of a commercial kit (Organon Teknika, Oss, The Netherlands) using the procedure described by Goverde and Veenkamp [8].

Results and discussion

Isolation of epithelial and stromal fraction

The isolation and purification of epithelial cells from human prostate has been described extensively by Oishi *et al.* [3]. This procedure yields a relatively large number of epithelial cells (about 20 million cells per g wet weight of prostatic tissue) and is, therefore, suitable for the production of epithelial cells in sufficient amount to perform the metabolic studies to be described. Acid phosphatase can be demonstrated in more than 95% of the cells [3] indicating that this fraction consists almost wholly of epithelial cells. Further evidence for the epithelial origin of the cells has been obtained from ultrastructural studies [3]. More than 95% of the cells exclude trypan blue.

Stromal tissue can be obtained quite easily from the remaining tissue fragments as described in the methods section. The purity of this fraction as estimated after histological examination and/or staining for acid phosphatase is variable, but always somewhat lower than that of the epithelial fraction (roughly 70–90%). Although 'stromal cells' (single cell suspension) have been obtained after treatment of 'stromal tissue' with 0.1% pronase, the results are not yet completely satisfactorily with respect to recovery and purity. Recovery is always below one million cells per g tissue. The percentage of acid phosphatase-negative cells is about 70–90%.

With the aim of finding a (positive) marker for the stromal part also, we have studied the distribution of hydroxyproline in the different fractions. Our results are somewhat disappointing in that they show that hydroxyproline is a poor marker for single stromal cells. The content of hydroxyproline in stromal cells (110 pg (= g $\times$ 10^{-12})/μg DNA) amounts to only twice the content in purified epithelial cells (50 pg/μg DNA). Much higher levels (37 ng(= g $\times$ 10^{-9})/μg DNA) are found, however, in stromal tissue, probably due to extracellular hydroxyproline.

Androgen metabolism

We have performed comparative studies on the metabolism of testosterone in isolated epithelial cells, in stromal tissue, in stromal cells and in total prostatic tissue. Since our objective was the study of the formation and turnover of the different metabolites as a function of time, we have used a relatively low (not saturating) concentration of testosterone, 50 nM, in these experiments.

We first studied the effect of exogenously added NADPH upon the extent of conversion of testosterone after a fixed period of incubation (3 hours) in the presence of different concentrations of NADPH. Figure 1 shows that NADPH has a pronounced effect on the amount of testosterone converted in epithelial cells (upper figure) as well as in stromal tissue (lower figure) from BPH. The effect was maximal at a concentration of 0.2 mM NADPH. At higher concentrations the stimulant effect seemed somewhat smaller. This result is rather surprising, especially with regard to the (apparent) morphological integrity of the cells, and suggests that (some of) the cells had been damaged during preparation or incubation. In all subsequent experiments we included 0.2 mM NADPH in the incubation medium.

Figure 2 shows the time course of the metabolism of testosterone in total

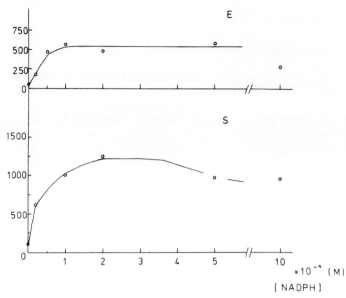

Fig. 1. Formation of 5α-reduced metabolites (androstanolone plus androstanediol) after incubation with 50 nM ³H-labelled testosterone for 3 hours at different concentrations of NADPH in separated epithelial cells (E) and stromal tissue (S) from human benign prostatic hyperplasia (BPH). Formation of metabolites is expressed in pM of steroid formed per 100 mg protein during 3 hours.

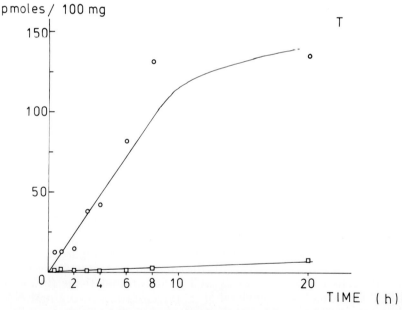

Fig. 2. Time course of metabolism of testosterone in whole prostatic tissue (BPH). Formation of metabolites is expressed in pM per 100 mg protein. ○ —— ○ = 5α-reduced metabolites (androstanolone plus androstanediol). □ —— □ = 17-oxidized metabolites (androstanedione plus androstenedione). About 20 mg of minced prostatic tissue were incubated with 50 nM ³H-labelled testosterone in the presence of 0.2 mM NADPH in a total volume of 1.0 ml.

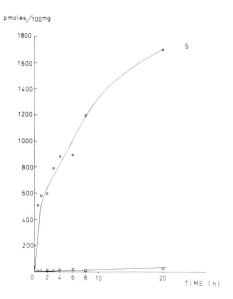

Fig. 3. Time course of metabolism of testosterone in separated stromal tissue from BPH. Formation of metabolites is expressed in pM per 100 mg protein. ○ —— ○ = 5α-reduced metabolites (androstanolone plus androstanediol). □ —— □ = 17-oxidized metabolites (androstanedione plus androstenedione). About 20 mg of stromal tissue was incubated with 50 nM ³H-labelled testosterone in the presence of 0.2 mM NADPH in a volume of 1.0 ml.

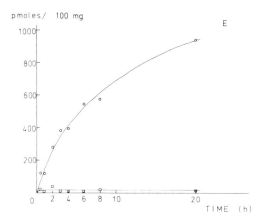

Fig. 4. Time course of metabolism of testosterone in separated epithelial cells from BPH-tissue. The tissue from which these cells were isolated is the same as that used for the preparation of the stromal fraction represented in Fig. 3. Formation of metabolites is expressed in pM per 100 mg protein. ○ —— ○ = 5α-reduced metabolites (androstanolone plus androstanediol). □ —— □: 17-oxidized metabolites (androstanedione plus androstenedione). About 12 million cells were incubated with 50 nM ³H-labelled testosterone in the presence of 0.2 mM NADPH in a volume of 1.0 ml.

prostatic tissue (BPH). The circles represent the 5α-reduced metabolites formed. These are composed mainly of androstanolone. Androstanediol accounts for 10–15% of the 5α-reduced fraction. The lower line (squares) represents the formation of 17-keto-metabolites (androstanedione, androstenedione and androsterone). It can be seen that, at least under the conditions we have used, their contribution to the total quantity of metabolites is very small (less than 5%). With BPH stromal tissue, as shown in figure 3, the same pattern of metabolites is observed: androstanolone is the major metabolite formed (85–90%), with some androstanediol and hardly any 17-oxidized compounds. In isolated BPH epithelial cells the metabolism of testosterone is very similar (Figure 4), with androstanolone as the main metabolite.

Although the metabolism of testosterone was qualitatively similar in BPH epithelial cells and stromal tissue, significant quantitative differences exist. In the stroma only 3% of testosterone is recovered after 20 hours of incubation whereas in the epithelial cells about half the testosterone is still unmetabolized after the same period. In Figure 5 we have compared the metabolites formed after 2 hours of incubation. The data are taken from time curves similar to those shown in Figures 2–4. It can be seen from Figure 5 that the quantity of metabolites formed after 2 hours is about 2.5 times higher in stromal tissue than in epithelial cells under these conditions when calculated on the basis of protein. It should be noted that the experimental conditions we have used do not allow an exact comparison of the (potential) enzymatic activities in the two fractions. Our data suggest, however, that the activity of 5α-reductase is higher in the stromal than in the epithelial part of the hypertrophied prostate, which is in agreement with the conclusions of Cowan et al. [9]. On the other hand, considering the high purity of our epithelial cell preparation it can be concluded that the epithelium also contains definite 5α-reductase activity.

The right-hand part of figure 5 shows the results obtained with stromal cells derived from BPH stromal tissue by treatment with 0.1% pronase. These

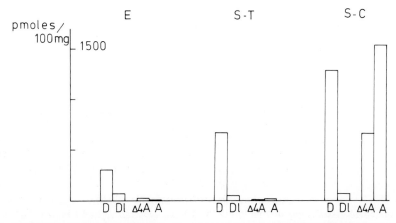

Fig. 5. Comparison of metabolites formed in separated epithelial cells (E), stromal tissue (S–T) and stromal cells (S–C) from BPH-tissue after incubation for 2 hours with 50 nM ³H-testosterone in the presence of 0.2 mM NADPH. D = androstanolone, Dl = androstanediol, Δ4A = androstenedione, A = androstanedione. The data are expressed in pM per 100 mg protein.

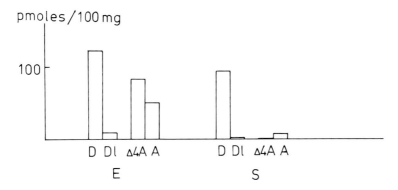

Fig. 6. Comparison of metabolites formed in separated epithelial cells (E) and stromal tissue (S) prostatic carcinomatous tissue after 2 hours of incubation with 50 nM ³H-testosterone in the presence of 0.1 mM NADPH. D = androstanolone, Dl = andro-stanediol, Δ4A = androstenedione, A = androstanedione. The data are expressed in pM per 100 mg protein.

cells not only appear to be more active as regards 5α-reductase, but also to have very high 17β-dehydrogenase activity. In general their pattern of metabolism resembles more metabolism in fibroblasts derived from BPH-tissue [4]. At present, it is not clear whether the differences in metabolism are due to selective isolation of a specific cell type present in 'stromal tissue' in small amounts or whether the enzyme activities are influenced by the action of proteolytic enzymes.

The results of a similar experiment performed with epithelial cells and stromal tissue from prostatic carcinoma are shown in figure 6. Two major qualitative differences between BPH and prostatic carcinoma can be observed. Firstly, the activity of 17β-dehydrogenase seems to be relatively higher in the case of carcinoma, especially in the epithelium. Secondly, metabolic activity seems to be higher in epithelium than in stroma of carcinoma tissue. This might indicate that the lower activity of 5α-reductase observed in prostatic carcinoma [10–12] is largely due to altered metabolism in the prostatic stroma. However, further experiments on a more quantitative basis will have to be done to substantiate these results.

Androgen receptor in separated epithelial cells

Extracts from isolated epithelial cells from BPH tissues prepared by sonication and heparin treatment as described in the methods section, were incubated with ³H-androstanolone in the presence or absence of a 1,000-fold excess of unlabelled compound for 18 hours at 10°C. The incubation mixture was subsequently subjected to protamine sulphate precipitation and/or agar gel electrophoresis. Figure 7 shows an example of such an assay by gel electrophoresis. It clearly demonstrates the presence of androgen receptor in isolated epithelial cells. The Table displays the number of receptor sites, measured by protamine sulphate precipitation, found in four different samples of isolated epithelial cells. When the results obtained by agar gel electrophoresis and those obtained by protamine sulphate precipitation are compared no significant differences can be found. The quantity of androgen receptors in our isolated epithelial cells seems to be slightly higher

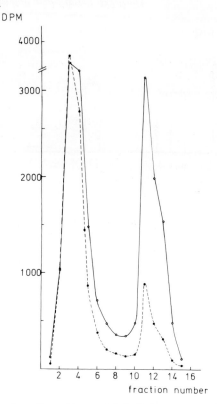

Fig. 7. Agar gel electrophoretic pattern of labelled extracts of isolated epithelial cells from BPH tissue. The extracts, obtained with 1 mg/ml heparin in phosphate buffer after sonication of the cells for 4 × 5 seconds (MSE 100 W Ultrasonic Disintegrator), were incubated for 18 hours at 10°C with 50 nM ³H-androstanolone ○ —— ○) or with 50 nM ³H-androstanolone in the presence of a 1,000-fold excess of the non-radioactive compound (● – – – ●). The sample was applied on the gel at the position of fraction 10. The receptor complex has moved to the anodic (right) side. The peak on the left represents unbound steroid.

Table   Androgen receptor content of isolated epithelial cells from BPH. Extraction of the receptor complex and labelling with ³H-androstanolone was performed as described in the methods section. The amount of receptor was quantitated by protamine sulphate precipitation [5].

Sample	Receptor sites/cell
1	2,500
2	2,900
3	3,000
4	3,600

than the quantity reported by Lieskovsky and Bruchovsky [13] for nuclear receptors in whole prostatic tissue. Since we have not been able to demonstrate androgen receptor in cytosol from epithelial cells, it is possible that this difference results from an asymmetric distribution of the receptor over the different cell types. Measurement of androgen receptor content in stroma is currently being undertaken in our laboratory.

Summary

Human prostatic tissues were fractionated by means of a method, previously described, employing mechanical pressure and differential sedimentation techniques. By this procedure a highly purified epithelial fraction was separated from the remaining stromal tissue. We have studied the metabolism of testosterone in both fractions. In addition, the receptor content of the purified epithelial cells has been measured.

As it was shown that the metabolism of testosterone in all fractions was stimulated by the addition of nadide phosphate, reduced form (NADPH), the samples, containing an amount of cells or tissue corresponding to 2–3 mg protein, were incubated with 50 nM (= M $\times$ 10^{-9}) ^{3}H-testosterone in the presence of 0.2 mM NADPH. Time-course experiments did not reveal any significant qualitative differences in metabolism in the individual fractions from BPH tissue. The main metabolites formed were androstanolone (DHT) together with smaller amounts of androstanediol (10–15% of the amount of DHT). The formation of 17-oxidized products was almost negligible. The results suggest, however, that important quantitative differences exist among the separated fractions: the activity of 5α-reductase seemed to be considerably higher in the stromal than in the epithelial fraction. The metabolism observed in a single cell suspension prepared from stromal tissue by enzyme treatment, was different from metabolism in the stromal tissue in quantitative as well as in qualitative respects. The significance of this observation is not yet fully understood. The activity of 5α-reductase in the separated fractions from carcinomatous tissue was found to be low compared to that in fractions from BPH tissue, especially in the stromal tissue fraction.

The presence of androgen receptor could be demonstrated in epithelial cells isolated from BPH tissue; the receptor content ranged from 2,500 to 3,600 sites per cell.

References

1. Cunha, G. R. and Lung, B. (1979): *In Vitro, 15,* 50–71.
2. Franks, L. M., Riddle, P. N., Carbonell, B. W. and Gey, G. O. (1970): *Journal of pathology, 100,* 113–119.
3. Oishi, K., Romijn, J. C. and Schröder, F. H. (1979): *J. Urol.* (submitted for publication).
4. Schweikert, H. U., Hein, H. J. and Schröder, F. H. (1979): *Invest. Urol.* (in press).
5. Foekens, J. A., Bolt-deVries, J., Romijn, J. C. and Mulder, E. (1979): Proceedings of this workshop.
6. Lowry, O. H., Rosebrough, N. J., Farr, A. L. and Randall, R. J. (1951): *J. Biol. Chem., 193,* 265–275.
7. Giles, K. W. and Myers, A. (1965): *Nature (London), 206,* 93.
8. Goverde, B. C. and Veenkamp, F. J. N. (1972): *Clin. Chim. Acta, 41,* 29–40.
9. Cowan, R. A., Cowan, S. K., Grant, J. K. and Elder, H. Y. (1977): *J. Endocrinol., 74,* 111–120.
10. Prout, G. R., Kliman, J., Daly, J. J., Maclaughlin, R. A. and Griffin, P. P. (1976): *J. Urol., 116,* 603–610.
11. Morfin, R. F., Leav, I., Charles, J. F., Cavazos, L. F., Ofner, P. and Flock, H. H. (1977): *Cancer (Philadelphia), 39,* 1517–1534.
12. Bruchovsky, N. and Lieskovsky, G. (1979): *J. Endocrinol., 80,* 289–301.
13. Lieskovsky, G. and Bruchovsky, N. (1979): *J. Urol., 121,* 54–58.

Testosterone plasma kinetics in patients with prostatic carcinoma treated with estradiol undecylate, cyproterone acetate and estramustine phosphate: a preliminary report

G. H. Jacobi and J. E. Altwein
Department of Urology, University of Mainz Medical School, Mainz, Federal Republic of Germany

Hormone treatment of patients with carcinoma of the prostate affects the metabolic disposition of testosterone to the target organ. This extra-prostatic action may be assessed by measuring the plasma kinetics of testosterone. To gain insight into the influence of therapeutically-administered hormones in patients with carcinoma of the prostate each patient needs to be studied before and after the trial period to avoid intraindividual variation of kinetic parameters. In this short article preliminary data from an uncompleted comparative investigation of estradiol undecylate (EU), cyproterone acetate (CA), and estramustine phosphate (EP) is presented.

Materials and methods

Patients

17 patients with untreated, histologically-proven and graded carcinoma of the prostate with an average age of 67 years consented to the study after full explanation of its purpose. Immediately prior to and during the study no other medication was taken that might influence androgen metabolism. Liver function tests were normal in all patients. Plasma kinetics of testosterone were measured in all patients pre- and post-treatment and patients thus served as their own controls.

Experimental procedure

After blood sampling for testosterone, luteinizing hormone (LH), follicle-stimulating hormone (FSH) and prolactin, 200 μCi (1,2-^{3}H)-testosterone was injected intravenously at 8.00 a.m. The patients fasted for 12 hours before and remained recumbent for 1 hour before and for the first 2 hours of the tests. The previous protocol [1] was altered in such a way that heparinized blood samples were drawn up to 48 hours. At that time the final part of the elimination curve (slope-β) was a straight line. The testing procedure was repeated after a 6-month regimen of EU (100 mg every 4 weeks, intramuscularly), CA (300 mg every week, i.m.) or a 5-day regimen of EP (300 mg every day, i.v.).

Chemical analysis

Serum hormones were determined according to Dotti et al. [2]. When this study is completed the endogenous hormones and sex hormone-binding globulin (SHBG) will be assessed in a single assay using stored samples and will be the subject of a later report. Extraction, separation by thin-layer chromatography and assay for radioactivity were performed as reported previously [3]. Hormone determinations were also performed as described before [1].

Kinetics

The effect of EU, CA and EP on the plasma kinetics of testosterone metabolism was studied using bolus injection of the tracer. The following kinetic parameters were investigated within a two compartment system [4] and calculated after graphical analysis from areas under activity curves according to Gurpide [5]: $t_{1/2}$ (= biological half-life (hours)); β (= slope of the final part of the elimination curve (hours^{-1})): V_d (= volume of distribution (litres)); MCR (= metabolic clearance rate (litres/day)) and PR (= production rate (nM (= M $\times$ 10^{-9}) $\times$ hours^{-1})).

Materials

(1,2-^{3}H)-testosterone (58 Ci/mM) was purchased from the Radiochemical Centre, Bucks., England. For details of other materials see reference [3].

Results and discussion

Estradiol undecylate

All 3 patients responded to a 6-month EU regimen with a suppression of testosterone, LH, FSH and a rise of prolactin (Table I). The disappearance of tritiated testosterone from plasma in one patient with a stage-D carcinoma of the prostate was decreased after 6 months EU exposure (Figure 1). Increase in biological half-life and flattening of the terminal part of the curve, expressed through reduction in slope-β, was encountered in all 3 patients (Table II), This is in agreement with a drop in MCR and PR in 2 of the 3 patients.

MCR is considered the best overall measurement of testosterone metabolism [6]. It is influenced by a variety of factors, e.g. production rate, plasma level, extent of binding to plasma proteins [7], volume of distribution and rate of metabolism [6]. Post-treatment decline in MCR was most pronounced in the patient with a high pre-treatment value (H.A., Table II), reflecting the oestrogen-induced SHBG rise [8]. In 2/3 of the patients the pre-treatment V_d was diminished. One might venture to theorize that EU resulted in less testosterone remaining in a smaller volume but being metabolized more efficiently. Thus less testosterone should reach the target organ, i.e., the prostate. The third patient (B.G., Table II) had a low pre-treatment value of MCR.

Table I Prostatic carcinoma: estradiol undecylate 100 mg every 4 weeks i.m. Endogenous hormones before and 6 months after treatment (4 weeks after last injection).

Patient	Age	Stage	Testosterone		LH		FSH		Prolactin	
		T N M[a]	(ng/100 ml)		(mIU/ml[b])		(mIU/ml[b])		(ng/ml)	
			pre	post	pre	post	pre	post	pre	post
A.H.	77	$T_4 N_2 M_1$	510	296	3	4	12	4	7	22
K.K.	65	$T_2 N_0 M_0$	329	109	5	2	6	2	12	20
B.G.	66	$T_3 N_0 M_0$	259	298	15	1	25	2	13	14

[a]TNM = Tumour Nodes Metastases
[b]IU = international units

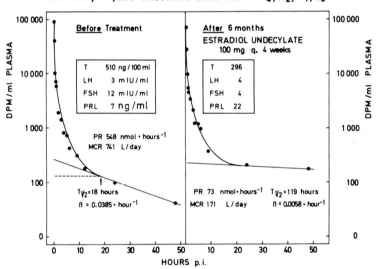

PAT. A.H., 77 years PROSTATIC CARCINOMA $T_4, N_2, M_1, G_3{}^a$

Fig. 1. Endogenous harmone levels and plasma testosterone elimination curves before and after 6-month treatment with 100 mg EU every 4 weeks. After injection of ^{3}H-testosterone, venous blood for analysis of testosterone and metabolites was drawn up to 48 hours. From the areas under the elimination curve the kinetic parameters MCR and $t_{1/2}$ were calculated graphically. $G_3{}^a$ = low degree of tumour differentiation.

Table II Prostatic carcinoma: estradiol undecylate 100 mg every 4 weeks i.m. Kinetic parameters of testosterone before and 6 months after treatment (4 weeks after last injection).

Patient	Age	$t_{1/2}$		Slope-β		V_d		MCR		PR	
		(hours)		(hours^{-1})		(litres)		(litres day^{-1})		(nM hour^{-1})	
		pre	post	pre	post	pre	post	pre	post	pre	post
A.H.	77	18	119	0.038	0.006	80.2	12.3	741	171	548	73
K.K.	65	40	92	0.017	0.008	54.1	11.6	224	173	107	28
B.G.	66	15	33	0.046	0.029	19.0	28.4	212	196	79	84

Cyproterone acetate

A 6-month trial with CA resulted in testosterone suppression in 3 of the 4 patients (Table III). LH and FSH levels showed no particular trends but prolactin rose in 3 of the 4 patients. The biological half-life of testosterone was increased in all 4 patients and the slope-β was depressed correspondingly (Table IV). The V_d rose in 3 of the 4 patients. With the exception of one patient (L.O., Table IV) MCR-changes through CA treatment were insignificant. This is partly explained by decreased SHBG, as observed by Bartsch *et al.* [8].

Estramustine phosphate

EP is a chemical combination of estradiol phosphate and nitrogen mustard. The extent of oestrogenic action is not yet settled. The disappearance of tritiated testosterone from plasma (Figure 2) is less influenced by EP than by oestrogens [9]. Applying the t-test for matched-paired data to the pre- and post-treatment values, the mean differences were not significant (Table V). In contrast, 2 patients in a study of Bird *et al.* [10] with carcinoma of the prostate treated over 5 days with ethinylestradiol (0.5 mg twice daily (b.i.d.)) responded with decreased clearance rates and volumes of distribution. The EP effect upon testosterone plasma kinetics is even less pronounced when compared with a 5-day regimen of low-dose oestrogen (e.g. 0.6 mg ethinylestradiol) studied previously [9].

Table III Prostatic carcinoma: cyproterone acetate 300 mg every week i.m. Endogenous hormones before and 6 months after treatment (1 week after last injection).

Patient	Age	Stage	Testosterone		LH		FSH		PRL	
		T N M[a]	(ng/100 ml)		(mIU/ml[b])		(mIU/ml[b])		(ng/ml)	
			pre	post	pre	post	pre	post	pre	post
Z.K.	70	$T_1 N_0 M_0$	660	167	2	3	4	7	11	19
L.O.	67	$T_4 N_0 M_0$	200	53	3	5	2	4	22	14
K.H.	59	$T_3 N_0 M_0$	470	291	5	2	7	4	7	12
P.H.	74	$T_2 N_0 M_0$	215	322	8	8	19	15	10	14

[a]TNM = Tumour Node Metastases
[b]IU = international units

Table IV Prostatic carcinoma: cyproterone acetate 300 mg every week i.m. Kinetic parameters of testosterone before and 6 months after treatment (1 week after last injection).

Patient	Age	$t_{1/2}$		Slope-β		V_d		MCR		PR	
		(hours)		(hours^{-1})		(litres)		(litres/day^{-1})		(nM hour^{-1})	
		pre	post	pre	post	pre	post	pre	post	pre	post
Z.K.	70	13	37	0.053	0.019	14.5	55.2	186	247	178	60
L.O.	67	10	48	0.069	0.014	28.6	49.1	476	170	138	13
K.H.	59	20	38	0.036	0.018	10.4	32.9	188	144	140	60
P.H.	74	42	44	0.018	0.016	45.5	33.9	190	136	95	63

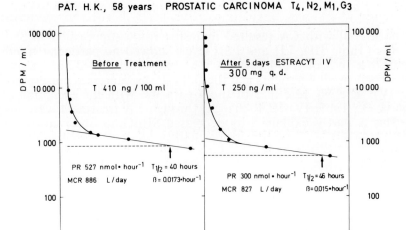

Fig. 2. Endogenous circulating testosterone and ³H-testosterone elimination curves in plasma before and after a 5-day regimen of 300 mg EP per day.

Table V Prostatic carcinoma: estramustine phosphate 300 mg i.v. every day for 5 days. Kinetic parameters before and after treatment (1 day after last injection).

Patient	Age	$t_{1/2}$ (hours)		Slope-β (hours^{-1})		V_d (litres)		MCR (litres. day^{-1})		PR (nM. hour^{-1})	
		pre	post	pre	post	pre	post	pre	post	pre	post
H.K.	58	40	46	0.017	0.015	19.9	20.8	886	827	527	300
H.H.	60	34	20	0.020	0.035	18.9	14.7	930	1,220	671	620
K.W.	71	132	55	0.005	0.013	23.7	21.9	280	660	199	335
R.J.	77	55	61	0.013	0.011	28.5	31.5	860	860	624	437
N.A.	77	61	34	0.011	0.020	23.4	15.3	641	755	463	378
S.G.	70	20	21	0.034	0.033	20.0	13.0	1,675	1,030	1,209	521
L.J.	48	12	11	0.058	0.063	98.4	91.8	1,361	1,390	989	704
R.J.	64	77	24	0.009	0.028	70.3	17.4	1,521	1,206	1,100	612
S.S.	75	62	38	0.011	0.018	33.2	11.2	889	495	645	249
B.H.	73	135	60	0.005	0.012	42.9	31.5	531	875	383	444
Mean difference D		25.8 n.s.		0.006 n.s.		11.0 n.s.		25.6 n.s.		221.0 n.s.	

n.s. = not significant

Fossa et al. [1] measured estradiol- and testosterone-levels in plasma in 3 previously untreated patients. One week after administration of 5–10 mg/kg EP per os estradiol rose (range 660–1,700 pg (= g × 10^{-12})/ml), whereas testosterone dropped (range 40–250 ng (= g × 10^{-9})/100 ml). After a 3-week regimen testosterone values in their 3 patients were in the range 10–40 ng/100 ml. Other investigators [12] noticed that although 10 to 15%

of EP is hydrolyzed in man to estradiol within 24 hours little of this estradiol is found in systemic circulation. Thus, after short-term administration, EP, even in a dose of 300 mg every day exerts only slight oestrogenic action as far as alteration of the kinetics of metabolism of testosterone in plasma is concerned. Determinations of total oestrogen secretion in 24-hour urine specimens and of circulating prolactin after EP administration indicate, however, a pronounced catabolism of this compound into degradation products still active oestrogenically. (These results will be the subject of a later report.)

Trial of a long-term treatment comparing EP with another N-alkylating agent such as cyclophosphamide, not combined with an oestrogenic compound, with regard to their effects on androgen kinetics, is warranted.

Summary

In 17 patients with untreated carcinoma of the prostate testosterone plasma kinetics were studied before and after estradiol undecylate (3 patients), cyproterone acetate (4 patients) and estramustine phosphate (10 patients). A 6-month regimen of estradiol undecylate resulted in an increased biological half-life and a decline in metabolic clearance rates. Cyproterone acetate impaired testosterone elimination moderately with a slight increase in biological half-life and insignificant changes in testosterone clearance rates. A 5-day regimen of a daily dose of 300 mg estramustine phosphate did not alter testosterone plasma kinetics significantly. Thus the oestrogenic action of this compound is even less than low-dose oestrogen application over the same period of time.

Acknowledgements

This study was supported by Grant no. Ja 277/2 from the Deutsche Forschungsgemeinschaft, Bonn – Bad Godesberg, Federal Republic of Germany.

References

1. Jacobi, G. H., Sinterhauf, K., Kurth, K. H. and Altwein, J. E. (1978): Bromocriptine and prostatic carcinoma: plasma kinetics, production and tissue uptake of ^{3}H-testosterone *in vivo*. *J. Urol., 119*, 240.
2. Dotti, C., Filippi, G., Castagnetti, C. and Franchini, R. (1975): Experimental determination of the operative parameters for a double antibody solid phase radioimmunoassay of luteinizing and follicle-stimulating hormones in serum. *Ric. Clin. Lab., 5*, 249.
3. Jacobi, G. H., Kurth, K. H. and Altwein, J. E. (1979): Effekt von Bromocriptin beim Prostatakarzinom: Testosteronstoffwechsel in Abhängigkeit vom Differenzierungsgrad. *Urologe A 18*, 91.
4. Tait, J. F., Tait, S. A. S., Little, B. and Laumas, K. R. (1961): The disappearance of 7-H^3-d-aldosterone in the plasma of normal subjects. *J. Clin. Invest., 40*, 72.
5. Gurpide, E. (1975): Tracer methods in hormone research. In: *Monographs on Endocrinology*, Vol. VIII, p. 171. Editors: F. Gross, A. Labhart, M. B. Lipsett, T. Mann, L. T. Samuels and J. Zander. Springer-Verlag, Berlin, Heidelberg, New York.
6. Tait, J. F. and Burstein, S. (1964): *In vivo* studies of steroid dynamics in man. In: *The Hormones*, Vol. V, p. 441. Editors: G. Pincus, K. V. Thimann and E. B. Astwood. Academic Press, New York.
7. Vermeulen, A. and Verdonck, L. (1968): Studies on the binding of testosterone to human plasma. *Steroids, 11*, 609.

8. Bartsch, W., Horst, H. J., Becker, H. and Nehse, G. (1977): Sex hormone-binding globulin-binding capacity, testosterone, 5α-dihydrotestosterone, oestradiol and prolactin in plasma of patients with prostatic carcinoma under various types of hormonal treatment. *Acta Endocrinol. (Copenhagen), 85*, 650.
9. Jacobi, G. H., Sinterhauf, K. and Altwein, J. E. (1978): Prostatic carcinoma: plasma kinetics and interaprostatic metabolism of testosterone in low-dose estrogen-treated patients *in vivo. Urology, 12*, 359.
10. Bird, C. E., Green, R. N., Calandra, R. S., Connolly, J. G. and Clark, A. F. (1971): Kinetics of ^{3}H-testosterone metabolism in patients with carcinoma of the prostate: effects of oestrogen administration. *Acta Endocrinol. (Copenhagen), 67*, 733.
11. Fossa, S. D., Fossa, J. and Aakvaag, A. (1977): Hormone changes in patients with prostatic carcinoma during treatment with estramustine phosphate. *J. Urol., 118*, 1013.
12. Kirdani, R. Y., Mittelman, A., Murphy, G. B. and Sandberg, A. A. (1975): Studies on phenolic steroids in human subjects. XIV. Fate of a nitrogen mustard of estradiol-17β. *J. Clin. Endocrinol. Metab., 41*, 305.

Discussion

P. Ekman (Stockholm, Sweden): Obviously data in the literature are controversial since several studies indicate that EP influences serum levels in a similar fashion to conventional oestrogen therapy. Compare, e.g., Fossa *et al., Vitamins & Hormones 33*, 1975.

J. E. Altwein: Fossa's paper (*J. Urol. 118*, 1013, 1977) commented that 'other investigators have not found estradiol in measurable quantities in the blood of patients receiving EP'. Fredholm *et al.* (*Acta Pharmacol. Toxicol., Supp. 35*, 28, 1974) have shown that EP has only one hundredth of the oestrogenic action of estradiol. Kjaer *et al.* (*Urology, 5*, 802, 1975) administered EP in a high dose (900 mg p.o.) over 14 days to 10 patients with carcinoma of the prostate. The average decrease in plasma testosterone was 43.8% (range 6–88%). Kadohma *et al.* (*J. Urol., 119*, 235, 1978) clarified the issue by demonstrating that EP is primarily hydrolyzed and its hydrolysis products are metabolized and/or conjugated in the liver. The estradiol (and carbamate?) released is metabolized readily and conjugated in the liver.

The lack of significant oestrogenic effects is a reflection of the efficacy with which the liver accomplished these metabolic transformations (Kadohma *et al.*). Our kinetic data are in keeping with these findings. Our unpublished data on the 24-hour urinary excretion of oestrogenic degradation products, such as oestrone-, estradiol-, and oestriol conjugates, which are found in a 40–50 fold excess after EP treatment, also support this fact. Such catabolites are, however, responsible for another 'oestrogenic' action, namely, the induced hyperprolactinemia generally encountered during administration of EP.

J. Thijssen (Utrecht, The Netherlands): Did you measure SHBG levels in your patients, because the differences in MCR observed by you could be explained by changes in SHBG?

J. E. Altwein: The differences in MCR are indeed reflected in part by variations in SHBG. As mentioned before, EP resulted in a marked appearance of degradation products still active oestrogenically, which are capable of increasing SHBG synthesis. We have determined SHBG before and after treatment (saturation analysis: Blank *et al., J. Steroid Biochem. 9,* 21, 1978) and found 3.6 to 7.8 mg/l (mean 4.9 mg/l) before and 5.1 to 11.3 mg/l (mean 7.8 mg/l) after EP. These SHBG values are, although scattered over a wide range, statistically significant at the 5% level. We will report the complete data, including the effects of EP on free and bound ratios of testosterone, after completion of this study.

J. Thijssen: Do you have an explanation for the large range in MCR for testosterone in your patients (from 136–1675 1/24 hours)?

J. E. Altwein: Since the MCR is influenced by several factors, e.g., production rate, plasma level, volume of distribution, rates of metabolism and extent of binding, the range may be large. Among the few available studies of the plasma kinetics of testosterone similarly wide ranges were encountered. Bird *et al.* (*Acta Endocrinol. 67,* 733, 1971), for example, recorded MCRs between 135 and 1343 1/24 hours. Furthermore, the extent (stage) of the underlying malignant disease will have some bearing, too. Because of this we studied each patient before and after treatment to permit statistical analysis for 'matched pairs'.

General Discussion

R. Ghanadian (London, United Kingdom): I should like to address a remark to Dr. Habib. You mentioned an increase in androstanolone (DHT) levels in BPH tissue and an increase in testosterone levels in cancer tissues and said that an increase had not been demonstrated in the serum level of DHT in BPH patients, in contrast to the work some years ago (supported by the data reported by Vermeulen and Desy and by Horton *et al.*) that DHT serum levels increase in patients with BPH. We have data on plasma levels of testosterone and DHT in 34 patients with prostatic carcinoma compared with those in normal subjects of the same age group.

We found that testosterone was increased in patients with prostatic carcinoma, and that the ratio of testosterone DHT is doubled as compared with that in normal subjects.

P. Ekman (Stockholm, Sweden): Since most of the differing opinions disclosed this morning obviously are mainly due to different assay techniques, might we not agree on some factors which could induce heterogeneity of assay results?

My suggestions are:
1. Since TUR material gives unreliable binding data, we should not use such material in future.
2. Since natural ligands have the disadvantage of binding to sex hormone-binding globulin (SHBG) and since we need exchange assays for elimination of endogenous steroid receptors and the natural ligands are less suitable, we should agree upon the use of synthetic steroids as ligands in receptor assays in future.

Two questions:
1. How long can we wait before we freeze tissue specimens without significant loss of receptor? According to our experience 1−7 hours is acceptable.
2. How long can we keep the samples at $-70°$C without loss of receptors? Our data indicate that a storage time of 6 months influences receptor content very little.

N. Bruchovsky (Edmonton, Canada): In view of Dr. Heyns' observation that oestrogens stimulate nuclear uptake of androgens and Dr. Mobbs' and Dr. Teulings' findings that oestrogens greatly increase the concentration of intracellular SHBG which, in turn, might result in increased androgen levels within tissue, does it make good sense to use continuous oestrogen therapy after an initial response has been obtained? Perhaps it would be wiser to discontinue oestrogen therapy following evidence of favourable response to avoid potentially adverse changes within the target cells during lengthy periods of treatment?

H. A. van Gilse (Rotterdam, The Netherlands): In answer to your suggestion that oestrogen treatment might be stopped in order to prevent an increase in androgen levels, clinical practice of about 25 years ago, when the biochemical background was not known, demonstrated that the results of oestrogen therapy were better and of longer duration if patients were treated permanently until progression occurred and if therapy was not stopped before that stage.

N. Bruchovsky: The question of whether survival is enhanced by oestrogen therapy remains controversial even when short-term regression of carcinoma is achieved. We feel that continuous therapy with oestrogens is not logical if the carcinoma develops a super-efficient mechanism for trapping DHT even in the presence of small circulating levels of testosterone. A major objective of therapy should be to delay emergence of an apparent hormone-resistant state. This might be accomplished by keeping the concentration of testosterone in blood at a level compatible with no growth rather than advance or regression of disease. With availability of radioimmuno-assays this type of clinical investigation would not be unreasonable.

J.-Å. Gustafsson, (Stockholm, Sweden): It is difficult to judge the significance of Dr. de Voogt's data since he does not give any details of the methodology used. However, I feel one should be careful in stating generally that cytoplasmic receptors are not valuable as predictive instruments in selecting patients for therapy. After all, we have seen today that various groups report widely varying results even with regard to the presence or absence of receptors in different kinds of prostatic tissues (e.g. oestrogen receptors in BPH). Evidently this must reflect major methodological problems. The most rational approach to this problem would be to distribute a standard to laboratories so that they could standardize their methods. Before this has been done care is needed in comparing results from various laboratories as regards correlation between receptor content and response to therapy. It appears better to express negativism on the present state of methodology rather than on the correlation between receptors and response. Promising innovations in the field of receptor methodology are represented by the use of electrofocusing of oestrogen receptors in fine needle aspiration biopsies of breast cancer tissue and the present efforts to develop radioimmunological assays of steroid receptors.

H. J. de Voogt (Leiden, The Netherlands): The methodology which I did not mention was the same as that used by Wagner. Dingjan has reported extensively on methodology in his Leiden thesis of 1978.

I agree with you that, at present, there is too much variation in methodology and that standardization should be an answer to this. However, my point was that the difficulties in obtaining enough tissue material and the heterogeneity of prostatic tissue in biopsy specimens together with the disappointing results as to correlation between response and endocrine therapy all lead to the conclusion that cytoplasmic steroid-receptor assay is probably not the most suitable assay for routine clinical use. This does not preclude its value as a scientific method in experimental research.

II
CLINICAL RELEVANCE OF STUDIES ON METABOLISM AND RECEPTOR-BINDING OF STEROID HORMONES FOR BPH AND PROSTATIC CARCINOMA

Studies on the in vitro binding and metabolism of testosterone in benign prostatic hypertrophy and carcinoma of the prostate: a correlation with endogenous androgen levels

F. K. Habib
Department of Surgery, University of Edinburgh Medical School, Edinburgh, Scotland

Introduction

With the exception of the pioneering studies of Huggins [1], the relationship of hormone to prostatic cancer is today, for the most part, inferentially based either on the results of basic research with androgens in animal systems [2–6] or on *in vitro* experiments carried out on normal and benign human prostatic tissue [7–10].

Although considerable insight has been gained from these studies in recent years, the relationship of benign prostatic hypertrophy (BPH) to cancer of the prostate (PCA) is still controversial [11]. The two conditions are common and both increase progressively with age; there are also reports suggesting that BPH may be a precursor of PCA [12]. Nonetheless, there are equally strong indications that carcinoma cells retain a variety of characteristics markedly different from those observed in benign tissue [13–14]. Identification of those characteristics is pertinent to the understanding of the biochemical events leading to the development of neoplasia in the human prostate. These new considerations at the endocrine level could be of profound relevance to the diagnosis and prognosis of the disease.

In this communication I would like to consider briefly the distribution of androgens in pathological prostates and highlight some of the differences observed in our laboratory between androgenic activity in benign and malignant tissues. Only minimal reference will be made to other groups who have also investigated these themes.

Materials and methods

The experiments described below were performed on human tissue obtained either from retropubic prostatectomy or transurethral resection. The technical procedures used for the extraction, separation and radioimmunoassay of endogenous steroids in prostatic tissues, the identification and quantitative analysis of metabolites in steroid treated specimens and the characterization of hormone binding proteins in subcellular fractions have all been described previously [15–17].

In view of the reported variations in the levels of androgen with age [18–19] and the rarity of normal prostates after the age of 60 [20], we assumed that all prostates in the age range under investigation (59–91 years) belonged either to the BPH or PCA categories. This was confirmed by parallel histological examinations. Normal samples were obtained from autopsy specimens pertaining to a marginally younger age group (40–52 years).

Results

a) Endogenous steroid hormones

The concentrations of endogenous steroids occurring in normal prostatic tissue, BPH and PCA are compared in Table I. The levels of androstanolone (DHT) measured in the pathological prostates (BPH or PCA) were noticeably high and significantly greater (in all cases $p < 0.01$) than the amounts detected in the normal gland. Moreover, comparisons between the BPH and PCA groups revealed twice as much DHT in the hypertrophied specimens with no significant overlap between the benign and malignant groups ($p < 0.01$). Testosterone, by contrast, was very elevated in the neoplastic specimens whereas the levels associated with normal and benign tissue were considerably lower ($p < 0.01$). We could not detect any significant differences between testosterone concentrations in normal and BPH specimens. There was an increase in concentration of androstenedione in tissues obtained from PCA compared with those from BPH.

Further inspection of the androgen data (Figure 1) revealed a strong positive correlation between testosterone and its 5α-reduced metabolite, DHT, in the hyperplastic (r = 0.82; $p < 0.01$) and neoplastic tissues (r = 0.77; $p < 0.01$). There was also a significant relationship between the primary androgen, testosterone, and its other metabolite, androstenedione, in BPH (r = 0.84; $p < 0.01$) and PCA (r = 0.87; $p < 0.01$) (Figure 2). Since testosterone and DHT were present in approximately equal concentrations in the normal gland we would anticipate a similar significant relationship between the two steroids in this tissue.

Table I Mean hormonal concentrations (pM (= M × 10⁻¹²)/g dry weight ± standard error of mean (SEM)) in prostatic tissue of patients with BPH and PCA compared with normal subjects.

Table I Mean hormonal concentrations (pM (= $M \times 10^{-12}$)/g dry weight ± standard error of mean (SEM)) in prostatic tissue of patients with BPH and PCA compared with normal subjects.

Group*		Testosterone	Androstanolone	Androstenedione	Androstanolone / Testosterone
Normal	(10)	12.6 ± 2.3	12.94 ± 1.9	Not determined	1.02
BPH	(20)	14.1 ± 2.4	45.5 ± 5.8	30.0 ± 7.6	3.22
PCA	(10)	39.6 ± 6.2	22.4 ± 2.4	42.0 ± 7.9	0.56

* Number in parentheses indicates number of patients in each group.

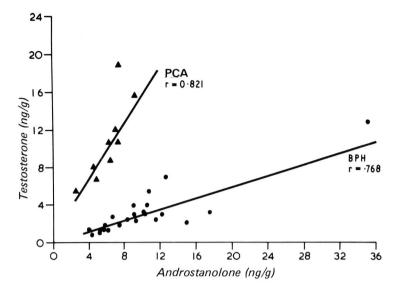

Fig. 1. Relationship between the concentration of testosterone and androstanolone in BPH and PCA. Regression lines are shown with correlation coefficient r. From [14].

We also used discriminant analysis and combined the androgen data into a single variable. The androgen tissue ratios for the three prostate groups are shown in Table I.

The ratio DHT/testosterone was, in all BPH cases, greater than 3.0 whereas in PCA the ratio was less than 0.6. Normal tissues maintained a value approximately equal to 1.0. The variations in androgen ratios further highlight the hormonal differences between the three types of tissue.

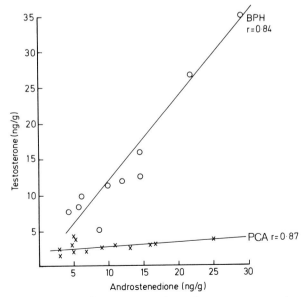

Fig. 2. Relationship between the concentration of testosterone and androstenedione in BPH and PCA. Regression line is shown with correlation coefficient r.

In addition to the androgen measurements we monitored hormone concentrations in the plasma of all patients included in this study to ascertain whether the hormonal changes observed in tissue were associated with any changes in levels of steroids in the circulating plasma pool. The data presented in Table II show no significant differences between testosterone, DHT and androstenedione concentrations in plasma obtained from the three groups of patients. The DHT/testosterone ratios were of the same order of magnitude suggesting that the bulk of the DHT measured in the blood results from direct peripheral conversion of testosterone. Contributions from the high DHT reserves of the hypertrophied prostate are, therefore, minimal and insignificant.

Table II Plasma androgen concentration (nM (= M $\times$ 10^{-9})/l ± SEM) in normal, BPH and PCA patients.

Group*	Testosterone	Androstanolone	Androstenedione	Androstanolone / Testosterone
Normal (10)	17.2 ± 2.9	2.4 ± 0.6	Not determined	0.14
BPH (20)	19.7 ± 2.6	2.6 ± 0.9	5.5 ± 1.7	0.13
PCA (10)	16.9 ± 2.8	2.4 ± 0.5	4.4 ± 1.1	0.14

* Number in parentheses indicates number of patients in each group.

The studies described so far on endogenous steroid levels in plasma and prostate lend further support to the growing evidence that male hormone action at the target site is not initiated by the circulating androgens but by products of the reductive and oxidative metabolism of these steroids in the responsive tissue.

b) Androgen metabolism

Testosterone is converted by the prostate gland to a variety of metabolites. The formation of these metabolites in different proportions may be associated with disorders of prostatic growth. In PCA tissue we have demonstrated the accumulation of testosterone but the relevance of this androgen to the pathogenesis of the disease in man is still not known.

The *in vitro* experiments described below were undertaken to obtain further information on the mechanism responsible for the differences in androgen composition of the normal and pathological prostate. Aliquots of freshly prepared cytosol were incubated with 2 nM of ^{3}H-testosterone in the presence of 0.5 mM nadide phosphate, reduced form (NADPH). Our preliminary experiments showed that 5α-reduction was very dependent upon the presence of the cofactor and that both 5α-reductase and 3α(β)-hydroxysteroid dehydrogenase were most active when the concentration of the cofactor was 5 $\times$ 10^{-3} M. NADPH did not hinder 17β-hydroxysteroid dehydrogenase activity. All incubations were carried out in triplicate by shaking in an atmosphere of 5% CO_2:95% O_2 for one hour at 37°C.

The metabolites produced by the 9 hypertrophied specimens are shown in Table III. DHT was the major androgen formed and its concentration ranged from 24.1 to 43.3% (mean 33.5%), whereas the 3α(β)-androstanediol varied between 3.4 and 6.3% (mean 5.2%). Androstenedione was not detectable in one of the specimens analysed. On average this steroid constituted 1.2% of the metabolites formed. These studies emphasize the predominance of the reductive products of testosterone in BPH tissues. Furthermore, the results in Table III indicate that the percentage of unconverted testosterone was always inversely proportional to the levels of DHT formed but that no similar relationship could be established with androstenedione. We also noticed that changes in 5α-reductase activity were always paralleled by concurrent changes in $3\alpha(\beta)$-dehydrogenase activity such that the ratio of mean activities of 5α-reductase to $3\alpha(\beta)$-dehydrogenase in BPH was always constant. In these experiments this constant was approximately equal to 6.9.

Table III   The in vitro metabolism of ^3H-testosterone by 9 cytosol specimens obtained from BPH tissue.

Specimen no.	Steroid recovered (% radioactivity recovered)			
	Testosterone unconverted	Androstanolone	$3\alpha(\beta)$-Androstanediol	Androstenedione
1	64.5	27.5	Not determined	2.6
2	52.9	38.9	5.6	1.9
3	69.3	24.1	3.4	1.27
4	51.0	41.2	5.9	1.37
5	68.4	25.5	Not determined	1.60
6	50.2	43.0	6.2	0.56
7	65.7	27.8	3.9	0.93
8	49.7	43.3	6.3	Not detected
9	60.8	30.2	4.1	0.76
Mean ± S.D.	59.2 ± 8.2	33.5 ± 7.9	5.0 ± 1.18	1.22 ± 0.66

The metabolism of testosterone by the poorly differentiated carcinoma of the prostate specimens is shown in Table IV. The pattern obtained is markedly different from that observed in BPH. A striking result was the complete absence of $3\alpha(\beta)$-hydroxysteroid dehydrogenase activity. The amounts of DHT formed were also low (mean 5.3%) whereas 17β-hydroxysteroid dehydrogenase activity was considerably enhanced. The androstenedione recovered accounted for 19.2% of the metabolites measured. The high levels of unconverted testosterone in neoplastic cytosol were noteworthy. These PCA experiments demonstrate a distinct shift in the metabolic pathways of testosterone as compared with BPH.

Table IV   The in vitro metabolism of ^3H-testosterone by PCA cytosols. All sampling was in triplicate. Values shown are means ± SD.

% Steroid recovered			
Testosterone unconverted	Androstanolone	$3\alpha(\beta)$-Androstanediol	Androstenedione
60.9 ± 2.6	5.3 ± 1.0	Not detected	19.2 ± 2.2

Discussion

The studies described in this paper confirm the existence of fundamental biochemical differences between PCA and BPH. Some of these differences have been reported elsewhere [14, 15, 17] and underline the potential value of hormone measurements as possible markers for monitoring the presence of tumours.

These results also suggest that assay of tissue androgen levels in the pathological prostate correlates well with hormone metabolism studies. A rise in endogenous DHT levels was always associated with high 5α-reductase activity whereas very low concentrations of the 5α-reduced metabolite reflected reduced enzymatic activity. Thus the excessively elevated testosterone levels measured in all cancer specimens were primarily induced by inhibition of 5α-reductase. This is clearly evident from our androgen metabolism studies. There are reports [21] indicating that prostatic 5α-reductase is dependent upon the proportion of stromal elements in the tissue. Unlike BPH, PCA is predominantly epithelial in nature but whether this would account for the changes in the enzymatic properties of the tissue still remains to be elucidated. We should not, however, discount the possibility that accumulation of testosterone in the malignant prostate coupled with a concomitant depletion of DHT may also arise from the presence of a tumour-specific testosterone receptor [22].

The higher levels of androstenedione measured in PCA further emphasize the quantitative differences in the metabolism of testosterone by hyperplastic and neoplastic tissue. The increases in 17β-hydroxysteroid dehydrogenase activity were characteristic of all neoplastic specimens. Supplementing the PCA cytosol preparations with NADPH did not restore 5α-reductase to its original activity or hinder the formation of androstenedione.

The results discussed in this paper could have implications for the treatment of prostatic disorders. It seems that several factors influence prostatic growth but probably androgen metabolism and the presence of receptor proteins are the most important. In view of the differences between BPH and PCA further studies of these parameters could be of use for selecting types of endocrine treatment and predicting clinical responsiveness to anti-androgen therapy.

Acknowledgements

The investigations described in this chapter were performed in the Division of Steroid Endocrinology at the University of Leeds and were supported by a research grant from the Yorkshire Cancer Research Campaign.

References

1. Huggins, C. and Clark, P. J. (1940): Quantitative studies of prostatic secretion. II The effect of castration and of oestrogen injection on the normal and on the hyperplastic prostate glands of dogs. *J. Exp. Med., 72,* 747–762.
2. Liao, S., Liang, T., Fang, S., Castaneda, E. and Shao, T. C. (1973): Steroid structure and androgenic activity. Specificities involved in the receptor binding and nuclear retention of various androgens. *J. Biol. Chem., 248,* 6154–6162.
3. Rennie, P. and Bruchovsky, N. (1973): Studies on the relationship between androgen receptor and the transport of androgens in rat prostate. *J. Biol. Chem., 248,* 3288–3297.

4. Voigt, W., Feldman, M. and Dunning, W. F. (1975): Sensitivity in prostatic cancer of Copenhagen rats. *Cancer Res., 35,* 1840–1846.
5. Krieg, M. and Voigt, K. D. (1977): Biochemical substrate of androgenic actions at a cellular level in prostate, Bulbo-cavernosus/Levator ani and in skeletal muscle. *Acta Endocrinol. (Copenhagen), 85,* 43–89.
6. Isaacs, J. T., Heston, W. D. W., Weissman, R. M. and Coffey, D. S. (1978): Animal models of the hormone – sensitive and insensitive prostatic adenocarcinomas, Dunning R-3327-H, R-3327-HI and R-3327-AT. *Cancer Res., 38,* 4353–4359.
7. Mainwaring, W. I. P. and Milroy, E. J. G. (1973): Characterization of the specific androgen receptors in the human prostate gland. *J. Endocrinol., 57,* 371–384.
8. Jacobi, G. H. and Wilson, J. D. (1977): Formation of 5α-androstane-3α,17β-diol by normal and hypertrophic human prostate. *J. Clin. Endocrinol. Metab., 44,* 107–115.
9. Morfin, R. F., Di Stefano, S., Bercovici, J. P. and Flock, H. H. (1978): Comparison of testosterone, 5α-dihydrotestosterone and 5α-androstane-3β,17β-diol metabolisms in human normal and hyperplastic prostates. *J. Steroid Biochem., 9,* 245–252.
10. Meikle, A. W., Stringham, J. D. and Olsen, D. C. (1978): Subnormal tissue 3α-androstanediol and androsterone in prostatic hyperplasia. *J. Clin. Endocrinol. Metab., 47,* 909–913.
11. Greenwald, P., Kirmiss, V., Polan, A. and Dick, V. S. (1974): Cancer of the prostate among men with benign prostatic hyperplasia. *J. Nat. Cancer Inst., 53,* 335–340.
12. Sommers, S. C. (1957): Endocrine changes with prostatic carcinoma. *Cancer, 10,* 345–358.
13. Krieg, M., Grobe, I., Voigt, K. D., Altenähr, E. and Klosterhalfen, H. (1978): Human prostatic carcinoma: significant differences in its androgen binding and metabolism compared to the human benign prostatic hypertrophy. *Acta Endocrinol. (Copenhagen), 88,* 397–407.
14. Habib, F. K., Mason, M. K., Smith, P. H. and Stitch, S. R. (1979): Prostatic cancer: Is the endocrine function of the gland dependent on zinc? *Brit. J. Cancer, 39,* 700–704.
15. Habib, F. K., Lee, I. R., Stitch, S. R. and Smith, P. H. (1976): Androgen levels in the plasma and prostatic tissues of patients with benign hypertrophy and carcinoma of the prostate. *J. Endocrinol., 71,* 99–107.
16. Srivastava, A. K., Stitch, S. R. and Habib, F. K. (1978): Oestrogen- and progesterone-binding proteins in benign and malignant human uterine tissue. In: *Endometrial Carcinoma,* pp. 289–300. Editors: M. G. Brush, R. J. B. King and J. R. W. Taylor, Bailliere, London.
17. Habib, F. K., Rafati, G., Robinson, M. R. G. and Stitch, S. R. (1979): Effects of tamoxifen on the binding and metabolism of testosterone by human prostatic tissue and plasma *in vitro. J. Endocrinol., 83,* 369–378.
18. Chisholm, G. D. and Ghanadian, R. (1976): Comparison between the changes in serum 5α-dihydrotestosterone and testosterone in normal men and patients with benign prostatic hypertrophy. *Fifth International Congress of Endocrinology, Hamburg,* Abstract 455.
19. Hammond, G. L., Kontturi, M., Vihko, P. and Vihko, R. (1978): Serum steroids in normal males and patients with prostatic diseases. *Clin. Endocrinol., 9,* 113–121.
20. Franks, L. M. (1974): Biology of the prostate and its tumours. In: *The treatment of prostatic hypertrophy and neoplasia,* pp. 1–26. Editor: J. E. Castro. Medical and Technical Publishing Co., Lancaster.
21. Cowan, R. A., Cowan, S. K., Grant, J. K. and Elder, H. Y. (1977): Biochemical investigation of separated epithelium and stroma from benign hyperplastic prostatic tissue. *J. Endocrinol., 74,* 111–120.
22. Habib, F. K., Robinson, M. R. G., Smith, P. H. and Stitch, S. R. (1979): Testosterone binding in carcinoma of the prostate. In: *Research on Steroids,* Vol. VIII, pp. 367–370. Editors: A. Klopper, L. Lerner, H. J. van der Molen and F. Sciarra, Academic Press, London.

Discussion

J.-Å. Gustafsson (Stockholm, Sweden): Would you please provide further details concerning the conditions under which you have performed your enzymatic measurements? Did you use cytosol or microsomal (?) preparations? Did you wash under substrate and cofactor saturation conditions? Did you determine apparent Km and Vmax (?) values, etc.? I feel that it is essential to make certain that one works under enzymological conditions when one wants to measure enzymatic activities.

F. K. Habib: In view of the shortage of time I have intentionally omitted any experimental details from my talk but you are absolutely right. Enzymatic studies should be carried out under enzymological conditions.

The bulk of the androgen metabolism studies described were carried out on the cytosol fraction obtained by high speed centrifugation (105,000 g) of prostatic homogenate. Aliquots (0.5 ml) of the cytosol were incubated with 2 nM ^{3}H-testosterone in the presence of 0.5 mM NADPH. Preliminary experiments had revealed that 5α-reductase and 3α(β)-hydroxysteroid dehydrogenase were most active when the concentration of the cofactor was 5×10^{-3} M. The incubations were carried out in an atmosphere of 5% CO_2 : 95% O_2 for one hour at 37°C. Specific details of the extraction method, chromatographic separation and identification of the metabolites have already been reported (see reference [17] in the text).

M. Krieg (Hamburg, FRG): What is the ratio of endogenous DHT concentration in PCA as compared to BPH?

F. K. Habib: Although the endogenous levels of DHT are high in both PCA and BPH tissues when compared to the concentration found in normal specimens, we have also noted that the levels of the 5α-reduced metabolite were twice as high in BPH as in PCA tissue.

I. Lasnitzki (Cambridge, U.K.): We found that testosterone metabolism shows a shift towards the oxidative pathway in patients aged between 70 and 80 years. Sex hormone-binding globulin (SHBG) levels also rise with advancing age. Did you take the age of the patients and their plasma SHBG levels into account when measuring the conversion of testosterone?

F. K. Habib: We have noticed a shift towards the oxidative pathway in carcinoma patients only, independent of the age of the patient. In BPH the bulk of the testosterone was always, irrespective of age, metabolized to DHT whereas the levels of androstenedione found were minute and in some cases not detectable.

I agree that the levels of SHBG go up with age but these do not seem to hinder the metabolic activities of the gland. In fact there is growing evidence to suggest that the hormone action at the target site is not initiated by the circulating androgens but by products of the reductive and oxidative metabolism of these steroids in the responsive tissue.

Human prostate hyperplasia and adenocarcinoma: steroid hormone receptor assays and therapy

J. P. Raynaud, M. M. Bouton and P. M. Martin*
Roussel Uclaf Research Centre, Romainville, and the J. Paoli and I. Calmettes Institute, Marseilles, France

Introduction

The assay, first of oestrogen, then of progestogen receptors in human breast and endometrial cancer specimens has afforded a simple and fairly accurate means of identifying patients who will not respond to endocrine therapy [1, 2]. Steroid hormone receptor assays on prostate adenocarcinoma samples may prove similarly useful in selecting potentially responsive patients and in determining appropriate hormonal treatment. In the present study we have measured not only androgen but also oestrogen and progestogen receptors in human prostate tissue since, as yet, the relative importance of these various receptors in hormonal regulation of the prostate is unknown.

Although the detection of steroid hormone receptors in human breast tissue is now a routine procedure, detection of these receptors in human prostate tissue, whether hyperplastic or adenocarcinomatous has encountered more serious methodological difficulties which have severely handicapped a large-scale routine study. The samples are often heavily contaminated with plasma sex hormone-binding globulin, endogenous androgens occupy most binding sites thus necessitating an efficient exchange technique and the enzyme systems, particularly in benign prostate hyperplasia (BPH), are extremely active and lead to steroid degradation even *in vitro*. All these factors contribute to difficulty in developing a simple and rapid receptor assay, which could advantageously replace more cumbersome physicochemical techniques such as agar-gel electrophoresis and salt precipitation.

As described in detail in several recent articles [1, 3–5] these difficulties can be largely overcome by the use of synthetic radioligands that bind minimally to specific plasma proteins, that are not degraded on *in vitro* incubation with cytosol and that are specific to one hormone class. However, as shown below, further improvements are still necessary since, of all the available radioligands, only the oestrogen moxestrol (RU 2858) meets all requirements [3]. Metribolone (RU 1881) binds both to androgen and progestogen receptors but this disadvantage can be overcome by the parallel use of triamcinolone acetonide [6, 7]. The relatively high non-specific binding of promegestone (RU 5020), used to measure progestogen receptor, precludes its use in cases where the total protein concentration is high and the binding site concentration very low.

Materials and methods

Test compounds

(6,7-³H)-RU 2858 (48 Ci/mmol), (6,7-³H)-RU 1881 (56 Ci/mmol), (6,7-³H)-RU 5020 (57 Ci/mmol) and (1α,2α-³H)-testosterone (54 Ci/mmol) were synthesized at the Roussel-Uclaf Research Centre. Purity (≥ 98%) was checked by thin-layer chromatography in the following solvent systems: benzene/ethyl acetate (7/3, v/v), methylene chloride/methanol (9/1, v/v), and carbon

Table I   Chemical names of the test-compounds.

Androstanolone	17β-Hydroxy-5α-androstan-3-one
Chlormadinone acetate	17α-Acetyloxy-6-chloro-pregna-4,6-diene-3,20-dione
Cyproterone acetate	17α-Acetyloxy-6-chloro-1,2-dihydro-(1β,2β)-3′H-cyclopropa-[1,2]pregna-1,4,6-triene-3,20-dione
Dexamethasone	9α-Fluoro-11β,17α,21-trihydroxy-16α-methyl-pregna-1,4-diene-3,20-dione
Ethynyl Oestradiol	19-Nor-17α-pregna-1,3,5(10)-trien-20-yne-3,17β-diol
Hydrocortisone	11β,17α,21-Trihydroxy-pregn-4-ene-3,20-dione
Hydroxyflutamide	2-Hydroxy-2-methyl-N-[(4-nitro-3-trifluoromethyl)phenyl]-propanamide
Megestrol acetate	17α-Acetyloxy-6-methyl-pregna-4,6-diene-3,20-dione
Metribolone (RU 1881)	17β-Hydroxy-17α-methyl-estra-4-9,11-trien-3-one
Moxestrol (RU 2858)	11β-Methoxy-19-nor-17α-pregna-1,3,5(10)-trien-20-yne-3,17β-diol
Norethisterone	17β-Hydroxy-19-nor-17α-pregn-4-en-20-yn-3-one
Norgestrel	13β-Ethyl-17β-hydroxy-18,19-dinor-17α-pregn-4-en-20-yn-3-one
Oestradiol	Estra-1,3,5(10)-triene-3,17β-diol
Oestriol	Estra-1,3,5(10)-triene-3, 16α,17β-triol
Progesterone	Pregn-4-ene-3,20-dione
Promegestone (RU 5020)	17α,21-Dimethyl-19-nor-pregna-4,9-diene-3,20-dione
RU 23908	5,5-Dimethyl-3-[4-nitro-3-(trifluoromethyl)phenyl]2,4-imidazolidinedione
RU 2956	17β-Hydroxy-2,2,17α-trimethyl-estra-4,9,11-trien-3-one
Testosterone	17β-Hydroxy-androst-4-en-3-one
Triamcinolone acetonide	9α-Fluroro-11β,21-dihydroxy-16α,17α[1-methylethylidene bis (oxy)]-pregna-1, 4-diene-3,20-dione

tetrachloride/acetone (7/3, v/v) for ^{3}H-RU 2858; benzene/ethyl acetate (5/5, v/v) for ^{3}H-RU 1881 and ^{3}H-testosterone; benzene/ethyl acetate (7/3, v/v) for ^{3}H-RU 5020. The non-radioactive steroids listed in Table I were used.

Experimental material

Samples of normal human prostate (from 2 road-accident victims, 20–25 years old), BPH and prostate adenocarcinoma were obtained from the Hôtel Dieu, Marseilles, and stored in liquid nitrogen (for less than 2 weeks) until use.

Adult Sprague-Dawley rats ($\sim$ 200 g) were obtained from Charles River (France) and were castrated 24 hours before sacrifice.

Cytosol preparation

Cytosol from prostate adenocarcinomas (cytosol A) and BPH (cytosol B) were prepared and analysed at the J. Paoli and I. Calmettes Institute in Marseilles and the Roussel-Uclaf Research Centre in Romainville, respectively. The tissues were powdered in the frozen state using a Thermovac tissue pulverizer and homogenized in 10 mM trometamol (tris)-HCl (pH 8.0 at 0°C) containing 1 mM edetic acid (EDTA), 12 mM α-monothioglycerol and 10% glycerol (1/5, w/v) for cytosol A and in 10 mM tris-HCl (pH 7.4 at room temperature) containing 1.5 mM EDTA, 1 mM dithioerythritol, 10% glycerol and 0.1 mM phenylmethylsulfonyl fluoride (PMSF) (Sigma) for Cytosol B in a motor-driven glass/glass or Teflon/glass conical homogenizer. Cytosol (supernatant) was prepared by centrifuging homogenate at 105,000 g for 45 minutes at 0–4°C in a 50 Ti rotor (Beckman L2 65B centrifuge).

Cytosol from rat material (cytosol C) was prepared from ventral prostates minced with scissors and homogenized with a motor-driven Teflon/glass homogenizer in 1:6 (w/v) 10 mM tris-HCl buffer (pH 7.4) containing 0.25 M sucrose and 0.1 mM PMSF, then centrifuged at 105,000 g for 60 minutes at 0–4°C.

Dextran-coated charcoal (DCC) adsorption assay

Cytosols were incubated with radioligand as described in the table and figure legends. For cytosol A, a 200 μl sample was stirred for 30 minutes at 0–4°C with 500 μl of DCC suspension (0.05% Dextran 80,000/0.5% charcoal (Norit A)/0.01% gelatin) and then centrifuged for 10 minutes at 1,000 g at 0–4°C. For cytosols B and C, a 100 μl sample was stirred for 10 minutes at 0–4°C in a microtitre plate (Greiner plates, System Cooke M 220–24 Å) with 100 μl of a DCC suspension (0.625% Dextran 80,000/1.25% charcoal (Norit A)) and then centrifuged for 10 minutes at 800 g at 0–4°C. In each case the concentration of bound radioligand was determined by measuring the radioactivity in an aliquot of supernatant. Radioligand bound in the presence of a large excess of unlabelled hormone is assumed to be nonspecifically bound. The difference in supernatant radioactivity in the presence or absence of unlabelled hormone is identified as the concentration of specifically-bound hormone.

Measurement of the inhibition of ³H-RU 2858-, ³H-RU 1881- and ³H-testosterone-binding

Aliquots of cytosols A, B, or C were incubated with 10 nM ³H-RU 2858, 25 nM ³H-RU 1881 or 5 nM ³H-testosterone and various concentrations of unlabelled competitor (premixed) under different conditions of incubation temperature and time. After incubation, bound labelled steroid (B) was measured by DCC adsorption. The ratio B/B_0, in which B_0 represents the concentration of bound radioligand in the absence of unlabelled steroid, was plotted against the concentration of unlabelled steroid added. The concentration of unlabelled steroid required for a 50% displacement of radioligand from its specific binding sites (after subtraction of non-specific binding) was determined. The ratio of the 50% displacement concentration for radioligand and competitor (multiplied by 100) gives the relative binding affinity (RBA) of the competitor.

Density gradient centrifugation

Cytosol A was incubated with (a) 10 nM ³H-RU 2858 for 18 hours at 0°C in the presence or absence of a 100-fold concentration of unlabelled RU 2858, (b) 10 nM ³H-RU 1881 for 18 hours at 0°C in the presence or absence of a 100-fold concentration of unlabelled RU 1881 and various concentrations of triamcinolone acetonide and (c) 10 nM ³H-RU 5020 for 18 hours at 0°C in the presence or absence of a 100-fold concentration of unlabelled RU 5020. The cytosol was treated with DCC to remove excess free steroid, layered on a sucrose density gradient and centrifuged as described in the figure legends (Beckman Spinco L2 65B centrifuge). The radioactivity of fractions collected from the top of the tubes was measured.

Results

Choice of radioligands for receptor assays

Owing to the known disadvantages of the use of natural hormones as radioligands (specific plasma binding, degradation on incubation with cytosol, and formation of a fast-dissociating receptor complex), labelled synthetic hormones were used to assay receptors. These radioligands do not bind, or bind minimally, to specific plasma proteins and are not degraded on *in vitro* incubation with cytosol [3–5]. Table II gives their hormone specificity as measured in routine screening tests [5, 8] and an indication of the kinetics of their interaction with the different cytosolic hormone receptors [9–11]. The oestrogen RU 2858, unlike estradiol, does not interfere with androgen binding in rat prostate. It binds solely to the oestrogen receptor of mouse uterus with which it forms a much more slowly-dissociating complex than estradiol as shown by the fact that, on changing incubation conditions from 2 hours at 0°C to 5 hours at 25°C, its relative binding affinity (RBA) increases from a value (12) less than that obtained for estradiol to a value (112) greater than the estradiol value. The progestogen RU 5020 competes less than progesterone for binding to the androgen, mineralocorticoid and glucocorticoid receptors in cytosol from rat prostate, kidney and thymus, respectively. It forms a more slowly-dissociating and therefore more stable complex with the progestogen receptor in rabbit uterus than progesterone

Table II Relative binding affinities (RBAs) measured during routine screening.

	ES		PG			AND		MIN		GLU	
	2 hr 0°	5 hr 25°	2 hr 0°	24 hr 0°	30 min 0°	2 hr 0°	24 hr 0°	4 hr 0°	24 hr 0°	4 hr 0°	24 hr 0°
Oestradiol	100	100	2.6 ± 0.9	0.9 ± 0.2	22 ± 2	7.9 ± 1.3	4.5 ± 0.8	0.9 ± 0.2	0.5 ± 0.2	1.1 ± 0.2	0.3 ± 0.03
RU 2858	12 ± 1	112 ± 8	0.7 ± 0.2	0.5 ± 0.1	0.25	<0.1	<0.1	0.1	<0.1	2.1	0.6 ± 0.1
Progesterone	<0.1	—	100	100	21 ± 3	5.5 ± 0.6	1.7 ± 0.3	84	22 ± 6	42 ± 3	17 ± 2
RU 5020	<0.1	—	222 ± 7	533 ± 40	11 ± 1	1.4 ± 0.4	1.9	8	2.5 ± 0.3	22 ± 3	6.5 ± 0.7
Testosterone	<0.1	—	1.2 ± 0.3	1.1 ± 0.3	100	100	100	9 ± 0.5	3.7 ± 1.0	0.9 ± 0.3	0.4 ± 0.2
RU 1881	<0.1	—	208 ± 18	191 ± 28	158 ± 26	203 ± 5	294 ± 26	132	38 ± 5	10	4.1 ± 0.5
Triamcinolone acetonide	<0.1	—	15 ± 4	12 ± 1	0.17	<0.1	—	31	8.0 ± 2.0	141 ± 20	174 ± 5

ES = Oestrogen receptor (mouse uterus), PG = Progestin receptor (rabbit uterus), AND = Androgen receptor (rat prostate), MIN = Mineralocorticoid receptor (rat kidney), GLU = Glucocorticoid receptor (rat thymus).

RBAs were measured as previously described [5] and in the presence of a specific glugocorticoid to assess mineralocorticoid binding in rat kidney [43]. Results are expressed as means ± S.E.M. or as the means of two determinations which differ by 15% or less. The RBA values for the endogenous hormones (oestradiol, progesterone, testosterone, aldosterone) and of the synthetic hormone dexamethasone were taken as equal to 100.

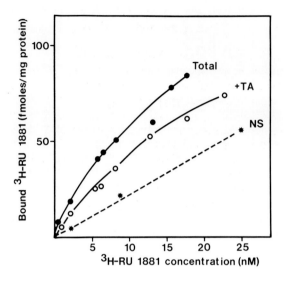

Fig. 1.   *Illustration of the assay of androgen and progestogen-binding sites in human benign hyperplastic prostate. Cytosol B (6.5 mg protein per ml) was incubated with ³H-RU 1881 for 16 hours at 15°C in the absence or presence of a 100-fold excess of triamcinolone acetonide (TA). (NS = non-specific binding).*

since its RBA is 5 times greater than the RBA of progesterone after 24 hours' incubation but only 2 times greater after 2 hours' incubation. The androgen RU 1881 binds markedly to the androgen receptor in rat prostate, the progestogen receptor in rabbit uterus and the mineralocorticoid receptor in rat kidney. From a comparison of RU 1881 RBA data after different incubation times, the androgen receptor complex would appear to be more stable than the progestogen receptor complex and much more stable than the mineralocorticoid receptor complex. RU 1881 can only be used effectively in the presence of an excess of a non-radioactive ligand such as triamcinolone acetonide which does not bind at all to the androgen receptor but which binds sufficiently to the progestogen, mineralocorticoid and glucocorticoid receptors to prevent ³H-RU 1881-binding to these receptors [6–8]. Other authors have suggested that when nuclear and not cytoplasmic RU 1881 binding is measured, only androgen-specific binding is recorded [12, 13].

³H-RU 2858 and ³H-RU 1881 (in the presence of triamcinolone acetonide) can be used effectively to assay cytosolic oestrogen and androgen receptors as previously described [1, 3, 6, 7, 14] and as illustrated by the saturation curves in figure 1 for a BPH specimen. However, the low dilution factor (1/5, w/v) and the relatively high non-specific binding of high specific activity ³H-RU 5020 make it preferable to measure, instead of RU 5020 binding, the sum total of progestogen plus corticoid binding sites. This is given by the difference between the total binding recorded with ³H-RU 1881 (androgen plus progestogen plus corticoid binding sites) and that recorded in the presence of triamcinolone acetonide (androgen binding sites only).

Characterization of oestrogen, androgen and progestogen receptors in human prostate adenocarcinoma cytosol by sucrose density gradient centrifugation

After incubation of cytosol from human prostate adenocarcinomas with ³H-RU 2858, complexes sedimenting in the 4S and 8S regions of a sucrose density gradient were formed (Fig. 2a; swinging bucket technique). These radioactivity peaks were suppressed on addition of excess unlabelled RU 2858. After incubation of cytosol from human prostate adenocarcinomas with ³H-RU 1881, complexes sedimenting in the 4S and 8S regions were also formed (Fig. 2b; swinging bucket technique). These radioactivity peaks were slightly lowered on additon of a 10-fold excess of triamcinolone acetonide and more considerably lowered on addition of a 100-fold excess. However, a 500-fold excess had no further effect. Thus, it would seem that the progestogen and corticoid binding sites present cannot be saturated by a 10-fold excess of triamcinolone acetonide but are saturated by a 100-fold excess. In the presence of a 100-fold excess of triamcinolone acetonide and unlabelled RU 1881 the radioactivity peaks were totally suppressed. After incubation of cytosol from human prostate adenocarcinomas with ³H-

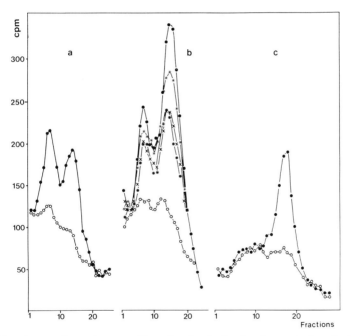

*Fig. 2. Density gradient ultracentrifugation (swinging bucket technique) of ³H-RU 2858-(a), ³H-RU 1881-(b) and ³H-RU 5020-(c) binding to human prostate adenocarcinoma cytosol freed from plasma contamination. Cytosol A was layered (150 μl) on a 5 to 25% linear sucrose gradient which was centrifuged at 50,000 rpm in an SW 60 rotor for 18 hours at 0–4°C. (a) Binding of 10 nM ³H-RU 2858 in the absence (●) or presence (○) of a 500-fold excess of unlabelled RU 2858. (b) Binding of 10 nM ³H-RU 1881 alone (●), in the presence of various concentrations of triamcinolone acetonide (10-fold, *; 100-fold, ×; 500 fold, *) and in the presence of a 100-fold excess of triamcinolone acetonide and unlabelled RU 1881 (○). (c) Binding of 10 nM ³H-RU 5020 in the absence (●) or presence (○) of a 100-fold excess of unlabelled RU 5020. Bovine serum albumin (BSA) sedimented in fractions 7–8.*

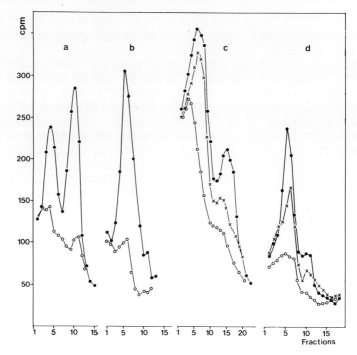

Fig. 3. Density gradient ultracentrifugation (vertical tube technique) of ³H-RU 2858-(a, b) and ³H-RU 1881-(c, d) binding to human prostate adenocarcinoma cytosol freed from plasma contamination. Cytosol A was layered on a 5 to 15% sucrose gradient (2.4 ml) which was centrifuged at 60,000 rpm in an SW 60 rotor for 5 hours at 0–4°C. (a, b) Binding of 10 nM ³H-RU 2858 in the absence (●) or presence (○) of a 500-fold excess of unlabelled RU 2858. (c, d) Binding of 10 nM ³H-RU 1881 alone (●), in the presence of a 100-fold excess of triamcinolone acetonide (✕) and in the presence of a 100-fold excess of triamcinolone acetonide and unlabelled RU 1881 (○). BSA sedimented in fractions 4–5.

RU 5020 a complex sedimenting in the 8S region of a sucrose gradient was formed in the presence (not shown) or absence (Fig. 2c; swinging bucket technique) of a complex in the 4S region. These radioactivity peaks were displaced by an excess of unlabelled RU 5020. When using vertical tube rotor gradient analysis [15] as a time-saving device (Figs 3a-d), 8S radioactivity peaks were obtained for both RU 2858 (Fig. 3a) and RU 1881 (Fig. 3c) binding but resolution was not always as good as with the swinging bucket technique (Figs 3b and 3d).

All these results point to the existence of specific oestrogen, androgen and progestogen receptors in cytosol from human prostate adenocarcinomas. In most cases the 4 S receptor was predominant since it is more stable [16].

Hormone binding specificity in cytosol from human prostate adenocarcinomas and human benign hyperplastic prostates

The hormone specificity of the oestrogen receptor in cytosol from human prostate adenocarcinomas is illustrated in figure 4a, which shows that, under short-time incubation conditions, oestradiol and ethynyl oestradiol compete more markedly for ³H-RU 2858 binding than unlabelled RU 2858 which,

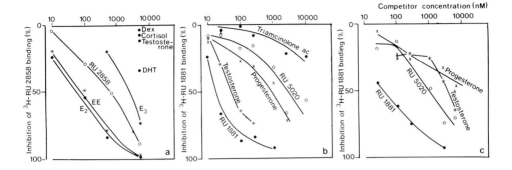

Fig. 4. Competition for ³H-RU 2858-(a) and ³H-RU 1881-(b, c) binding in cytosol from human prostate adenocarcinoma (a, b) and human benign hyperplastic prostate (c). Cytosol A (8 mg protein per ml) was incubated for 4 hours at 0°C with ³H-RU 2858. Cytosols A and B (6.5 mg protein per ml) were incubated for 16 hours at 15°C with ³H-RU 1881 in the presence of increasing concentrations of unlabelled steroids. Bound radioligand was measured by DCC adsorption (E = oestradiol, EE = ethynyl oestradiol, E₃ = oestriol, DHT = androstanolone, Dex = dexamethasone).

however, competes more markedly than oestriol. At a concentration of 5000 nM, androstanolone prevented binding by 35%. Dexamethasone, hydrocortisone and testosterone had virtually no effect at this concentration.

In cytosol from castrated rat prostate reputed to contain no specific progestogen receptor, only androgens but not progestogens compete markedly for ³H-RU 1881 binding [17, 18]. On the other hand, in cytosol from human prostate adenocarcinomas (Fig. 4b) and human benign hyperplastic prostates (Fig. 4c), both androgens and progestogens (e.g., RU 5020) competed for ³H-RU 1881 binding, suggesting the presence of either two distinct receptors (androgen and progestogen) or of a modified androgen receptor.

Relevance of steroid hormone receptors in human prostate cytosol to anti-hormone treatment

Table III summarizes the hormone receptor assay results for patients with prostate adenocarcinoma or hyperplasia who had not undergone any hormone therapy. Of the two normal prostate samples, both contained androgen receptor and neither oestrogen receptor. Of the 19 cranial BPH samples, 15 contained both androgen and progestogen-cum-corticoid receptors. Of the 11 caudal prostate samples, only one contained androgen receptor and none progestogen-cum-corticoid receptor. Of the 3 cranial and 3 caudal BPH samples tested, none contained oestrogen receptor. Nineteen adenocarcinoma specimens were tested for the presence of receptors: 5 contained androgen receptor only, 8 contained both androgen and oestrogen receptors and 4 both androgen and progestogen-cum-corticoid receptors. Only 2 samples did not contain androgen receptors, but contained oestrogen and progestogen-cum-corticoid receptors.

If these receptors identified in human prostate adenocarcinomas are functional and are involved in tumour growth, then anti-hormonal treatment may prove useful. Both steroid and non-steroid anti-androgens (e.g. cyproterone acetate and flutamide) have been tested in this indication and a pos-

Table III Exchange assay results: receptor-positive samples.

Normal prostate (2 specimens)	$E^+ = 0/2$
	$A^+ = 2/2$
Hyperplastic prostate	
— cranial lobe (19 specimens)	$E^+ = 0/3$
	$A^+P^+ = 15/19$
	$A^-P^- = 4/19$
— caudal lobe (11 specimens)	$E^+ = 0/3$
	$A^+P^- = 1/11$
	$A^-P^- = 10/11$
Prostate adenocarcinoma (19 specimens)	$A^+E^-P^- = 5/19$
	$E^+A^+ = 8/19$
	$E^+P^+ = 2/19$
	$A^+P^+ = 4/19$

E^+: oestrogen receptor positive assayed with ^{3}H-RU 2858 (5 hours incubation at 25°C)
A^+: androgen receptor positive assayed with ^{3}H-RU 1881 in the presence of a 100-fold excess of triamcinolone acetonide (16 hours incubation at 15°C)
P^+: progestogen-cum-corticoid receptor positive assayed by difference

sible mechanism for their anti-androgenic action is proposed here. Although it has been known for a long time that steroid anti-androgens can compete effectively for binding to the androgen receptor, the action of non-steroid anti-androgens has remained rather obscure since only high concentrations of these compounds or of their active metabolites are able to compete. Recently, however, it has been shown that by reducing incubation time, marked competition can occur, as illustrated by the results in figure 5 and Table IV. On the basis of these results it is in fact suggested that, as in the case of certain steroid and non-steroid anti-oestrogens, a very fleeting complex is formed with the cytosolic receptor [10, 11, 19, 20]. The values of the RBAs at short-incubation times (30 minutes) suggest that the association between non-steroid anti-androgen and receptor is fast. Higher RBAs have been obtained after even shorter incubation times (unpublished data). The RBAs after longer incubation times (2 or 24 hours) suggest that, in the absence of degradation, the complex formed dissociates extremely rapidly compared to the dissociation rate of the endogenous hormone receptor complex.

Several progestogens, in particular megestrol acetate and chlormadinone acetate, have also been used in the treatment of hormone-dependent prostatic disorders. As shown in Table IV these compounds are also able to compete for androgen receptor binding after short incubation times to an extent which is comparable to the competition of the steroid anti-androgens RU 2956 and cyproterone acetate. Furthermore, their RBAs decrease similarly with incubation time suggesting that they might also be potent anti-androgens. The kinetics of the androgen receptor binding of the progestogen RU 5020, also a pregnane derivative, were, on the other hand, similar to those of the nonsteroid anti-androgens, hydroxyflutamide and RU 23908. In contrast, the estrane progestogens, norethisterone and, in particular,

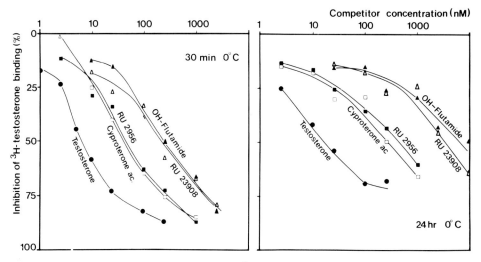

Fig. 5. Competition by anti-androgens for ³H-testosterone-binding in castrated rat ventral prostate cytosol after incubation for 30 minutes at 0°C (a) and 24 hours at 0°C (b). Bound radioligand was measured by DCC adsorption.

Table IV Relative binding affinities for the cytosolic androgen receptor in rat prostate.

	30 minutes 0°C	2 hours 0°C	24 hours 0°C
RU 1881	158 ± 26	203 ± 5	294 ± 26
Androstanolone	94 ± 10	120 ± 3	180 ± 39
Testosterone	100	100	100
RU 2956	55 ± 13	14 ± 2	3.6 ± 0.5
Cyproterone acetate	51	16 ± 1	5.4
Hydroxyflutamide	8.2	1.1	0.2
RU 23908	9.1	1.1	0.4
RU 5020	11 ± 1	1.4 ± 0.4	1.9
Progesterone	21 ± 3	5.5 ± 0.6	1.7 ± 0.3
Megestrol acetate	67 ± 15	19 ± 4	7.9 ± 1.2
Chlormadinone acetate	81 ± 20	20 ± 4	14 ± 3
Norethisterone	76 ± 12	43 ± 3	26
Norgestrel	110 ± 23	87 ± 23	73 ± 20

Mean ± SEM or means of two determinations differing by less than 15%.

norgestrel, competed effectively for androgen-receptor binding even after 24 hours incubation, thus explaining their known androgenic side-effects.

Discussion

It is now well-accepted that synthetic radioligands can be advantageously used to detect, study and assay steroid hormone receptors in normal and pathological human tissues. We have shown in the present study that RU 2858 and RU 5020 form more stable, i.e., more slowly-dissociating, complexes with the cytosolic oestrogen and progestogen receptors, respectively, than the endogenous hormones and that the specificity of their binding, as regards hormone class, equals if not betters that of the endogenous hormones in routine screening tests. RU 1881 binds to the androgen, progestogen and mineralocorticoid cytosolic receptors. However, the androgen binding is the most stable and, according to previous reports [12, 13], nuclear RU 1881 binding has predominantly androgen specificity. In cytosol, interference of RU 1881 progestogen and mineralocorticoid binding can be reduced by addition of an excess of triamcinolone acetonide which does not compete for androgen binding but competes for progestogen and corticoid binding [6–8]. These specificity studies have been performed under conditions minimizing secondary tissue binding [5, 8] but specificity profiles nevertheless depend upon tissue and also upon incubation conditions. Thus, RU 5020 competes more than progesterone for glucocorticoid binding in the rat liver [1, 5, 8] but less than progesterone in the rat thymus. In both cases, however, the RU 5020 glucocorticoid binding is less stable than the progestogen binding and, consequently, assays with RU 5020 in these or other tissues should use long incubation times to maximize progestogen binding and minimize glucocorticoid binding. Similar long incubation times favour the androgen binding of RU 1881. Differences in specificity according to tissue could be due to differences in plasma contamination but all three radioligands (RU 2858, RU 5020 and RU 1881) bind minimally to specific plasma proteins under our assay conditions [1, 3–5]. Moreover, none are degraded on *in vitro* incubation with cytosol under these conditions [4]. In the above studies, on account of the high protein content (low dilution factor) of the cytosols and of the low receptor concentrations present, progestogen binding was not assayed with labelled RU 5020 which has relatively high nonspecific binding [1, 4, 5] but by the difference in RU 1881 binding in the presence or absence of triamcinolone acetonide. This difference represents progestogen, mineralocorticoid and glucocorticoid binding and is referred to here as 'progestogen-cum-corticoid' binding.

The presence of an androgen receptor in the human prostate was first established using labelled androstanolone or testosterone and techniques attempting to distinguish tissue binding from interfering plasma binding [21–23]. The majority of recent studies have used RU 1881. Androgen receptors have been detected with this radioligand in rat prostate, in human prostate, whether normal, hyperplastic or adenocarcinomatous [12, 13, 17, 18, 24–31], and in dog prostate [32], a convenient animal model for the study of prostate disorders and anti-androgen treatment. The systematic detection and evaluation of other receptors has received less attention, although the lack of RU 1881 specificity has led to the demonstration of the prevalence of a progestogen or progestogen-like receptor in human BPH and adenocarcinoma. In our study, the presence of progestogen-cum-corticoid binding was very frequent in BPH (15 out of 19 samples) but much less so in adenocarcinomas (6 out of 19 samples) and, like androgen binding, was found only in the cranial prostatic lobe of BPH patients. According to several specificity studies, this binding has the characteristics of uterine progestogen binding and is, therefore, taken to be a true progestogen-like binding rather than modified androgen binding. Whether its appearance is directly linked to ageing and hyperplasia is a point which requires further study in a larger number of patients, preferably using a microassay technique as already described for the measurement of the androgen receptor [31].

The prevalence of oestrogen receptor in human prostate is rather more controversial. By the use of RU 2858 which eliminates the problems of specific plasma binding encountered in earlier studies with oestradiol [33 -35], we have detected oestrogen receptor in 10 out of 19 adenocarcinomas always, however, in association with androgen and/or progestogen-cum-corticoid receptor, but none in the 3 BPH samples tested. Recently other teams have also detected oestrogen receptor using RU 2858. In particular, Bashirelahi *et al.* [36] have confirmed their earlier observations with oestradiol on human prostate [35], and Pertshuk *et al.* [28] have shown the presence of oestrogen receptor in both BPH and adenocarcinoma samples using a fluorescence technique. On the other hand, Ekman *et al.* [30] did not detect oestrogen receptor in cancer patients previously treated with oestrogen derivatives and, in agreement with our results, Emmott *et al.* [37] found no oestrogen receptor in BPH patients.

In breast cancer, the first criterion of responsiveness to hormone therapy was the presence of oestrogen receptor. To improve the prognostic this was followed by the parallel measurement of progestogen receptor [1], since in most target tissues oestrogen administration increases the number of available progestogen-binding sites; the presence of progestogen receptor above a certain basal level would be an indicator of a functional oestrogen receptor and consequently of the pertinence of hormone therapy, e.g. of anti-oestrogen therapy. In the ageing male, plasma testosterone levels are reduced whereas oestrogen levels increase. If oestrogens increase the number of progestogen binding sites in the prostate, one would expect to find oestrogen receptors in the majority of samples containing progestogen receptor. However, none of the 3 BPH samples and only 2 of the 6 adenocarcinoma samples containing progestogen receptor also contained oestrogen receptor, implying impaired hormonal regulation. A thorough study of progestogen receptor induction in the prostate and more assay data are required in order to reach a conclusion. Furthermore, a distinction between receptors in the stroma and epithelium might shed even more light since, according to a report [24], the progestogen-like receptor binding of RU 1881 is a feature of the prostatic stroma rather than of the epithelium.

A recent study on the hyperplastic dog prostate [38] which contains oestrogen receptor has shown that oestradiol can be involved in the regulation of the activity of the cytoplasmic androgen receptor. Although we did not detect any oestrogen receptor in the 3 human BPH samples tested a relationship may exist between oestrogen and androgen receptors in human prostate adenocarcinoma since 8 of the 17 samples containing androgen receptor also contained oestrogen receptor. At least two recent studies [39, 40] have attempted to correlate, with some success, the duration of hormonal response in men with prostatic cancer with cytoplasmic or nuclear androgen receptor content. If this androgen receptor is under oestrogen control a correlation with oestrogen-receptor content may prove as fruitful if not more so. Furthermore, as in breast cancer, this oestrogen receptor could then be the target of anti-hormone therapy.

Available hormone therapy for prostate cancer consists of compounds classified as oestrogens, progestogens or anti-androgens. BPH has been treated with large doses of progestogens. However, until more is known about the aetiology of these diseases, in particular about their hormone dependence, the choice of treatment will remain empirical and patients who do not respond to one form of hormone therapy may yet respond to another. Furthermore, much remains to be understood about the possible mechanisms of action of the hormones used. In the present study, we have shown that nonsteroid anti-androgens currently tested in the treatment of prostate cancer (e.g. flutamide) are able to compete effectively for androgen receptor binding, just as steroid anti-androgens (e.g. cyproterone acetate and RU 2956) do, as long as incubation times are kept short. They bind strongly after very short incubation times, but only weakly after longer incubation times, thus indicating that, in the absence of *in vitro* degradation, they associate fast with the receptor to form a short-lived complex unable to induce a full biological response [11, 19, 20]. By occupying the available binding sites they furthermore prevent the endogenous hormone from inducing its response, thus giving rise to the anti-hormonal effect [10] which may account for their relative therapeutic efficacy. This mechanism is similar to that already described for steroid and non-steroid anti-oestrogens [10, 11, 41]. The main progestogens used in the treatment of hormone-responsive prostate disorders are megestrol acetate and chlormadinone acetate which, like other pregnane derivatives (e.g. RU 5020) but unlike androstane progestogens (e.g. norethisterone and norgestrel), have virtually no androgenic activity as indicated by their low androgen-receptor binding after 2 hours incubation and by their inability to stimulate prostate growth in the castrated rat and to inhibit luteinizing hormone (LH)-induced luteinizing hormone-releasing hormone (LHRH) release in rat anterior pituitary cells in culture [8, 42, 43]. On the other hand, these pregnane progestogens can, under certain circumstances, act as anti-androgens [44, 45] perhaps because they can compete effectively for androgen-receptor binding after short incubation times. According to the binding data given above, the kinetics of the androgen-receptor binding of the 'progestogens' megestrol acetate and chlormadinone acetate and of the steroid 'anti-androgens' cyproterone acetate and RU 2956 are highly similar, as are the kinetics of the progestogen RU 5020 and of the non-steroid 'anti-androgens', hydroxyflutamide and RU 23908. Furthermore, these pregnane progestogens are potent anti-oestrogens as indicated by their inhibition of oestradiol-induced increase in uterine weight in the mouse [43] and of replenishment of cytoplasmic oestrogen receptor in the mouse uterus [10, 46]. Thus in the treatment of prostate cancer, or even BPH, they may interfere with the androgen receptor, with the oestrogen receptor or even with the progestogen-like receptor brought into evidence by the use of RU 1881. Whether this receptor has the characteristics of a true progestogen receptor (e.g. whether it can be induced by oestrogens and translocated into the nucleus) remains to be proved.

Finally, as regards treatment by oestrogen derivatives such as estramustine phosphate, the reader is referred to other articles in this volume.

In spite of the potential benefits of hormone therapy, it should not be forgotten that steroid-hormone receptors are present in all target tissues, albeit to different extents, and that anti-hormones interfere, consequently, not only with binding to peripheral but also to central receptors. Thus the anti-androgens flutamide and RU 23908 in the treatment of prostate cancer lead by gonadotrophin stimulation to increased endogenous androgen secretion which counteracts the peripheral anti-androgen effect [20, 47]. The additional partial suppression of pituitary function is thus necessary to obtain a full peripheral anti-hormonal effect.

Acknowledgments

We are extremely grateful to Professor J. Ducassou and Dr. G. Serment of the Department of Urology of the Hôtel Dieu, Marseilles, for supplying samples of human prostate. The competent technical assistance of A. M. Tremblet is gratefully acknowledged.

References

1. McGuire, W. L., Raynaud, J. P. and Baulieu, E. E. (Eds.) (1977): Progesterone Receptors in Normal and Neoplastic Tissues. *Prog. Cancer Res. Ther.*, Vol. IV. Raven Press, New York.
2. Byar, D. P., Sears, M. E. and McGuire, W. L. (1979): Relationship between estrogen receptor values and clinical data in predicting the response to endocrine therapy for patients with advanced breast cancer. *Eur. J. Cancer, 15,* 299.
3. Raynaud, J. P., Martin, P. M., Bouton, M. M. and Ojasoo, T. (1978): 11β-Methoxy-17-ethynyl-1,3,5(10)-estratriene-3,17β-diol (Moxestrol), a tag for estrogen receptor-binding sites in human tissues. *Cancer Res., 38,* 3044.
4. Raynaud, J. P., Ojasoo, T. and Vaché, V. (1979): Unusual steroids in measuring steroid receptors. In: *Steroid Receptors and the Management of Cancer.* Editors: E. B. Thompson and M. E. Lippman. CRC Press, Cleveland.
5. Ojasoo, T. and Raynaud, J. P. (1978): Unique steroid congeners for receptor studies. *Cancer Res., 38,* 4186.
6. Zava, D. T., Landrum, B., Horwitz, K. B. and McGuire, W. L. (1979): Androgen receptor assay with (3H)methyltrienolone (R 1881) in the presence of progesterone receptors. *Endocrinology, 104,* 1007.
7. Asselin, J., Melançon, R. Gourdeau, T., Labrie, F., Bonne, C. and Raynaud, J. P. (1979): Specific binding of 3H-methyltrienolone to both progestin and androgen binding components in human benign prostatic hypertrophy (BPH). *J. Steroid Biochem., 10,* 483.
8. Raynaud, J. P., Ojasoo, T., Bouton, M. M. and Philibert, D. (1979): Receptor binding as a tool in the development of new bioactive steroids. In: *Drug Design*, Vol. VIII, p. 169. Editor: E. J. Ariens. Academic Press, New York.
9. Bouton, M. M. and Raynaud, J. P. (1978): The relevance of kinetic parameters in the determination of specific binding to the estrogen receptor. *J. Steroid Biochem., 9,* 9.
10. Raynaud, J. P. (1978): The mechanism of action of anti-hormones. In: *Advances in Pharmacology and Therapeutics*, Vol. I, Receptors, p. 259. Editor: J. Jacob. Pergamon Press, Oxford.
11. Bouton, M. M., Bonne, C. and Raynaud, J. P. (1978): 'In vitro' screening for anti-hormones. *J. Steroid Biochem., 9,* 836.
12. Menon, M., Tananis, C. E., Hicks, L. L., Hawkins, E. F., McLoughlin, M. G. and Walsh, P. C. (1978): Characterization of the binding of a potent synthetic androgen, methyltrienolone, to human tissues. *J. Clin. Invest., 61,* 150.
13. Shain, S. A. and Boesel, R. W. (1978): Human prostate steroid hormone receptor quantitation. Current methodology and possible utility as a clinical discriminant in carcinoma. *Invest. Urol., 16,* 169.
14. Bonne, C. and Raynaud, J. P. (1976): Assay of androgen binding sites by exchange with methyltrienolone (R 1881). *Steroids, 27,* 497.
15. Jordan, V. C. and Prestwich, G. (1977): Binding of (3H)tamoxifen in rat uterine cytosols: a comparison of swinging bucket and vertical tube rotor sucrose density gradient analysis. *Mol. Cell. Endocrinol., 8,* 179.
16. Namkung, P. C., Moe, R. E. and Petra, P. H. (1979): Stability of estrogen receptors in frozen human breast tumor tissue. *Cancer Res., 39,* 1124.
17. Asselin, J., Labrie, F., Gourdeau, Y., Bonne, C. and Raynaud, J. P. (1976): Binding of (3H)methyltrienolone (R 1881) in rat prostate and human benign prostatic hypertrophy (BPH). *Steroids, 28,* 449.

18. Dubé, J. Y., Chapdelaine, P., Tremblay, R. R., Bonne, C. and Raynaud, J. P. (1976): Comparative binding specificity of methyltrienolone in human and rat prostate. *Horm. Res., 7,* 341.
19. Raynaud, J. P., Bonne, C. and Lagacé, L. (1978): On the mechanism of action of non-steroidal anti-androgens. *Endocrinology, Suppl. 102,* 304.
20. Raynaud, J. P., Bonne, C., Bouton, M. M., Kelly, P. and Lagacé, L. (1979): Action of a non-steroid anti-androgen, RU 23908, in peripheral and central tissues. *J. Steroid Biochem., 11,* 93.
21. Geller, J., Cantor, T. and Albert, J. (1975): Evidence for a specific dihydrotestosterone-binding cytosol receptor in the human prostate. *J. Clin. Endocrinol. Metab., 41,* 854.
22. Hansson, V., Tveter, K. J., Attramadal, A. and Torgersen, O. (1971): Androgenic receptors in human benign nodular prostatic hyperplasia. *Acta Endocrinol. (Copenhagen), 68,* 79.
23. Mainwaring, W. I. P. and Milroy, E. J. G. (1973): Characterization of the specific androgen receptors in the human prostate gland. *J. Endocrinol., 57,* 371.
24. Cowan, R. A., Cowan, S. K. and Grant, J. K. (1977): Binding of methyltrienolone (R 1881) to a progesterone receptor-like component of human prostatic cytosol. *J. Endocrinol., 74,* 281.
25. Walsh, P. C., Greco, J. M., Tananis, C. E., Hicks, L. L., McLoughlin, M. G. and Menon, M. (1977): The binding of a potent synthetic androgen methyltrienolone (R1881) to cytosol preparations of human prostatic cancer. *Trans. Am. Assoc. Genito-urinary Surgeons, 69.*
26. Snochowski, M., Pousette, Å., Ekman, P., Bression, D., Andersson, L., Högberg, B. and Gustafsson, J. Å. (1977): Characterization and measurement of the androgen receptor in human benign prostatic hyperplasia and prostatic carcinoma. *J. Clin. Endocrinol. Metab., 45,* 920.
27. Gustafsson, J. Å., Ekman, P., Pousette, Å., Snochowski, M. and Högberg, B. (1978): Demonstration of progestin receptor in human benign prostatic hyperplasia and prostatic carcinoma. *Invest. Urol., 15,* 361.
28. Pertshuk, L. P., Zava, D. T., Gaetjens, E., Macchia, R. J., Brigati, D. J. and Kim, D. S. (1978): Detection of androgen and estrogen receptors in human prostatic carcinoma and hyperplasia by fluorescence microscopy. *Res. Commun. Chem. Pathol. Pharmacol., 22,* 427.
29. Sirett, D. A. N. and Grant, J. K. (1978): Androgen binding in cytosols and nuclei of human benign hyperplastic prostate tissue. *J. Endocrinol., 77,* 101.
30. Ekman, P., Snochowski, M., Dahlberg, E. and Gustafsson, J. Å. (1979): Steroid receptors in metastatic carcinoma of the human prostate. *Eur. J. Cancer, 15,* 257.
31. Hicks, L. L. and Walsh, P. C. (1979): A microassay for the measurement of androgen receptors in human prostatic tissue. *Steroids, 33,* 389.
32. Shain, S. A. and Boesel, R. W. (1978): Androgen receptor content of the normal and hyperplastic canine prostate. *J. Clin. Invest., 61,* 654.
33. Fraser, H. M., Mitchell, A. J. H., Anderson, C. K. and Oakey, R. E. (1974): The interaction of dihydrotestosterone and oestradiol-17 with macromolecules in human hyperplastic prostate tissue. *Acta Endocrinol. (Copenhagen), 76,* 773.
34. Hawkins, E. F., Nijs, M., Brassinne, C. and Tagnon, H. J. (1975): Steroid receptors in the human prostate. 1. Estradiol-17 binding in benign prostatic hypertrophy. *Steroids, 26,* 458.
35. Bashirelahi, N., O'Toole, J. H. and Young, J. D. (1976): A specific 17-estradiol receptor in human benign hypertrophic prostate. *Biochem. Med., 15,* 254.
36. Bashirelahi, N., Kneussl, E. S. and Young, J. D., (1978): Androgen and estrogen receptors in human prostate. In: *Abstracts, 60th Annual Endocrine Society Meeting,* p. 297, no. 444.
37. Emmott, R. C., Murphy, J. B., Hicks, L. L. and Walsh, P. C. (1979): Estrogen receptors in human benign prostatic hyperplasia (BPH). In: *Abstracts, Meeting of the American Urological Association, New York.*
38. Moore, R. J., Gazak, J. M. and Wilson, J. D. (1979): Regulation of cytoplasmic

dihydrotestosterone binding in dog prostate by 17-estradiol. *J. Clin. Invest., 63,* 351.

39. Gustafsson, J. Å., Ekman, P., Snochowski, M., Zetterberg, A., Pousette, Å. and Högberg, B. (1978): Correlation between clinical response to hormone therapy and steroid receptor content in prostatic cancer. *Cancer Res., 38,* 4345.
40. Walsh, P. C., Hicks, L. L., Reiner, W. G. and Trachtenberg, J. (1979): The use of androgen receptors to predict the duration of hormonal response in prostatic cancer. In: *Abstracts, Meeting of the American Urological Association, New York.*
41. Nicholson, R. I., Syne, J. S., Daniel, C. P. and Griffiths, K. (1979): The binding of tamoxifen to estrogen receptor proteins under equilibrium and non-equilibrium conditions. *Eur. J. Cancer, 15,* 317.
42. Labrie, F., Ferland, L., Lagacé, L., Drouin, J., Asselin, J., Azadian-Boulanger, G. and Raynaud, J. P. (1977): High inhibitory activity of R 5020, a pure progestin, at the hypothalamo-adenohypophyseal level on gonadotropin secretion. *Fertil. Steril., 28,* 1104.
43. Raynaud, J. P., Bouton, M. M., Moguilewsky, M., Ojasoo, T., Philibert, D., Beck, G., Labrie, F. and Mornon, J. P. (1980): Steroid hormone receptors and pharmacology. *J. Steroid Biochem., 12,* 143.
44. Mowszowicz, I., Bieber, D. E., Chung, K. W., Bullock, L. P. and Bardin, C. W. (1974): Synandrogenic and antiandrogenic effect of progestins: Comparison with nonprogestational antiandrogens. *Endocrinology, 95,* 1589.
45. Bullock, L. P. and Bardin, C. W. (1977): Androgenic, synandrogenic, and antiandrogenic actions of progestins. *Ann. N.Y. Acad. Sci., 286,* 321.
46. Bouton, M. M., Martin, P. M. and Raynaud, J. P. (1979): The anti-estrogenic activity of progestins. *Cancer Treat. Rep., 63,* 1151.
47. Neri, R. O. (1977): Studies on the biology and mechanism of action of nonsteroidal antiandrogens. In: *Androgens and Antiandrogens,* p. 179. Editors: L. Martini and M. Motta. Raven Press, New York.

Discussion

F. Rommerts (Rotterdam, The Netherlands): What is known about effects of antiandrogens on aromatase enzyme systems?

J.-P. Raynaud: To my knowledge very little is known about the effects of anti-androgens on aromatase enzyme systems. According to Schwarzel *et al.* (*Endocrinology,* 1973, *92,* 866), cyproterone would seem to have a weak effect on aromatization.

P. Ekman (Stockholm, Sweden): Is it true that you can only store the specimens for two weeks without losing considerable amount of receptor? According to our experiments we can store the specimens for at least six months in −70°C without loss of receptor content.

J.-P. Raynaud: Receptor content seems to depend upon the conditions of storage. According to data we published in 1977 (*Prog. Cancer Res. Therap., 4)* on oestrogen- and progestogen-receptor activity in human breast tumours, less than 50% of progestogen binding is recovered after 2 months storage of tissue samples at −40°C and about 80% after 2 months storage in liquid nitrogen. Upon storage of cytosol, degradation was even greater and depended upon the homogenization buffer. Similar degradation has been observed with prostate tissue receptors.

Studies on the effects of various anti-androgenic substances on the human prostate in vitro

E. K. Symes and E. Milroy
Courtauld Institute of Biochemistry and Department of Urology, The Middlesex Hospital, London, United Kingdom

Introduction

The development of compounds that specifically inhibit abnormal growth of the prostate would be of value in the clinical management of carcinoma and benign hyperplasia of the prostate. As normal growth of the prostate is under the control of androgens attention has focused on compounds (anti-androgens) that interfere with the cellular hormonal response mechanism.

The testing of possibly useful compounds presents some problems as there are no particularly appropriate animal models [1]. In most species, though not the dog, tumours of the prostate rarely arise spontaneously. However, not only does the pathology of the dog tumour differ considerably from the human but so also does the biochemical mechanism [2]. To circumvent this problem we have been examining the effects of anti-androgens on the human prostate *in vitro* using benign hyperplastic material.

Oestrogenic compounds, particularly diethylstilboestrol, have been widely used in the treatment of carcinoma of the prostate. Our studies have included an investigation of the cellular effects of some oestrogen agonists and antagonists.

Materials and methods

Chemicals

(^{14}C)-androstanolone (> 50 mCi/mM) and (1,2,6,7^{3}H)-testosterone (80–105 Ci/mM) were purchased from the Radiochemical Centre, Amersham, Bucks, U.K. Non-radioactive steroids were supplied by Steraloids Ltd., Croydon, U.K. Tamoxifen was generously donated by Dr. J. Patterson, Imperial Chemical Industries, Pharmaceuticals Division, Alderley Park, Cheshire, U.K., cyproterone acetate by Schering Pharmaceuticals, Burgess Hill, Sussex, U.K., and flutamide and hydroxyflutamide by Dr. R. Neri, Schering Corporation, U.S.A. All other chemicals were of the highest available purity.

Nuclear uptake of androgen

The method has already been published in detail [3]. In brief, 0.5 mm slices of tissue were incubated in Krebs-Ringer bicarbonate buffer containing ^{3}H-testosterone (1.5 × 10^{-9} M) and, where appropriate, unlabelled steroids. After incubation for 90 minutes at 37°C the tissue slices (1.5–2.0 g) were washed and then frozen at −70°C. Subsequently the nuclei were prepared from these tissue specimens and purified. The purity of the nuclear preparations was determined by light microscopy and comparison of the optical density at 260 and 280 nm (= m × 10^{-9}). Any samples contaminated with cytoplasm were discarded. Steroids were extracted from the nuclei and total radioactivity determined.

Characterisation of nuclear radioactivity

Where appropriate steroids were separated by paper chromatography in a Bush A system [4]. In excess of 80% of total radioactivity was found in association with testosterone or androstanolone in all studies. ^{14}C-Androstanolone was added prior to extraction of steroids from nuclei to allow correction for procedural losses.

5α-reductase

A post nuclear supernatant was prepared. Fresh tissue was cut into small pieces and tris buffer pH 7.0 (0.01 M) containing EDTA (5 × 10^{-5} M), MgCl$_2$ (5 × 10^{-3} M), β-mercaptoethanol (0.5 × 10^{-3} M) and NaCl (0.05 M) was added (1 : 5 w/v). The tissue was homogenized using a motor driven Silverson homogenizer. The homogenate was centrifuged at 100 g for 10 minutes and the supernatant used as a source of enzyme.

The enzyme was assayed in tris buffer containing ^{3}H-testosterone as substrate, and a reduced NADPH generating system. The optimized assay conditions were as follows: ^{3}H-testosterone (100 Ci/mM) 2.7 × 10^{-9} M, glucose-6-phosphate 10^{-3} M, glucose-6-phosphate dehydrogenase 10^{-6} g/ml, NADPH$^+$ 10^{-4} M, 0.5 ml of 100 g supernatant (equivalent to 100 mg of tissue), tris buffer to 2.5 ml final volume. Incubation was carried out at 37°C for 8 minutes. The reaction was stopped by the addition of absolute ethanol (2 volumes). 50 μg of both authentic testosterone and androstanolone and 5 × 10^3 disintegrations per minute (dpm) of (^{14}C)-androstanolone were added. After removal of ethanol by evaporation steroids were extracted into chloroform (2 × 2 volumes). The combined extracts were dried and the product androstanolone was separated by paper chromatography in a Bush A system. The area corresponding to androstanolone was identified by staining a narrow band at the edge of the chromatogram with Zimmerman reagent (0.5% metadinitrobenzene: benzyltrimethylammonium hydroxide, 2 : 1 v/v). Androstanolone was eluted from the chromatogram, dried, and the radioactivity determined. The ^{14}C counts were used to correct for procedural losses.

Results

The uptake of radioactivity into the nucleus after incubation *in vitro* has

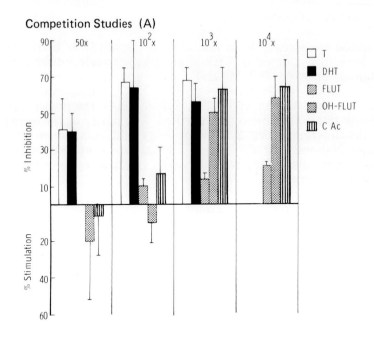

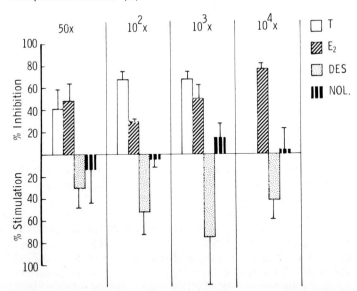

Fig. 1. Competition Studies: nuclear counts were determined from incubations in the presence of ^{3}H-testosterone and increasing concentrations of cold competitors. Mean and standard error of mean plotted. Percentage inhibition or stimulation = 100 × (counts/ minute (cpm)/mg deoxyribonucleicacid (DNA) in presence of ^{3}H-testosterone alone) − (cpm/mg DNA in presence of ^{3}H testosterone + competitor)/(cpm/mg DNA in presence of ^{3}H-testosterone alone). T = testosterone; DHT = androstanolone; FLUT = flutamide; OH-FLUT = hydroxyflutamide; C Ac = cyproterone acetate; E_2 = 17β-oestradiol; DES = diethylstilboestrol; NOL = tamoxifen.

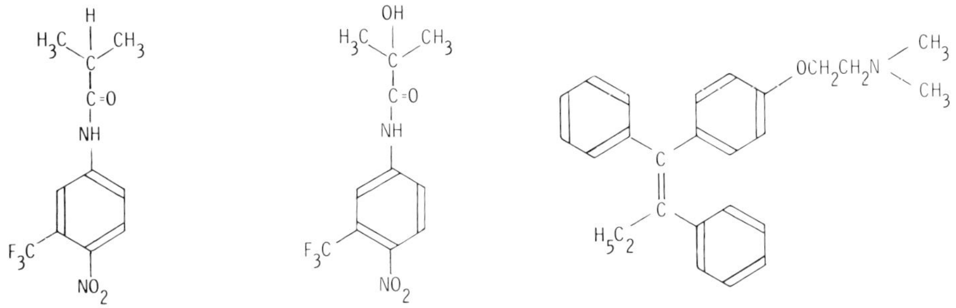

FLUTAMIDE
(SCH 13521)

HYDROXY-FLUTAMIDE

TAMOXIFEN
(IcI 46,474)

Fig. 2.

already been shown by us to reflect the expected underlying biochemical mechanism [3]. The major steroid detected in the nucleus after incubation in the presence of testosterone is androstanolone and the observed steroid specificity is consistent with an androgen receptor protein-mediated process. The results displayed in figure 1A show that the anti-androgen cyproterone acetate competes in this system although with less affinity than the natural androgens. The nonsteroidal anti-androgen flutamide does not compete but a metabolite, hydroxyflutamide, does.

The action of oestradiol, diethylstilboestrol and an oestrogen antagonist, taxomifen, has been studied. Each compound behaved very differently (figure 1B). Oestradiol competed actively in the system, diethylstilboestrol caused enhancement of uptake while tamoxifen had no effect. The chemical structures of the compounds examined are shown in figure 2.

Alterations in the metabolism of testosterone, particularly its conversion to androstanolone, could affect tissue response. For instance it has been reported that oestradiol produces some inhibition of the enzyme 5α-reductase [5]. The origins of the counts in the nucleus were examined after incubation in the presence of flutamide and diethylstilboestrol. No significant decrease in the ratio of androstanolone to testosterone could be detected (Table). Further confirmation that diethylstilboestrol is unlikely to affect testosterone metabolism was obtained from an independent analysis of the effect of diethylstilboestrol on 5α-reductase. As shown in figure 3 diethylstilboestrol behaved very similarly to oestradiol, inhibiting the enzyme only at very high concentrations.

The 5α-reductase assay conditions were based on those published by Bruchovsky and Wilson [6]. A post nuclear supernatant was used as source of the enzyme. Although it is known that 5α-reductase is located in both nuclear and microsomal fractions the total homogenate contained large fibrous lumps that made reproducible aliquots difficult to obtain. Since both the nuclear and microsomal enzymes have similar properties and sufficient activity was associated with the supernatant the procedure was acceptable. The Michaelis constant (Km) of the enzyme was approximately 1.5×10^{-8} M. The inhibitory constant (Ki) for diethylstilboestrol was estimated at 10^{-5} M.

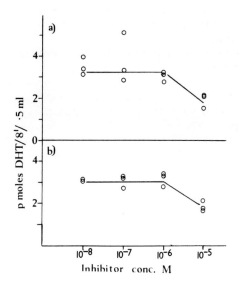

Fig. 3.   *Effect of increasing concentrations of (a) diethylstilboestrol and (b) oestradiol on 5α-reductase activity.*

Table   *Total nuclear counts from incubations in the presence of various concentrations of diethylstilboestrol and flutamide were analysed by paper chromatography. The ratio of counts associated with androstanolone: those associated with testosterone is quoted. More than 80% of counts were associated with testosterone and androstanolone, in all cases.*

Test substances and concentrations	Androstanolone/testosterone ratio	
	First experiment	Second experiment
Diethylstilboestrol		
10^{-7} M	4.78	—
10^{-6} M	1.72	3.02
10^{-5} M	1.06	1.63
Flutamide		
10^{-5} M	5.3	—
None	2.08	1.55

Discussion

The biochemical events involved in the growth response of the prostate to testosterone are thought to be:

1) initial hormonal uptake;
2) conversion of testosterone to androstanolone;
3) binding to cytoplasmic receptor protein;
4) activation and translocation to the nucleus;
5) interactions in the nucleus leading ultimately to growth and division.

The test system we have developed encompasses the first few steps in this series of events, thus interference by possible anti-androgens at any of these stages may be detected.

Our initial studies were concerned with the cellular action of the known anti-androgens cyproterone acetate and flutamide. Cyproterone acetate competed for uptake, a result consistent with its known affinity for the androgen receptor. Flutamide, however, did not compete for uptake nor did it affect the metabolism of testosterone. Discrepancy between the *in vivo* and *in vitro* action has been reported before [5] and it is believed that flutamide is converted to an active metabolite *in vivo* [7]. The metabolite we have studied, hydroxyflutamide, competes for uptake.

Manipulation of the hormonal environment is a common approach to the treatment of carcinoma of the prostate. The most widely used agent is diethylstilboestrol. Like oestradiol, this compound inhibits the pituitary gonadal axis resulting in suppression of testosterone production. Some authorities [8, 9] feel that there may be local effects of diethylstilboestrol on the prostate tumour cells which might justify administering a higher dose than that required to suppress testosterone secretion [10]. We have studied the *in vitro* effects of diethylstilboestrol. Unlike oestradiol, which competes for nuclear uptake, diethylstilboestrol showed a significant enhancement of uptake. The action of oestradiol is consistent with its observed affinity for the androgen receptor [11, 12]. The stimulant effect observed with diethyl-stilboestrol is presumably related to an increase in available hormone for translocation to the nucleus. Three possible mechanisms that could account for this phenomenon are 1) activation of 5α-reductase, 2) inhibition of hy-droxysteroid dehydrogenases, 3) displacement from other binding sites. Our results indicate that diethylstilboestrol affects 5α-reductase only at very high concentrations and that this effect is inhibitory. The possibility of displace-ment from other sites is of interest particularly in view of the reports of large quantities of a low affinity binding protein in rat ventral prostate [13].

Our data demonstrate that very high concentrations of diethylstilboestrol are necessary to produce significant reduction in 5α-reductase activity. The administration of at least 2 g/day of diethylstilboestrol would be required to reach these concentrations, assuming complete absorption and similar clearance [14]. In practice, less than 10% of orally administered diethyl-stilboestrol is absorbed [15]. Large doses would be unacceptable because of the inevitable cardiovascular complications and liver toxicity. We can dem-onstrate no local effect on androgen response systems that would justify an increase in the dose of diethylstilboestrol above that required to suppress testosterone production.

It has recently been suggested that tamoxifen, used with considerable success in the treatment of carcinoma of the breast [16], might be a useful agent in the treatment of prostatic carcinoma but unless this compound in-terfered with cellular androgen response mechanism it would not be possible to envisage a favourable effect in suppressing prostatic growth. We have not been able to demonstrate any effect of tamoxifen on the nuclear uptake of androgen in human benign prostatic hyperplastic material *in vitro*.

Acknowledgement

Part of this work was carried out with the help of grant Biochem. 46 from the Cancer Research Campaign.

References

1. Mainwaring, W. I. P. (1976): In: *Steroid Hormone Action and Cancer*, p. 152. Editors: K. M. J. Menon and J. R. Reel. Plenum Publishing Corp., New York.
2. Evans, C. R. and Pierrepoint, C. G. (1975): *J. Endocrinol., 64*, 539.
3. Symes, E. K., Milroy, E. J. G. and Mainwaring, W. I. P. (1978): *J. Urol., 120*, 180.
4. Bush, I. E. (1952): *Biochem. J., 50*, 370.
5. Mainwaring, W. I. P., Mangan, F. R., Feherty, P. A. and Freifeld, M. (1974): *Mol. Cell. Endocrinol., 1*, 113.
6. Bruchovsky, N. and Wilson, J. D. (1968): *J. Biol. Chem., 243*, 2912.
7. Katchen, B. and Buxbaum, S. (1975): *J. Clin. Endocrinol. Metab., 41*, 373.
8. Fergusson, J. D. (1958): *Br. J. Urol., 30*, 397.
9. Susan, L. P., Roth, R. B. and Adkins, W. C. (1976): *Urology, 7*, 598.
10. Robinson, M. R. G. and Thomas, B. S. (1971): *Br. Med. J., 4*, 391.
11. Fraser, H. M., Mitchell, A. J. H., Anderson, C. K. and Oakey, R. E. (1974): *Acta Endocrinol. (Copenhagen), 76*, 773.
12. Barley, J., Ginsburg, M., Greenstein, B. D., MacLusky, N. J. and Thomas, P. J. (1975): *Brain Res., 100*, 383.
13. Heyns, W. and De Moor, P. (1977): *Eur. J. Biochem., 78*, 221.
14. Symes, E. K. and Milroy, E. (1978): *Br. J. Urol., 50*, 562.
15. Fischer, L. J., Weissinger, J. L., Rickert, D. E. and Hintze, K. L. (1976): *J. Toxicol. Environ. Health, 1*, 587.
16. Mouridsen, H., Palshof, T., Patterson, J. and Battersby, L. (1978): *Cancer Treatment Rev., 5*, 131.

Discussion

N. Bruchovsky (Edmonton, Alberta, Canada): Could you determine whether DES stimulates uptake of androgen receptor or free androgen by analysing nuclear extracts by gel-filtration chromatography?

E. K. Symes: Yes, such an approach should be feasible. We have not attempted this but we have demonstrated that the increased androgen uptake is due to uptake of androstanolone.

M. Krieg (Hamburg, Federal Republic of Germany): Would you agree that, in general, there is a great similarity between the competition effect you have reported at the nuclear level with data reported by others concerning the cytosolic receptor?

E. K. Symes: I would agree with you. However, since the nuclear uptake of the steroid is thought to depend on its initial binding to cytoplasmic receptor and subsequent translocation as the receptor-steroid complex these results could be anticipated. What is more striking is the similarity in behaviour of these compounds in both human and rat model systems, suggesting that, at least in terms of assessing the anti-androgenic properties of compounds, the rat prostate may be an appropriate model.

B. G. Mobbs (Toronto, Canada): I'd like to make a comment on the high concentration of free androgen you find in the nuclei. Is it possible that the permeability of the nuclear membrane is altered during storage at $-70°C$ resulting in leakage of androgen into the nucleus from the cytoplasm?

E. K. Symes: I have not studied this possibility. However, the experiments I quoted on the distribution between free and bound nuclear androgen were done on material that had only been briefly at $-70°C$ during transport (about 30 minutes).

Lack of correlation between androgen receptor content and clinical response to treatment with diethylstilboestrol (DES) in human prostate carcinoma

R. K. Wagner
Max Planck Institute for Cell Biology, Wilhelmshaven, Federal Republic of Germany

Pharmacological doses of oestrogens have proved valuable in reversing the growth of over 70% of prostate carcinomas [1]. It is generally agreed that oestrogens act primarily by suppression of the hypothalamic-hypophyseal system to reduce circulating androgens, but a direct action on prostate carcinoma tissue has also been proposed:

1. Goodwin *et al.* [2] showed that treatment with diethylstilboestrol (DES) reduced secretion in androgen-maintained hypophysectomized dogs;

2. Lasnitzki [3], using mouse prostate glands grown in tissue culture, also demonstrated that DES can act directly on the prostate.

While the indirect action of DES via the reduction of androgen levels is mediated by the androgen receptor system, no such mechanism is known for the direct antiproliferative DES effect. If the androgen receptor system regulated both effects, then a correlation should exist between the presence of androgen receptor in prostatic carcinoma and response to treatment with DES.

We have, therefore, carried out a preliminary study in which the receptor pattern in prostate carcinomas was compared with the response of these tumours to DES therapy.

Before treatment needle biopsies were taken from the tumours for histological examination and receptor determination. Homogenates from 200—350 mg tissue were prepared by a Microdis-membrator after addition of 3 volumes of 0.01 M tris-HCl buffer pH 7.5. After ultracentrifugation the particle-free supernatants (cytosols) were incubated for 2 hours at 0—2°C with 5×10^{-9} M tritiated androstanolone (DHT) or oestradiol in the presence or absence of a 250-fold excess of the respective non-radioactive steroids. The cytoplasmic androgen- and oestrogen-receptor content was determined by agar electrophoresis at low temperature [4], a procedure which clearly separates cytosol receptors from sex hormone-binding globulin (SHBG), a strong DHT-binding plasma protein contaminating human target tissue cytosols.

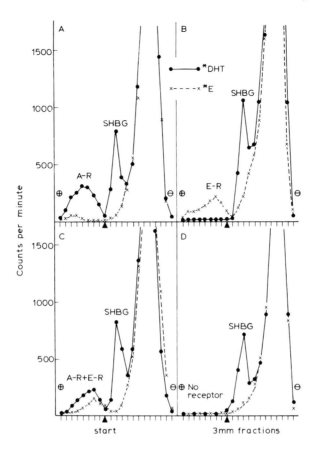

Fig. 1. *Different receptor patterns in human prostate carcinomas (agar gel electrophoresis). A-R = androgen receptor, E-R = oestrogen receptor, SHBG = sex hormone-binding globulin, *DHT = tritiated androstanolone, *E = tritiated oestradiol.*

So far we have investigated 18 human prostatic cancers and found 4 different receptor patterns as demonstrated in figure 1. In 3 carcinomas we found exclusively androgen receptor (Fig. 3A). Three carcinomas contained only oestrogen receptor (Fig. 3B). Seven carcinomas contained, like the normal prostate gland and like benign hypertrophic prostate, androgen and oestrogen receptors (Fig. 3C). In 5 carcinomas neither type of receptor was found (Fig. 3D). An invariable component of all prostate cancer cytosols was SHBG, forming a distinct peak between the receptor area and free DHT.

Figure 2 shows a control experiment in which we investigated muscle cytosol from rectus abdominis muscle, obtained during prostatectomy operations. While there was no specific binding in the receptor area of the agar plates, SHBG was present in all muscle cytosols.

Figure 3 shows a time-course experiment, performed using agar electrophoresis, in which we studied the dissociation pattern of several high affinity steroid hormone-protein complexes during agar electrophoretic analysis. While the oestradiol-oestrogen receptor complex virtually does not dissociate it can be seen that 48% of the DHT-androgen receptor com-

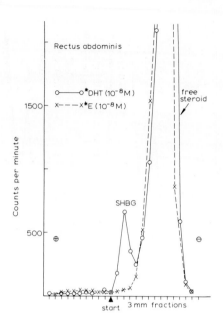

Fig. 2. Electrophoretic analysis of human muscle cytosol (rectus abdominis). *DHT = tritiated androstanolone, *E = tritiated oestradiol, SHBG = sex hormone-binding globulin.

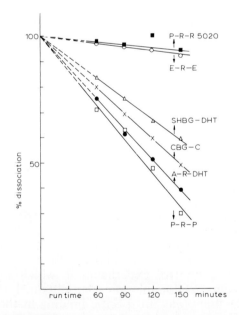

Fig. 3. Dissociation of high affinity steroid hormone-protein complexes during agar electrophoretic analysis. P-R-R5020 = progesterone receptor – R5020 complex, E-R-E = oestrogen receptor – -oestradiol complex, SHBG-DHT = sex hormone-binding globulin – androstanolone complex, CBG-C = corticosteroid-binding globulin – hydrocortisone complex, A-R-DHT = androgen receptor – androstanolone complex, P-R-P = progesterone receptor – progesterone complex.

Table I Androgen and oestrogen receptor in 11 human prostate carcinomas and clinical effect of DES treatment.

Patient	Age (years)	Androgen receptor	Oestrogen receptor	Duration of DES-therapy (months)	Tumour-nodes-metastases classification		Objective remission obtained	Current status
		(fM/mg tissue protein)			Prior to therapy	After therapy		
1) A.W.	68	300	0	6	T4, N4, M1c	T3, NO, M1b	Yes	Continuing remission
2) S.W.	79	0	80	12	T3, NX, M1b	T2, NX, MO	Yes	Continuing remission
3) K.H.	72	50	60	15	T3, NX, M1a	T2, NX, MO	Yes	Continuing remission
4) B.R.	70	0	40	11	T2, NO, MO	T1, NO, MO	Yes	Continuing remission
5) B.R.	70	20	20	9	T4, N3, M1c	T3, N2, MO	Yes	Continuing remission
6) H.W.	63	0	0	14	T1, NX, MO	T1, NO, MO	?	Unchanged
7) G.J.	69	0	0	24	T3, NX, MO	T3, NO, MO	No	Unchanged
8) K.B.	58	0	0	12	T3, NO, M1c	T3, NO, M1c	No	Unchanged
9) G.K.	63	50	20	32	T1, NO, MO	T2, N4, M1d	No	Relapse
10) F.E.	71	30	20	7	T2, NX, M1a	T3, NX, Mb	No	Relapse
11) K.A.	70	80	40	8	T3, N2, M1c	T4, N3, M1d	No	Relapse (died after 8 months of uremia)

Initial therapy: 10 days i.v. injections of 600 mg fosfestrol per day, followed by 10 days of injection of 300 mg fosfestrol. Maintenance therapy: the drug was given orally at 720 mg daily for 3 months. The dose was then slowly reduced to 360 or 240 mg daily, depending on clinical response and level of acid phosphatase in plasma.

plexes dissociate during a 2 hour analysis. Thus only about 50% of the
androgen receptor content actually present in the cytosols could be assessed
in the experiments presented in this study.

In our clinical study 11 patients with advanced prostate cancer were treated
with high doses of DES. The pattern of therapy is shown in the legend to
Table I. The tumours were classified before and at intervals during therapy
according to the tumour-nodes-metastases (TNM) classification. The size
of the original tumour was documented and bone and soft tissue metastases
recorded by roentgenologic, scintigraphic and lymphographic studies. The
receptor values are given in fM (= M $\times$ 10^{-15}) per mg tissue protein. In
case 1 we measured the receptors in an inguinal lymph node metastasis. In
all the other cases needle biopsies were used.

From the results in Table I it can be seen that no correlation could be
observed between androgen receptor and the response of the tumours to
DES treatment, nor was there any correlation with oestrogen receptor. Of
the 5 cases which regressed (cases 1–5) only three contained measurable
amounts of androgen receptor. Two contained only oestrogen receptor and
2 both receptors. In the next 3 carcinomas (cases 6–8) which were clinically
unchanged, neither receptor could be detected. These cases are difficult to

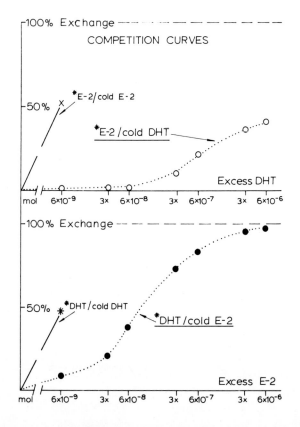

*Fig. 4. Competition of nonradioactive androstanolone (DHT) with tritiated oestradiol
(*E) on oestrogen receptor binding site (upper panel) and competition of nonradioactive oestradiol (E) with tritiated androstanolone (*DHT) on androgen receptor binding
site (lower panel).*

Table II

Compound	50% competitory dose, x fold excess to DHT	Compound	50% competitory dose, x fold excess to DHT
DHT	1	Progesterone	40
Testosterone	12	Chlormad. ac.	43
Norethisterone	15	Norethist. ac.	85
E-2	16	Cyproterone	300
Cyproterone ac.	18	17-α-Hydroxy-19-Nor-Prog	600
D-Norgestrel	25	L-Norgestrel	>10^6

evaluate, since it is not known whether or not the observed cessation in growth was an effect of the DES therapy.

The remaining 3 carcinomas (cases 9–11) were not influenced at all by DES treatment and grew progressively, although considerable amounts of androgen receptor and also oestrogen receptor were found in all 3 instances. The results in the latter 3 cases provide particularly strong evidence against the hypothesis that the effect of DES-treatment is mediated via the androgen receptor system.

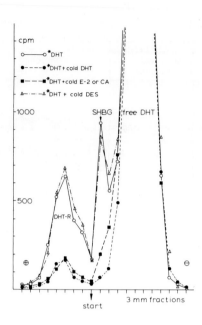

Fig. 5. Competition of several natural and synthetic steroid hormones with androstano-lone on the androgen receptor binding site. *DHT = tritiated androstanolone, DHT = androstanolone, E = oestradiol, CA = cyproterone acetate, DES = diethylstilboestrol, R = receptor, SHBG = sex hormone-binding globulin.

What might be the explanation for these results? The suppression of an-drogen production after DES administration may not be the main effect of this therapy. The direct antiproliferative effect of DES could cause the objective remissions observed.

From the following experiments it would be postulated that the direct DES effect might also be regulated through the androgen receptor system. In 1971 we showed that oestradiol has considerable affinity for the androgen receptor binding site [5]. From the competition curve in the lower panel of figure 4 it can be seen that only a 16-fold excess of non-radioactive oestra-diol causes a 50% reduction in DHT-binding to androgen receptor. Un-fortunately we did not test DES at that time. Table II shows that the anti-androgenic compound cyproterone acetate, which is also effective in treating prostatic cancer, also competes to a considerable extent with DHT at the androgen receptor binding site. Thus the beneficial effect of high oestradiol and cyproterone acetate doses on some prostate carcinomas could be ex-plained by an additional peripheral effect. These compounds apparently suppress the growth-promoting effect of endogenous androgens by a block-ade of the androgen receptor.

However, much to our surprise this concept is not valid for DES, as shown in figure 5. A human prostate cytosol was incubated with tritiated DHT in the absence or presence of a 250-fold excess of non-radioactive DHT (control), oestradiol, cyproterone acetate or DES. While cold DHT, oestra-diol and cyproterone acetate compete well with radiolabelled DHT for the androgen receptor binding site, diethylstilboestrol does not compete at all.

This finding clearly demonstrates that the direct, peripheral effect of DES on prostate carcinoma cells cannot be explained by a blockade of the androgen receptor. Thus, the lack of a correlation between androgen receptor values and clinical response to DES-treatment in our clinical study may be due to an 'intrinsic' cytotoxic effect of DES not mediated by the androgen receptor.

References

1. Huggins, C., Stevens, R. E. and Hodges, C. V. (1941): Studies on prostatic cancer. *Arch. Surg., 43,* 209.
2. Goodwin, D. A., Rasmussen-Taxdal, D. S., Ferreira, A. A. and Scott, W. W. (1961): Estrogen inhibition of androgen-maintained prostatic secretion in the hypophysec-tomized dog. *J. Urol., 86,* 134.
3. Lasnitzki, I. (1963): *Natl. Cancer Inst. Monogr., 12,* 381.
4. Wagner, R. K. (1978): Extracellular and intracellular steroid binding proteins. Proper-ties, discrimination, assay and clinical applications. *Acta Endocrinol., 88, Suppl. 218,* 1–78.
5. Jungblut, P. W., Hughes, S. F., Görlich, L., Gowers, U. and Wagner, R. K. (1971): Simultaneous occurrence of individual oestrogen- and androgen receptors in female and male target organs. *Hoppe-Seyler's Z. Physiol. Chem., 352,* 1603.

Discussion

F. Rommerts (Rotterdam, The Netherlands): In one of your slides you showed that the androgen receptor binding activity was 50% decreased at low temperature in about 2 hours, and that this was approximately similar to the decrease in binding activity of SHBG. Is this dissociation of the com-plex or breakdown of the protein?

R. K. Wagner: In both cases this phenomenon is due to the dissociation of specific hormone-protein complexes and not to protein degradation, since we could show that the androgen receptor and also SHBG can be recharged with DHT.

This experiment demonstrates that the DHT-androgen receptor and the progesterone-progestogen receptor complex has a much higher tendency to dissociate than the oestradiol-oestrogen receptor or promegestone (R5020)-progestogen receptor complex. This is not intrinsic to agar electrophoresis since we have observed a similar dissociation pattern during polyacrylamide electrophoresis and density gradient centrifugation. Recently we have also tested the synthetic androgen metribolone (R1881) and found that this compound dissociates during analysis from the androgen receptor binding site at a similar rate to DHT.

M. Krieg (Hamburg, FRG): The dissociation of DHT from the receptor during the running time depends strongly on the concentration of protein in the cytosol. You can avoid substantial dissociation by applying cytosol with higher protein concentration to the electrophoresis, because then the DHT, dissociated from albumin, will reload the receptor. We for instance found a dissociation within 1 hour running time of about 10% using a cytosolic pro-tein concentration of about 12 mg/ml.

R. K. Wagner: Under saturation conditions we found that dissociation is not dependent on the cytosol concentration of the specific protein, since the dissociation rate strongly depends on the dissociation constant of the spe-cific complex investigated.

In our experiments we have used 1 + 3 cytosols (1 part tissue and 3 volumes buffer) with a protein concentration between 4 and 5 mg/ml, which have a small tendency towards non-specific steroid hormone binding. If cytosols with large protein concentrations are used (> 10 mg/ml) a higher percentage of steroid is non-specifically bound (mainly to albumin). This hormone fraction is liberated during electrophoresis and is carried towards the cathode by the electroendosmotic buffer flow. On its way to the cathode it can indeed reload free receptor molecules which migrate in the anodic direction.

S. Liao (Chicago, Illinois, U.S.A.): Your result showing that oestradiol but not DES competes with DHT for binding to androgen receptor is very interesting. But have you checked whether DES is not oxidized during the incubation to isodienstral which is not oestrogenic and is not expected to compete?

R. K. Wagner: In this experiment the stability of DES was not tested directly, e.g., by chromatography, but indirectly: in the same experiment the oestrogen receptor was simultaneously measured and DES was used as a competitor for non-specific oestradiol binding. In all cytosols where oestrogen receptor was present we obtained competition. Thus DES was apparently stable under the conditions applied.

R. Ghanadian (London, U.K.): Due to the technique you have used, in which measurement of the total receptor population is not possible, I think your conclusion regarding correlation between the receptor and response to treatment is not justified. It is particularly important to note also that your data is on the cytosol receptor and not the nuclear one which is significantly higher.

R. K. Wagner: I wonder why the situation in human prostate carcinoma should be different from that in human mammary carcinoma where a correlation between cytoplasmic receptor values and clinical data after hormonal treatment has been found. Apart from the biochemical reasons outlined in my paper there may be other complicating factors: the major drawback concerning work with prostate carcinomas is the difficulty in obtaining cancer tissue for receptor analysis free of adjacent tissue. With needle biopsies, e.g., one can never be sure, since part of the sample may be contaminated with normal or benign prostate hypertrophy tissue, which regularly contains androgen and oestrogen receptors. In my opinion, the safest way would be the investigation of metastatic tissue including bone metastases. However, for ethical reasons, this could only be done in a very limited number of cases.

J. E. Altwein (Mainz, FRG): Was prolactin in the 10 fosfestrol-treated patients measured? Prolactin increment could be responsible for relapse.

R. K. Wagner: No, in this study we have not measured prolactin.

Is there a correlation between androgen receptor content and response to endocrine therapy in prostatic cancer?

N. Pfitzenmaier, W. Schmid and L. Röhl
Urological Clinic, University of Heidelberg and Department of Cell Biology, German Cancer Research Centre, Heidelberg, Federal Republic of Germany

Growth of carcinoma of the prostate is stimulated by testosterone and androstanolone (DHT). Most patients with known prostatic cancer are treated with hormones, but only about 65% of tumours respond to endocrine regimens. On the other hand, oestrogen treatment and/or androgen depletion by orchiectomy are not considered unproblematic, because of cardiovascular side effects and for psychological reasons.

Materials and methods

In a prospective study in 43 patients with prostatic carcinomas of varying histological grades of malignancy and including all clinical stages, hormonal responsiveness of the tumours was evaluated in relation to DHT-receptor content of the cytoplasm.

Eighteen of the tumours were well-differentiated adenocarcinomas, 16 were moderately-differentiated and 9 were low grade or anaplastic carcinomas of the prostate.

Each carcinoma was classified following the tumour-nodes-metastases (TNM) system according to Union Internationale Contre le Cancer (UICC) criteria. One of the patients had a stage T_1, 3 a stage T_2, 10 a stage T_4 and the majority (29) a stage T_3 carcinoma of the prostate. In all patients, clinical examination revealed either lymph node involvement and/or bone or soft tissue metastases.

Pretherapeutic tumour specimens were obtained by transperineal needle biopsy.

DHT-receptor determination was performed by means of agar-gel electrophoresis according to Wagner [1]. All patients were treated by orchiectomy and monthly injections of 80 mg polyestradiol, i.m.

Tumour regression, classified as response, was verified clinically, radiographically (intravenous pyelogram), by bone scan and, finally, by needle biopsy 3–6 months following treatment.

Results and conclusions

DHT receptors were found in 33 cases. In 10 cases no receptor could be identified.

Though cytoplasmic androgen receptors were found in most cases in the tumour specimens obtained by needle biopsy before endocrine treatment, 8 of the carcinomas which had no receptors showed a good (2) or at least a moderate (6) clinical response to the endocrine regimen. Two receptor-negative tumours showed no response to therapy (see Table).

Table   Clinical and histological response to endocrine therapy in 43 cases. Receptor-negative cases are shown in parenthesis.

Clinical		Histological	
		No tumour material in biopsy specimen	4 (1)
Good	29 (2)	Good	19 (1)
Moderate	12 (6)	Moderate	14 (4)
None	2 (2)	None	6 (4)

There was no correlation between tumour grading and receptor content.

For the evaluation of histological response we could only consider 39 out of 43 tumours because in 4 cases we did not obtain representative tumour material on control biopsy.

Nineteen carcinomas showed a good response, histologically. Eighteen of these were receptor-positive. Fourteen showed moderate response and 6 (4 of them receptor-negative) no response.

In conclusion, our results seem to demonstrate that there is no significant correlation between receptor content and response to endocrine therapy. These results are quite comparable with the findings of other authors [2, 3]. Summarizing our results we feel that androgen receptor-guided therapy of carcinoma of the prostate is not as meaningful as we initially expected it to be. Pretreatment evaluation of androgen receptor in the cytoplasm of prostatic cancer tissue does not therefore allow significantly better prediction of response to endocrine treatment of carcinoma of the prostate.

References

1. Wagner, R. K. (1972): *Hoppe-Seyler's Z. Physiol. Chem. 353*, 1235.
2. Dingjan, P. G. (1978): *Steroïd-hormoon receptoren in humaan prostaatweefsel.* Thesis. Dutch Efficiency Bureau, Pijnacker.
3. Wagner, R. K. (1980): Lack of correlation between androgen receptor content and clinical response to treatment with diethylstilboestrol in human prostate carcinoma. This volume, 190–198.

Discussion

H.-U. Schweikert (Bonn, Federal Republic of Germany): I wonder if you have tried to develop a micromethod which would allow measurement of both cytoplasmic and nuclear receptors in prostate biopsy specimens, since measuring both kinds of receptors might improve prediction of hormonal response in the treatment of prostatic carcinoma.

N. Pfitzenmaier: We have already used a micromethod for the determination of cytoplasmic androgen receptor. The material assayed was gained by needle biopsy. Normally 3 samples are taken. The total amount of cancer tissue is 200 to 250 mg. Such an amount of material is sufficient for determining androgen receptor content of the cytoplasm by agar-gel electrophoresis.

I think you are right that the additional determination of the nuclear androgen receptors may improve prediction of hormonal response in the treatment of prostatic cancer, but at this moment the agar-gel electrophoresis method is impractical for this because about 10–100 times as much prostatic cancer material is required as for determination of cytoplasmic receptor content.

Nuclear androgen receptor content may be determined in the near future by an exchange assay which Dr. Schmid of the German Cancer Research Centre is preparing.

Steroid receptors and endocrine therapy of prostatic carcinoma

G. Concolino*, A. Marocchi*, G. Ricci*, M. Liberti**, F. Di Silverio*** and U. Bracci**
*Institute of General Clinical Medicine and Medical Therapy V and **Institute of Clinical Urology of the University of Rome, Rome, Italy; ***Institute of Clinical Urology of the University of Chieti, Chieti, Italy

Demonstration of the androgen dependence of prostatic carcinoma was established as early as 1941 [1]. Since then the endocrine factors involved in the growth of prostatic tissue of experimental animals and of human beings have been extensively investigated [2–4].

From identification of steroid receptor molecules and knowledge of the mechanism of action of steroid hormones androgen receptors (AR) have been demonstrated in normal prostatic tissue as well as in benign prostatic hypertrophy and prostatic carcinoma [5–8]. More recently, the presence of oestrogen receptors (ER) in prostatic tissue has also been reported [9–12].

These receptors may represent the biochemical basis of the hormone dependence of benign or malignant prostatic diseases and receptor studies could, therefore, like studies of ER and progesterone receptors (PR) in breast cancer, be useful for choice of treatment in patients with prostatic cancer. Endocrine therapy (orchiectomy, administration of oestrogens or antioestrogens) could be selected for patients with tumour growth still under the influence of hormonal factors. For these reasons, patients who underwent transvesical resection of a prostatic tumour because of retention of urine were studied and the presence of AR, ER and PR in the tumour analysed with respect to clinical follow-up after hormonal treatment.

Materials and methods

Tissue specimens

Tissues analysed for receptor content were not collected by needle biopsy but through transvesical resection. Tissue specimens were processed immediately or stored at $-20°C$.

Chemicals

^{3}H-R1881 (R1881 = metribolone), 58.2 Ci/mM, was kindly supplied by Dr. J. P. Raynaud of Roussel-Uclaf. 2,4,6,7-^{3}H-estradiol (^{3}II-E), 100 Ci/mM, and ^{3}H-R5020 (17,21-dimethyl-19-norpregna-4,9-diene-3,20-dione), 51.4 Ci/mM, were purchased from the New England Nuclear Corporation. Tissue specimens were minced with scissors, weighed and homogenized at 0°C in three volumes of TEG buffer (0.025 M tris (trometamol)-HC1, pH 7.4; 0.0015 M EDTA (edetic acid), 0.01 M thioglycerol and 10% glycerol). The homogenate was centrifuged at 10,000 g for 30 minutes at 2°C. 20 nM (= M $\times$ 10^{-9}) cold androstanolone (DHT), estradiol (E) and R5020 were added to the supernatant which was then centrifuged at 200,000 g for 90 minutes at 2°C. The resulting supernatant, cytosol, was used for protein concentration, applying the method of Lowry [13]. Layne's method [14] was applied to the crude supernatant. Free hormones were then removed by adding a suspension of dextran-coated charcoal (0.5% charcoal (Norit A), 0.05% dextran in TEG buffer) for 15 minutes at 0°C and centrifuging at 1,600 g for 30 minutes at 2°C. The cytosol was then incubated overnight at 15°C with 20 nM ^{3}H-R1881 in the presence or absence of 100-fold excess of cold R1881, with 20 nM ^{3}H-E with or without a 100-fold excess of cold diethylstilbestrol (DES) for 5 hours at 25°C and then overnight at 4°C or with 20 nM ^{3}H-R5020 for 1 hour at 20°C and then overnight at 0°C in the presence or absence of a 100-fold excess of cold R5020. After exchange assay [15], total receptors were estimated using either the dextran-coated charcoal technique [16] or agar gel electrophoresis at high voltage [17] and protamine sulphate precipitation [18].

Quantitative studies for AR were carried out by incubating cytosol-DHT with increasing concentrations of ^{3}H-R1881 in the presence or absence of cold R1881. After overnight incubation at 15°C, unbound steroid was removed by adding a suspension of dextran-coated charcoal in TEG buffer.

Results

As shown in Table I, ER were found in only 3 and PR in 7 of the 15 prostatic cancers examined. AR were found in 24 of the 30 cancers studied. The concentration of ER binding sites was found to be 110.0 and 111.0 fM (= M $\times$ 10^{-15})/mg protein in 2 cancers (total receptors) and 1.4 fM/mg protein in 1 cancer (free receptors). The concentration of total PR ranged

Table I Steroid receptors in human prostatic carcinoma.

Receptors	Number of cancers in which receptors found/ number of cancers examined	Receptor concentration (fM/mg protein)	K_d $(10^{-9}M)$
ER	3/15	110–111 (total receptors, 2 cancers) 1.4 (free receptors, 1 cancer)	– – –
PR (total)	7/15	14–80	– – –
AR (total)	24/30	17–37	0.25–1.75

Table II Steroid receptors and clinical response to therapy with CA following orchiectomy and transvesical resection.

Patient	Initials	Age (years)	T N M[a]	AR	ER	PR	Months of treatment	Response
1	G.M.	74	$T_2N_0M_0$	+	−	n.d.	84	Remission
2	C.F.	70	$T_3N_0M_0$	+	−	n.d.	24	Partial objective regression
3	V.V.	63	$T_3N_0M_1$	+	−	n.d.	25	Objectively stable
4	C.C.	71	$T_4N_1M_1$	−	+	n.d.	9	Objectively stable
5	B.O.	64	$T_0N_0M_0$	+	−	n.d.	24	Objectively stable
6	D.M.	74	$T_3N_0M_0$	+	−	n.d.	12	Remission
7	C.F.	72	$T_2N_0M_{1a}$	+	−	+	8	Partial objective regression
8	C.G.	77	$T_2N_0M_0$	−	−	+	7	Objectively stable
9	F.S.	59	$T_1N_0M_0$	+	+	−	17	Objectively stable
10	M.C.	62	$T_4N_0M_0$	−	+	+	22	Objectively stable
11	Z.L.	68	$T_3N_0M_0$	+	−	+	28	Partial objective regression

a   = Tumour-nodes-metastases classification (Union Internationale Contre le Cancer, Geneva, 1974).
n.d. = not detected.

between 14 and 80 fM/mg protein while that of total AR was slightly lower, between 17 and 37 fM/mg protein. It is worth mentioning that the concentration of AR in neoplastic tissues was found to be comparable with that in normal prostatic tissue [19, 20].

Saturation analysis was performed for AR and the dissociation constant (K_d) measured. AR binding was high, K_d being of the order of $10^{-8}-10^{-9}$ M.

Of the patients studied, only 11 are reported in Table II, for the purpose of evaluating clinical follow-up of the patients in relation to receptor studies. It is interesting to note that PR were found in patients 8 and 10, whose prostatic cancers were found to be devoid of AR.

In evaluating response, *remission* was recorded when only subjective and clinical criteria of judgement of response were used, data for objective evaluation not being available. *Partial objective regression* and *objectively stable* refer to the use of objective criteria including changes in bone metastases, tumour mass and prostatic acid phosphatase.

Discussion

Endocrine therapy is well-established in the management of prostatic carcinoma. Nevertheless, prostatic cancer is composed of a heterogeneous population of cells that may differ in their hormonal requirements to reproduce and grow.

Orchiectomy seems to be the preferred form of therapy for prostatic carcinoma since more than 95 per cent of circulating plasma testosterone, which exerts its biological effects on the prostate after its conversion to DHT [2] and binding of DHT to cytosolic and nuclear receptors [21, 22], is produced by the testes. Oestrogens, which can suppress luteinizing hormone-release from the pituitary and block testicular testosterone secretion [23, 24], may however produce serious side-effects such as cardiovascular complications [25]. The clinical advantages of progestational therapy of prostatic carcinoma are not yet established [26]. The use of antiandrogens, like cyproterone acetate (CA) and flutamide or its hydroxylated derivative [27], which are able to compete with DHT at the receptor level, seems to be a suitable form of treatment of prostatic carcinoma.

The presence of hormone-insensitive cancers, however, which primarily need chemotherapy rather than endocrine therapy, led us to investigate parameters predictive of the hormone dependence of human prostatic cancers. Two main routes have been followed:

1. Initially, after the favourable results obtained with CA [28], this compound was administered to patients in order to discover if tumour growth could be arrested and tumour mass decreased. In the cases responding, hormonal treatment was started with orchiectomy followed by administration of CA 50 mg twice a day (Table III).

Table III Hormonal treatment (orchiectomy followed by 50 mg CA twice daily) in hormone-dependent prostatic cancer.

Patient	Initials	Age (years)	T N M	Months of treatment	Response
1	C.S.	65	$T_2 N_0 M_0$	24	Partial objective regression
2	G.C.	56	$T_3 N_0 M_0$	20	Remission
3	M.F.	76	$T_3 N_0 M_0$	15	Partial objective regression
4	M.P.	70	$T_4 N_0 M_0$	12	Partial objective regression
5	P.E.	74	$T_2 N_0 M_0$	16	Partial objective regression
6	P.G.	65	$T_2 N_0 M_0$	15	Partial objective regression
7	S.E.	68	$T_2 N_0 M_0$	12	Remission
8	S.P.	60	$T_2 N_0 M_0$	20	Partial objective regression
9	T.G.	74	$T_4 N_0 M_0$	12	Partial objective regression
10	F.S.	62	$T_3 N_0 M_0$	16	Remission

2. More recently, receptor studies have been performed on specimens of prostatic cancer and hormone dependence estimated on the basis of presence or absence of receptors. ER and PR have been studied, along with AR. While AR were found in 24 out of 30 cancers examined, ER were present in only 3 and PR in 7 out of the 15 cancers also tested for these two receptors.

As can be seen from Table II, of 11 patients studied two with AR^+ cancer (patients 1 and 6) showed remission after 84 and 12 months of treatment. Three patients with AR^+ cancer (patients 2, 7 and 11) showed partial objective regression after 24, 8 and 28 months of hormonal treatment. Six patients showed an objectively stable tumour after 7–25 months of treatment. Of these 6 patients, only 3 had an AR^+ tumour, while 2 had an $AR^- PR^+$ cancer and 1 an $AR^- ER^+$ tumour. Furthermore, of the 3 patients with metastatic disease only one (patient 7), with $AR^+ PR^+$ cancer, had partial objective regression, while the other two (patient 3 with $AR^+ ER^-$ cancer and patient 4 with $AR^- ER^+$ cancer) had an objectively stable response.

Although longer follow-up is required, it is interesting to emphasize that receptor studies may represent a suitable way to evaluate hormone responsiveness of prostatic carcinoma. Besides the possibility of using various forms of endocrine therapy, either additive with administration of oestrogens or medroxyprogesterone acetate, or ablative with orchiectomy, adrenalectomy or hypophysectomy, the association of CA with orchiectomy seems, in our opinion, to be the most advisable form of treatment, capable of blocking also uptake of androgens of extratesticular origin by prostatic cells. Whether CA acts in patients with hormone-responsive cancer only as an antiandrogen, or as a progestational compound able to interfere with tumour growth through an indirect action, lowering blood testosterone levels [29], or through a direct effect on neoplastic tissues when PR are present, needs to be further investigated.

References

1. Huggins, C. and Hodges, C. V. (1941): Studies on prostatic cancer. I. The effect of castration, of oestrogen and of androgen injection on serum phosphatases in metastatic carcinoma of the prostate. *Cancer Res., 1,* 293.
2. Bruchovsky, N. and Wilson, J. D. (1968): The conversion of testosterone to 5-alpha-androstan-17β-ol-3-one by rat prostate *in vivo* and *in vitro. J. Biol. Chem. 243,* 2012.
3. Grayhack, J. T. (1963): Pituitary factors influencing growth of the prostate. *Natl. Cancer Inst. Monogr., 12,* 189.
4. Baulieu, E. E., Lasnitzki, I. and Robel, P. (1968): Testosterone, prostate gland and hormone action. *Biochem. Biophys. Res. Commun., 32,* 575.
5. Mainwaring, W. I. P. (1969): The binding of (1,2-^{3}H)-testosterone within nuclei of rat prostate. *J. Endocrinol., 44,* 323.
6. Liao, S., Liang, T. and Tymoczko, J. L. (1971): Structural recognitions in the interactions of androgens and receptor proteins and in their association with nuclear acceptor components. *J. Steroid Biochem., 3,* 401.
7. Mainwaring, W. I. P. and Milroy, E. J. G. (1973): Characterization of the specific androgen receptors in the human prostate gland. *J. Endocrinol., 57,* 371.
8. Davies, P. and Griffiths, K. (1975): Similarities between 5-alpha-dihydrotestosterone receptor complexes from human and rat prostatic tissue: effect on RNA polymerase activity. *Mol. Cell. Endocrin., 3,* 143.
9. Bashirelahi, N., O'Toole, J. H. and Young, J. D. (1976): A specific 17β-estradiol receptor in human benign hypertrophic prostate. *Biochem. Med., 15,* 254.
10. Kirdani, R. Y. (1978): Prostatic estrogen receptors. *Prostatic Cancer Newsletter, 5,* 4.
11. Concolino, G., Di Silverio, F., Marocchi, A. and Tenaglia, R. (1978): Recettori steroidei nel carcinoma prostatico umano. *Atti Soc. Ital. Biochim. Clin., 7,* 512.
12. Markland, F. S., Chopp, R. T., Cosgrove, M. D. and Howard, E. B. (1978): Characterization of steroid hormone receptors in the Dunning R-3327 rat prostatic adenocarcinoma. *Cancer Res. 38,* 2818.
13. Lowry, O. H., Rosebrough, N. J., Farr, A. L. and Randall, R. J. (1951): Protein measurements with Folin phenol reagent. *J. Biol. Chem., 193,* 265.
14. Layne, E. (1957): Spectrophotometric and turbidimetric methods for measuring proteins. In: *Methods in Enzymology,* chapter 3, p. 447. Editors: S. P. Colowick and N. O. Kaplan. Academic Press, New York.
15. Anderson, J. N., Clark, J. H. and Peck, E. J., Jr. (1972): Oestrogen and nuclear binding sites. *Biochem. J., 126,* 561.
16. Korenman, S. G. and Dukes, B. A. (1970): Specific oestrogen binding by the cytoplasma of human breast carcinoma. *J. Clin. Endocrinol. Metab., 30,* 639.
17. Wagner, R. K. (1972): Characterization and assay of steroid hormone receptors and steroid-binding serum proteins by agar gel electrophoresis at low temperature. *Hoppe-Seylers Z. Physiol. Chem., 353,* 1235.
18. Chamness, G. C. and McGuire, W. L. (1972): Oestrogen receptor in the rat uterus, physiological form and artifacts. *Biochemistry, 11,* 2466.
19. Bonne, C. and Raynaud, J. P. (1976): Assay of androgen binding sites by exchange with methyltrienolone (R1881). *Steroids, 27,* 497.
20. Concolino, G., Marocchi, A., Di Silverio, F. and Liberti, M. (1977): Androgen receptor in human prostatic cancer: our experience with methyltrienolone. *J. Steroid Biochem., 8,* xviii (abstract).

21. Davies, P., Thomas, P. and Griffiths, K. (1977): Measurement of free and occupied cytoplasmic and nuclear androgen receptor sites in rat ventral prostate gland. *J. Endocrinol., 74,* 393.
22. Lieskovsky, G. and Bruchovsky, N. (1979): Assay of nuclear androgen receptor in human prostate. *J. Urol., 121,* 54.
23. Adler, A., Burger, H., Davis, J., Dulmanis, A., Hudson, B., Safarty, G. and Straffon, W. (1968): Carcinoma of prostate: response of plasma luteinizing hormone and testosterone to oestrogen therapy. *Br. Med. J., 1,* 28.
24. Shearer, R. J., Hendry, W. F., Sommerville, I. F. and Fergusson, J. D. (1973): Plasma testosterone: an accurate monitor of hormone treatment in prostatic cancer. *Brit. J. Urol., 45,* 667.
25. Byar, D. P. (1973): The Veterans' Administration Cooperative Urological Research Group's studies of cancer of the prostate. *Cancer, 32,* 1126.
26. Sander, S., Nissen-Meyer, R. and Aakvaag, A. (1978): On gestagen treatment of advanced prostatic carcinoma. *Scand. J. Urol. Nephrol., 12,* 119.
27. Symes, E. K., Milroy, E. J. G. and Mainwaring, W. I. P. (1978): The nuclear uptake of androgen by human benign prostate *in vitro*: action of antiandrogens. *J. Urol., 120,* 180.
28. Bracci, U. and Di Silverio, R. (1975): Il nostro attuale orientamento nella cura del cancro della prostata. *Giornale di Gerontologia, 23,* 287.
29. Sciarra, F., Sorcini, G., Di Silverio, F. and Gagliardi, V. (1971): Testosterone and 4-androstenedione concentration in peripheral and spermatic venous blood of patients with prostatic adenocarcinoma. *J. Steroid Biochem., 2,* 313.

Clinical significance of steroid receptor assay in the human prostate

P. Ekman
Department of Urology, Karolinska Hospital, and Department of Chemistry, Karolinska Institute, Stockholm, Sweden

Introduction

The discovery of steroid hormone receptors has substantially increased our knowledge of hormone action and the elaboration of reproducible assay methods for receptor measurement has been of great importance in steroid hormone research. From a clinical standpoint, the most important implication so far seems to be the possibility of predicting the sensivity of a cancer in a steroid target organ to endocrine therapy. Lack of steroid receptors in a cancer tissue indicates that endocrine therapy will be less likely to defeat the tumour, while the presence of steroid receptors suggests that the cancer is susceptible to endocrine manipulation [1, 2]. A correlation between tissue content of steroid receptors and response to hormonal therapy in advanced breast cancer was first described by Jensen and co-workers [3]. It is reasonable to suggest that a similar correlation exists in human prostatic carcinoma.

The prostate gland is strictly dependent on androgens for its normal function and development. After castration the gland atrophies rapidly but regains its normal function following androgen administration [4]. Androgens are of importance also for abnormal development of the human prostate, since cancer or hyperplasia hardly ever occurs in males castrated before the age of 40 [5].

The human prostate may be subdivided into a central or periurethral part and a peripheral or dorsal part [6]. The peripheral prostate seems to be a distinctly male structure, while the central parts constitute an ambisexual organ, possibly influenced by oestrogens in addition to androgens [7]. Benign prostatic hyperplasia (BPH) is extremely rare in the peripheral parts of the gland – Moore found only one case in 700 hyperplasias examined [8]. Prostatic carcinoma, on the other hand, starts almost exclusively in the peripheral prostate; the incidence of periurethral cancer debut is estimated as 2–3% [9].

The two diseases seem also to be different endocrinologically. While oestrogens have been widely used to antagonize the growth of prostatic carcinoma they are of no benefit in the treatment of BPH. Oestrogen administration has rather been reported to stimulate prostatic enlargement [10, 11]. Several investigations have been performed concerning the androgen/oestrogen ratio in patients with BPH. Some authors have described an increase in circulating oestrogens in patients with BPH when compared to age-matched controls [12, 13] but others have failed to find such a correlation [14]. In 1976 Walsh and Wilson showed that BPH could be induced in castrated dogs using $3\alpha,17\beta$-androstanediol, but not with testosterone (T) or androstanolone (dihydrotestosterone, DHT). The effect was augmented by the simultaneous administration of estradiol [15].

Our knowledge of factors responsible for the development of pathologic changes in the prostate is still very limited. The study of intracellular steroid action may afford valuable data to increase our understanding of processes involved in tumour development in the prostate.

Endocrine treatment has been a predominant form of therapy for prostatic carcinoma, partly because most patients suffering from prostatic cancer are in advanced stages of the disease when first diagnosed [16], and partly because many patients are of an age and in a general condition making radical surgery hazardous [17]. 75–80% of all prostatic carcinomas respond to oestrogen therapy [18] but a considerable number of relapses occur sooner or later despite continued hormonal treatment. Oestrogen therapy is also associated with a high rate of cardiovascular complications [19] and castration has become more widely used as a primary form of therapy in prostatic carcinoma. Castration seems to be at least as effective as oestrogen treatment in controlling the growth of prostatic carcinoma [20].

Other forms of endocrine therapy for prostatic carcinoma are administration of progestational anti-androgens like cyproterone acetate [21], megestrol acetate and medroxyprogesterone [22, 23]. Glucocorticoids have been of benefit in some cases with advanced prostatic carcinoma [24].

So far, however, no methods have existed to predict which cancers will respond to endocrine therapy and which should preferably be given alternative forms of treatment such as radiotherapy or cytotoxic drugs.

While oestrogens are ineffective in the treatment of BPH, progestogens seem to be of value in some cases [7]. Steroid receptor assays may become of value in BPH as well as in prostatic carcinoma in the selection of patients likely to benefit from endocrine treatment.

Studies on the androgen receptor in the human prostate have been hampered for several reasons. One major problem has been tissue contamination with a plasma protein, T-binding globulin (TBG) [25, 26], which binds T and DHT with affinity similar to that of the receptor. A variety of methods have been tried to overcome this obstacle (see references 27 and 28). The human prostate contains large amounts of endogenous DHT and therefore many receptor sites may be saturated [29]. Exchange assays are complicated by the slow dissociation of the steroid-receptor complex at low temperature [30] and the instability of the receptor at higher temperature [31].

Furthermore, the use of natural ligands, such as DHT, is limited due to their rapid metabolism [32, 33] even at low temperatures.

In view of the disadvantages of using natural steroids as ligands in receptor assays the introduction of radiolabelled synthetic steroids has been of great importance for steroid receptor research. Metribolone (MT), a synthetic androgen, has the great advantage of binding to intracellular receptors but not to TBG [33, 34]. In addition, it is resistant to metabolic conversion [33] and exchanges with receptor-bound endogenous steroid to the extent of about 70% during 20 hours incubation at 0°C [33, 35].

This paper reviews our results from steroid receptor assays of 'normal', hyperplastic and carcinomatous human prostatic tissue and discusses the possible clinical importance of steroid receptor assay in the human prostate.

Materials

Benign prostatic hyperplasia

Forty hyperplastic human prostate specimens were obtained by transvesical adenoma enucleations. Analysis of experimentally electroresected parts of enucleated tissues revealed a high degree of protein denaturation and, therefore, this type of material was not used in the study [36, 37].

'Normal' prostates

One specimen containing 'normal' peripheral prostatic tissue was accidentally removed from the 'surgical capsule' during an adenoma enucleation; nine further 'normal' prostates were obtained during cystectomy operations for bladder carcinoma. Attempts were made to divide the prostates into peripheral and central parts according to McNeal [6] for separate determinations of steroid receptor profiles. Occasionally benign prostatic hyperplasia was found.

Cancer specimens

Primary prostatic carcinoma was obtained by punch needle biopsies using the instrument designed by Veenema [38]. In most cases 3 to 4 biopsies were taken, yielding a total specimen weight of 50 to 200 mg, which was sufficient for the quantitation of one steroid receptor. In order to obtain material pure enough most biopsies were performed on bulky cancers, i.e., cancers in advanced stages.

Parts of each specimen were taken for histological examination. All biopsies contaminated with normal or hyperplastic tissue were excluded. Thirty-four representative tumours have so far been analysed. Thirty of the biopsies were obtained prior to onset of any therapy whereas four of the specimens were removed from patients who had already been given endocrine treatment for their prostatic carcinoma.

Eight soft tissue metastases of prostatic carcinoma were also analysed with regard to their steroid receptor profiles. One was removed from the right inguinal region, one from the abdominal wall and one from the retroperitoneal region. All the others were obtained from the left supraclavicular fossa. Five of the metastases were removed from patients relapsing during endocrine therapy.

Ligands

For androgen receptor measurements the steroid MT (R 1881) [34] was used. Oestrogen receptors were measured using R 2858 [39] as ligand and progestin receptor content was analysed using R 5020 [40]. For glucocorticoid receptor measurements dexamethasone was used [41].

Methods

All experiments in the present study were performed on cytosol preparations from human prostatic tissue. Approximately 1 g of tissue (per steroid receptor assay) was homogenized in three volumes of buffer (5 nM (= $M \times 10^{-9}$) tris-HCl, 1 mM EDTA, 0.1 mM dithioerythritol (DTE), 10% (w/v) glycerol, pH 7.4) using an Ultra Turrax homogenizer. Homogenization was performed 3 times for 5 seconds, allowing 30 seconds of cooling in an ice bath between each run. The small cancer biopsies, however, were gently homogenized with a Teflon-glass Potter-Elvehjem homogenizer. After centrifugation at 105,000 g for 60 minutes the supernatant containing the cytosol was collected for further studies.

For receptor quantitation incubations were carried out with (^{3}H)-labelled ligands in the presence or absence of a 100-fold excess of unlabelled ligand. 'Specific' (high-affinity, low-capacity) binding was defined as the binding of (^{3}H)-labelled steroid in the absence of unlabelled steroid minus the binding of (^{3}H)-labelled steroid in the presence of unlabelled steroid. The incubations were generally performed using six different concentrations of each ligand to allow construction of Scatchard plots [42]. All incubations were performed in duplicate. Due to the limited amount of material available in the cancer biopsies (50–200 mg) the number of incubations for the Scatchard analysis had to be reduced in most cases. In addition, the cytosol of the cancer biopsies had to be diluted between 6 and 30 times.

After incubation the samples were treated with dextran-coated charcoal (DCC; 0.5% (w/v) charcoal and 0.1% (w/v) Dextran 70 suspended in the buffer described above) to eliminate free, unbound steroids. Aliquots were taken for counting of radioactivity in an Intertechnique SL 30 scintillation spectrometer.

The maximum number of binding sites (B_{max}) and apparent dissociation constant (K_d) were calculated from Scatchard plots after correction for non-specific binding [43]. A programme was developed for a Nord-computer for calculation of relevant statistical data for the Scatchard plots. B_{max}-values were calculated with 95% confidence limits and K_d-values with standard deviations. Non-detectable levels of binding were said to exist when the slope of the Scatchard plot was not significantly ($p < 0.05$) different from zero. Binding was correlated to wet weight of tissue, to DNA and to protein content.

Twenty-nine of the biopsies from primary prostatic carcinomas were obtained from patients who were later given endocrine therapy. It was possible in this way to compare the effect of endocrine therapy and tumour content of steroid receptors. Eight of the patients with poorly differentiated tumours and no detectable metastases were initially given radiotherapy in a tumour dose of 5,400 rads. The effect of irradiation was evaluated prior to initiation of hormonal therapy which was started two months after cessation of the radiotherapy in five of the cases.

Eleven patients were subjected to bilateral orchiectomy as a primary form of endocrine treatment; four of these patients were also given hormonal drug therapy. Patients receiving drug therapy were either given polyestradiol phosphate, 80–160 mg/month, in combination with ethinylestradiol, 100–150 µg/day [44] or estramustine phosphate, 420–840 mg/day [45].

A positive effect of therapy was evaluated according to the following parameters:

1. decrease of elevated acid phosphatase levels to less than 50% of the pretreatment values;
2. a decreased size of the tumour as estimated by rectal palpation according to the tumour-nodes-metastases (TNM) staging system [46];
3. squamous cell metaplasia [47] as examined by fine needle aspiration biopsy or failure to demonstrate remaining active cancer cells in the tumour;
4. withdrawal of an indwelling catheter;
5. sclerosis of previously osteolytic metastases; relief of skeletal pains lasting for more than 3 months.

The patients were examined regularly and the physician was not informed of the results of the receptor assay when judging whether improvement had occurred or not. Improvement, when occurring, was evident within three months after onset of therapy.

In order to obtain sufficient amounts of cancer material, patients with cancers stage T 3 and T 4 were mainly selected. Since most of the patients were in advanced stages of the disease there were no problems in deciding whether the condition of a certain patient was improved (+), unchanged (0) or deteriorated (−). An unchanged state was regarded as unsuccessful treatment.

Results

BPH

All specimens (40/40) contained high-affinity, low-capacity binding proteins for MT. Twenty-nine out of thirty-nine were also 'progestin receptor-positive'. The mean value for MT-binding was 570 fM $(= M \times 10^{-15})$/mg deoxyribonucleic acid (DNA) and for R 5020-binding 420 fm/mg DNA. The progestin receptor was found to be less stable to repeated freezing and thawing [28], possibly due to its presence in free, unprotected form. No specimens contained oestrogen receptors (0/26) or glucocorticoid receptors (0/16) in the cytosol preparations (Table I).

'Normal' prostatic tissue

The receptor profiles in 'normal' prostatic tissue varied more than in BPH. All specimens — peripheral parts, central parts as well as the excised hyperplastic parts from the same specimens — contained high-affinity, low-capac-

Table I   *Steroid receptor contents in cytosol from BPH.* B_{max} *fM (= M × 10⁻¹⁵)/mg DNA. Mean values ± standard deviations (s.d.).*

MT	R 5020	R 2858	Dexamethasone
566 ± 317	420 ± 316	n.d.[1]	n.d.
(40/40)[2]	(29/39)	(0/26)	(0/16)

[1] n.d. = not detectable (slope of Scatchard plot not significantly $(p < 0.05)$ different from zero).
[2] the first figure within parenthesis refers to the number of samples used for calculation of mean value and the second figure refers to total number of samples analysed in the group.

Table II Receptor contents in cytosol from 'normal' human prostates B$_{max}$ fM/mg DNA.

Case	Type of tissue	MT	R 5020	R 2858	Dexamethasone
A.	Peripheral	236	223	n.d.[1]	n.d.
B.	Peripheral	467	n.d.	n.d.	n.d.
C.	Peripheral	300	209	n.d.	n.d.
D.	Peripheral	485	236	n.d.	n.d.
E.	Peripheral	345	n.d.	n.d.	n.d.
F.	Peripheral	1,080	n.d.	417	n.d.
G.	Peripheral	1,120	n.d.	430	n.d.
H.	Peripheral	836	n.d.	554	n.d.
D.	Central	730	n.d.	n.d.	n.d.
F.	Central	845	n.d.	311	n.d.
G.	Central	1,170	n.d.	148	n.d.
J.	Central + Peripheral	545	602	n.d.	n.d.
K.	Central + Peripheral	703	611	n.d.	n.d.
Mean values ± S.D.		682 ± 316	376 ± 210	372 ± 152	n.d.
A.	Hyperplasia	892	179	n.d.	n.d.
B.	Hyperplasia	1,020	167	n.d.	n.d.
C.	Hyperplasia	1,270	835	n.d.	n.d.
E.	Hyperplasia	714	1,080	n.d.	n.d.

[1] n.d. = not detectable (slope of Scatchard plot not significantly ($p < 0.05$) different from zero).

ity binding proteins for MT. Mean value for B$_{max}$ was 680 fM/mg DNA in the 'normal' specimens which does not differ significantly from mean B$_{max}$-value for BPH (570 fM/mg DNA). This is in agreement with experiences in animal studies [48]. Half of the 'normal' tissues were 'progestin-receptor-negative'. In five of the specimens high-affinity, low-capacity binding for oestrogens was found (mean value for B$_{max}$ was 320 fM/mg DNA) whereas all specimens were glucocorticoid 'receptor-negative' (Table II).

Primary prostatic carcinoma

Twenty-five of the biopsies were 'positive' for MT-binding with binding data varying from 51 to 318 fM/mg DNA. In 9 cases no high-affinity, low-capacity binding was demonstrable (Table III). Twenty-one of the 'receptor-positive' cases were given endocrine therapy and 18 of them had a clear tumour regression within three months of treatment (correlation $\simeq$ 85%). Two of the 'receptor-positive' non-responders had the lowest receptor levels in the series.

Eight of the 'receptor-negative' cases were also treated by endocrine manipulation but only three of them showed any tumour regression (correlation $\simeq$ 65% (Table IV).

Table III Receptor content and relevant clinical data in 34 primary prostatic carcinomas (for further parameters see reference [38]).

Patient number	Degree of differen- tiation	Receptor content fM/mg DNA	Treatment	Acid phosphatase (ncat (= cat × 10^{-9})/ litre)		Tumour size on palpation		Aspiration biopsy after 6–12 months of therapy	General effect of therapy
				Before therapy	After 3 months therapy	Before therapy	After 3 months therapy		
1	M[1]	318	Orchiectomy	570	54	T 2	T 0	n.p.[2]	+
2[4,5]	L	307	Irradiation						n.e.[3]
3[4]	L	230	Orchiectomy	154	17	T 4	T 2	n.p.	+
4	L	218	Estramustine phosphate	622	11	T 4	T 2	No cancer left	+
5	L	212	Oestrogens	33	16	T 3	T 1	Metaplasia	+
6	L	202	Orchiectomy	20	14	T 3	T 0	No cancer left	+
7	M	168	Estramustine phosphate	18	11	T 4	T 2	Metaplasia	+
8	L	166	Estramustine phosphate	8,700	89	T 4	T 2	No effect	+
9	M	152	Estramustine phosphate	26	17	T 2	T 2	No effect	0
10[4]	L	132	Estramustine phosphate	93	18	T 2	T 0	n.p.	+
11	M	127	Estramustine phosphate	1,597	164	T 3	T 2	n.p.	+
12	H	123	Electro-resection						n.e.[3]
13	L	120	Oestrogens	30	14	T 3	T 0	Metaplasia	+
14	M	115	Orchiectomy Estramustine phosphate	650	24	T 2	T 1	Metaplasia	+
15	L	114	Orchiectomy Estramustine phosphate	64	8	T 3	T 2	n.p.	+
16[4]	L	108	Irradiation						n.e.[3]
17	M	106	Oestrogens	413	49	T 3	T 2	n.p.	+

Table III *(continuatio).*

Patient number	Degree of differentiation	Receptor content fM/mg DNA	Treatment	Acid phosphatase (ncat $(= \text{cat} \times 10^{-9})$/litre)		Tumour size on palpation		Aspiration biopsy after 6–12 months of therapy	General effect of therapy
				Before therapy	After 3 months therapy	Before therapy	After 3 months therapy		
18	L	105	Electro-resection / Estramustine phosphate	650	17	T 4	T 2	n.p.	+
19	L	84	Estramustine phosphate	155	24	T 3	T 2	n.p.	+
20[4]	L	84	Estramustine phosphate	84	29	T 3	T 2	n.p.	+
21	L	77	Orchiectomy / Estramustine phosphate	456	7	T 3	T 0	n.p.	+
22[5]	L	76	Orchiectomy	47	22	T 3	T 1	n.p.	+
23	M	70	Estramustine phosphate	14	9	T 3	T 3	No effect	0
24[4]	L	58	Irradiation						n.e.[3]
25	L	51	Estramustine phosphate	2,750	4,690	T 3	T 4	n.p.	—(dead)
26[5]	L	n.d.[6]	Estramustine phosphate	14	25	T 3	T 4	n.p.	—(dead)
27[4]	L	n.d.[6]	Estramustine phosphate	39	25	T 3	T 3	No effect	—(dead)
28	L	n.d.[6]	Orchiectomy	18	13	T 2	T 4	n.p.	—
29[4]	L	n.d.[6]	Irradiation						n.e.[3]
30	L	n.d.[6]	Orchiectomy / Oestrogens	21	18	T 2	T 2	n.p.	0
31[5]	M	n.d.[6]	Orchiectomy	25	26	T 3	T 3	n.p.	0
32	M	n.d.[6]	Orchiectomy	227	44	T 3	T 2	n.p.	+
33	M	n.d.[6]	Oestrogens	223	15	T 4	T 3	n.p.	+
34	M	n.d.[6]	Oestrogens	9,460	34	T 3	T 2	No cancer left	+

[1] H = high, M = moderate, L = low
[2] Not performed
[3] Not given endocrine therapy and therefore not evaluated
[4] Patients given radiotherapy as primary treatment
[5] Patients given endocrine therapy prior to removal of tissue sample
[6] n.d. = not detectable (slope of Scatchard plot not significantly ($p < 0.05$) different from zero)

Table IV   Correlation between receptor content and response to endocrine therapy.

MT binding	Number of patients responding to endocrine therapy	Total number of patients given endocrine therapy	Percent responders
'Positive'	18	21	86
'Negative'	3	8	37

Prostatic cancer metastases

The steroid receptor profiles in metastases of human prostatic carcinoma varied extensively. Seven out of eight were 'positive' for MT-binding with B_{max}-values varying from 8,000 to 20 fM/mg DNA. Three were 'progestin-receptor-positive' whereas no metastasis contained high-affinity, low-capacity binding for oestrogens. Five of the metastases contained considerable amounts of glucocorticoid receptors (Table V).

Table V Steroid receptor profiles in cytosol of prostatic carcinoma metastases B_{max} fM/mg DNA.

Patient number	Previously treated with	MT	R 5020	R 2858	Dexamethasone
I	Estramustine phosphate	8,150	402	n.d.[1]	1,350
II	–	3,440	92	n.d.	2,270
III	Estramustine phosphate/Oestrogens	2,870	n.d.	n.d.	n.d.
IV	Orchiectomy	1,790	n.d.	n.d.	254
V	–	1,319	54	n.d.	401
VI	Oestrogens	674	n.d.	n.d.	942
VII	–	21	n.d.	n.d.	n.d.
VIII	Oestrogens/Estramustine phosphate	n.d.	n.d.	n.d.	n.d.

[1]   n.d. = not detectable (slope of Scatchard plot not significantly ($p < 0.05$) different from zero).

Discussion

It is still too early to estimate the future clinical importance of steroid receptor assays in the management of human prostatic disorders. As outlined in the introduction, receptor assays are considerably more difficult to perform in human prostates than, e.g., in breast cancers. Reports in the literature are usually based on few observations and reflect several matters of controversy. Some problems that remain to be solved are:

(i) Does the human prostate contain high-affinity, low-capacity binding proteins for oestrogens or not [49, 50, 51, 52. 53]?

(ii) Can MT be used as ligand for estimation of androgen receptors in cytosol also containing progestin receptors [28, 35, 54, 55]?

(iii) Will receptor assays become of clinical value in the prediction of tumour response to endocrine therapy in prostatic carcinoma [37, 56, 57]?

The present study also includes matters of controversy and some of the remarks should be regarded as speculation since the material upon which they are based is limited.

'Normal' tissue

Receptor assays in 'normal' human prostatic tissue disclose a rather heterogenous pattern. However, it should be borne in mind that normal human prostatic glands can probably only be found in males aged 15–35 years [58]. The normal-sized prostate of elderly men usually displays many alterations characteristic of senescence – atrophic parts, sclerosis and cyst formations [59, 60].

When attempting to find possible differences in prostatic cell properties and serum hormone levels between patients with or without prostatic disease, however, it would appear reasonable to use age-matched controls, even though their prostate glands are no longer truly normal. Another problem is that the histological pattern of early benign hyperplasia often is indistinguishable from that of the normal prostate [8] and therefore all comparisons of assay results from 'normal' and pathological prostatic tissue must be made with great caution. Attempts were made to divide the excised whole prostates according to McNeal [6] into an outer peripheral part and an inner central part. This is difficult to perform with accuracy and histological examination offers no help in distinguishing the parts from each other. The problems outlined may to some extent explain the somewhat varying results obtained when examining the receptor profiles of 'normal' prostatic tissue.

Influence of irradiation

Nine of the 'normal' prostates were obtained from patients who had received 3,600 rads of irradiation to the genito-urinary region prior to cystectomy for bladder carcinoma. This may further restrict the correctness of defining these specimens as normal. However, the results of receptor assays of the prostates containing hyperplastic parts disclosed no differences as to receptor profiles or B_{max}-values when compared with those of non-irradiated BPH specimens. It might be assumed that the influence of this dose of irradiation on the receptor proteins can be neglected. This may be of importance when considering the value of additive endocrine therapy following irradiation for prostatic carcinoma. This report includes four cases that were 'positive' with regard to MT-binding and who were initially given radiotherapy (5,400 rads) due to localized poorly differentiated prostatic carcinoma. The radiotherapy was ineffective in all cases – three of them in fact had tumour progression and metastatic spread during radiotherapy. Nevertheless, they all had a significant tumour regression following endocrine manipulations.

Cross-reactivity of MT

Despite all the advantages of using MT as compared to natural ligands like DHT in androgen receptor assays, the fact that MT binds both to the androgen and the progestin receptor tends to limit its usefulness [34, 61, 62]. As shown in this study most human benign prostatic hyperplasias contain considerable amounts of progestin receptor and therefore quantitation of androgen receptor content using MT receptor assay data is difficult.

One possibility of avoiding the cross-reactivity of MT is to saturate the progestin receptors with unlabelled ligand but this usually seems to lead to a considerable underestimation of the androgen receptor content. Attempts in this direction have been reviewed in a previous paper [28]. However, recent data indicate that incubation in the presence of a 500- to 1,000-fold excess of triamcinolone acetonide (TAC) may eliminate contamination with progestin receptors [63].

Shain and co-workers [54] have suggested the use of incubation overnight at 15°C instead of 0°C. The advantages are meant to be a more complete exchange of radio-labelled steroid with endogenously-bound steroid and degradation of the progestin receptor with elimination of this source of error as a result. However, on performing parallel incubations overnight at 0°C versus 15°C with the same human prostate cytosols which contained no detectable amounts of progestin receptor, we found binding data varying between 300 and 800 fM/mg DNA at 0°C, whereas only non-specific binding and no high-affinity, low-capacity binding was demonstrable for MT at 15°C. Obviously the higher rate of androgen receptor degradation at 15°C [33] creates new sources of error.

In conclusion, it seems to be difficult using MT as ligand to measure androgen receptor content adequately in cytosols also containing progestin receptors. However, the good correlation reported in this paper between the concentration of high-affinity, low-capacity binding sites for MT in cytosol and the response to endocrine therapy seems to justify the use of MT as ligand in receptor assays aimed at evaluating the hormonal sensitivity of prostatic carcinoma.

Aspects of the pathogenesis of benign prostatic hyperplasia

To increase our knowledge of pathogenic processes responsible for the development of prostatic hyperplasia and carcinoma numerous investigations have been performed on the content of steroid hormone metabolites in serum and urine. As mentioned before, available data are somewhat contradictory although many reports indicate a role for oestrogens in enhancing the development of BPH [12, 13, 15].

Oestrogen receptors have been reported in human BPH by a few investigators [49–51] but others have failed to show their existence [52, 53]. This study has also failed to demonstrate the presence of oestrogen receptors in cytosol from human BPH specimens. Despite the lack of ligand specificity studies it seems highly probable, however, that some specimens of 'normal' human prostatic tissue did contain oestrogen receptors in the cytosol preparation. The finding was verified by repeated assays using R 2858 as well as estradiol and diethylstilboestrol (DES) as ligand, with isoelectric focusing in polyacrylamide gel slabs and with the DCC-technique [28].

It has been shown that oestrogens can induce the synthesis of progestin receptors [64]. It may be speculated that the occurrence of progestin receptors in BPH is an oestrogenic effect. In this connection it is of interest that progestin anti-androgens appear to be useful for antagonizing the growth of BPH [7]. The reason why cytosolic oestrogen receptors are not demonstrable in hyperplastic prostates is unclear. It may be due to intracellular accumulation of oestrogen receptor-complexes. Oestrogen receptor assays in nuclear preparations of human BPH should clarify this.

Steroid receptor assay as a predictive test for endocrine therapy

An important finding in the present study is the good correlation between steroid receptor content in prostatic carcinoma and short term response to endocrine therapy. The lower correlation figure for the 'receptor-negative' cases (65% versus 85%) can probably to some extent be explained on methodological grounds, since usually very small amounts of tissue were available for the assays.

Some of the patients in this study were subjected to radiotherapy as a primary form of treatment. Based on very few observations it seems as though 'receptor-positive' cases were less sensitive to irradiation than 'receptor-negative' cases.

It would appear that steroid receptor quantitation offers a useful tool for individualization of therapy for prostatic carcinoma. However, no information is gained about the long term prognosis of the individual case. A few of the 'receptor-positive' responders have relapsed within ½– 1½ years and it would be of great interest to investigate whether or not changes occur in the steroid receptor profile in tumours no longer controlled by endocrine therapy. In this connection it seems 'disappointing' that four of the five metastases removed from patients relapsing during endocrine therapy contained considerable amounts of androgen receptor. Only half of them had repeated tumour regression when the therapy was changed to alternative endocrine manipulation. There was no correlation between receptor amounts demonstrated in the cytosol of the primary tumours and duration of response to endocrine therapy.

Heterogeneity of prostatic carcinoma

Forsgren and co-workers [65] showed a certain heterogeneity of rat ventral prostate epithelial cells with regard to content of prostatic secretion protein (PSP). It is quite conceivable that human prostatic carcinoma is even more heterogeneous with regard to steroid receptor content in the individual cells. It is well known that biopsies of prostatic carcinoma obtained from patients during oestrogen therapy may reveal squamous cell metaplasia on histological examination [47] as an effect of hormone therapy, but also often mixed up with considerable remaining amounts of active cancer cells.

Many patients relapsing after varying periods of effective oestrogen therapy improve again after castration. Forty per cent of patients with cancers no longer controlled by 'conventional' oestrogen therapy are subjectively improved and 20% have objective regression of metastases when treated by estramustine phosphate [66]. The exact mechanism of action of estramustine phosphate is not known. To a considerable extent, however, it can probably be ascribed to the steroidal component. Estramustine phosphate reduces the levels of circulating androgen and luteinizing hormone (LH) as efficiently as 'conventional' oestrogen therapy [45]. The drug does not seem to be superior to oestrogens in the primary therapy of prostatic carcinoma [67], and the side effects are the same. Recent data also indicate that some patients relapsing while on therapy with estramustine phosphate benefit from a change to 'conventional' oestrogen therapy (Hedlund, personal communication).

We still cannot explain these phenomena, but it is possible that the tumours develop resistance to one type of hormonal therapy while remaining susceptible to other endocrine manipulations. Steroid receptor assay of these tumours may increase our understanding but the results of the receptor assays of the metastases discussed in this paper give no clear answer to the question. It is also remarkable that no metastasis contained any high-affinity, low-capacity binding for oestrogens.

Other endocrine therapies

Progestins are not as effective in depression of testicular androgen production as oestrogens but have still been used with success in the treatment of prostatic carcinoma [21, 22, 23]. Part of the antitumour effect of progestins may be mediated via intracellular receptors and possibly, therefore, three of the patients whose metastases contained progestin receptors would benefit from progestin therapy.

Five of the 8 cancer metastases contained considerable amounts of glucocorticoid receptor, which is noteworthy since the prostate gland seems to lack high-affinity, low-capacity binding for glucocorticoids [28, 68]. The glucocorticoid receptor content cannot be ascribed to contamination with lymphatic tissue which in all cases constituted less than 2% of the total cell mass [69]. Corticosteroids have been used with success in the treatment of advanced prostatic carcinoma [24]. The effect has been thought mainly to be indirect via a depression of adrenal androgen production, but obviously a direct effect on the cancer cells is also possible.

Conclusions

In conclusion, steroid receptor assay may become of value in increasing our knowledge of processes responsible for tumour changes in the prostate gland, in selecting patients for endocrine versus non-endocrine therapy and possibly, also, in selecting different forms of endocrine treatment.

However, the value of receptor assays in predicting tumour response to endocrine therapy in prostatic carcinoma is still a matter of debate. A uniform opinion will probably not be achieved until improved and standardized techniques for tissue collection, receptor assay and evaluation of tumour response are introduced, nuclear receptor assays are included and possibly not until purified receptors, radio-immunoassay and immunofluorescent techniques have become available.

It should also be borne in mind that endocrine therapy does not cure a patient of his prostatic carcinoma but only controls tumour progression for various periods of time. Whether or not steroid receptor assays can be used to improve survival rates in prostatic carcinoma remains to be evaluated.

Acknowledgements

The help of Dr. Marek Snochowski, visiting scientist from the Polish Academy of Sciences, in elaborating the assay methods used in the study is gratefully acknowledged. Ms. Barbro Näsman has skilfully performed most of the assays. Dr. Jean-Pierre Raynaud has generously given labelled and unlabelled metribolone, R 5020 and R 2858. This work was supported by grants from Riksföreningen mot cancer, Leo Research foundation, Swedish Society of Medical Sciences and the Sven and Ebba-Christina Hagberg foundation.

References

1. Baulieu, E. E. (1975): Steroid receptors and hormone receptivity: New approaches in pharmacology and therapeutics. *Triangle, 14*, 47.
2. Horwitz, K. B., McGuire, W. L., Peirson, O. H. and Segaloff, A. (1975): Predicting responses to endocrine therapy in human breast cancer. A hypothesis. *Science, 189*, 726.
3. Jensen, E. V., Block, B. E., Smith, S., Kyser, K. and De Sombre, E. R. (1971): Estrogen receptors and breast cancer response to adrenalectomy. In: *National Cancer Institute Monograph – Prediction of responses in cancer therapy, Vol. 34*, p. 55.
4. Bruchovski, N., Lesser, B., van Doorn, E. and Craven, S. (1975): Hormonal effects on cell proliferation in rat prostate. *Vitam. Horm. (N.Y.), 33*, 61.
5. Moore, R. A. (1944): Benign hypertrophy and carcinoma of the prostate. Occurrence and experimental production in animals. *Surgery, 16*, 152.
6. McNeal, J. E. (1972): The prostate and prostatic urethra: A morphological synthesis. *J. Urol., 107*, 1008.
7. Geller, J. (1974): Medical treatment of benign prostatic hypertrophy. In: *The Treatment of Prostatic Hypertrophy and Neoplasia*, p. 27. Editor: J. E. Castro. MTP Publishing Company, Lancaster.
8. Moore, R. A. (1943): Benign hypertrophy of the prostate. A morphological study. *J. Urol., 50*, 680.
9. Dube, V. E., Farrow, G. M. and Greene, L. F. (1973): Prostatic carcinoma of ductal origin. *Cancer, 32*, 402.
10. Korenchevsky, V. and Dennison, M. (1934): Effect of oestrone on normal and castrated male rats. *Biochem. J., 28*, 1474.
11. Fingerhut, B. and Veenema, R. K. (1966): Histology and radioautography of induced benign enlargement of the mouse prostate. *Invest. Urol., 4*, 112.
12. Pirk, K. M. and Doerr, P. (1973): Age related changes and interrelationships between plasma testosterone, oestradiol and testosterone-binding globulin in normal adult males. *Acta Endocrinol. (Copenhagen), 74*, 792.
13. Sköldefors, H., Blomstedt, B. and Carlström, K. (1978): Serum hormone levels in benign prostatic hyperplasia. *Scand. J. Urol. Nephrol., 12*, 111.
14. Harper, M. E., Peeling, W. B., Cowley, T., Brownsey, B. G., Phillips, M. E. A., Groom, G., Fahmy, D. R. and Griffiths, K. (1976): Plasma steroid and protein hormone concentrations in patients with prostatic carcinoma before and during oestrogen therapy. *Acta Endocrinol. (Copenhagen), 81*, 409.
15. Walsh, P. C. and Wilson, J. C. (1976): The induction of prostatic hypertrophy in the dog with androstanediol. *J. Clin. Invest., 57*, 1093.
16. Gleason, D. F. and the Veterans Administration Cooperative Urological Research Group (1977): Histological grading and clinical staging of prostatic carcinoma. In: *Urological Pathology: The Prostate*, p. 171. Editor: M. Tannenbaum. Lea & Febiger, Philadelphia.
17. Correa, R. J., Gibbons, R. P., Cummings, K. B. and Mason, J. T. (1977): Total prostatectomy for stage B carcinoma of the prostate. *J. Urol., 117*, 328.
18. Fergusson, J. D. (1972): Secondary endocrine therapy. In: *Endocrine Therapy in Malignant Disease*, p. 263. Editor: B. A. Stoll. Saunders Company, London.
19. Veterans Administrative Cooperative Urological Research Group (1967): Treatment and survival of patients with cancer of the prostate. *Surg. Gynecol. Obstet., 124*, 1011.
20. Fergusson, J. D. (1972): Castration and oestrogen therapy. In: *Endocrine Therapy in Malignant Disease*, p. 247. Editor: B. A. Stoll. Saunders Company, London.
21. Geller, J., Vazakas, G., Fruchtman, B., Newman, H., Nakao, K. and Loh, A. (1968): The effect of cyproterone acetate on advanced carcinoma of the prostate. *Surg. Gynecol. Obstet., 127*, 748.
22. Rafla, S. and Johnson, R. (1974): The treatment of advanced prostatic carcinoma with medroxyprogesterone. *Curr. Ther. Res., Clin. Exp., 16*, 261.
23. Johnson, D. E., Kaesler, K. E. and Ayala, A. G. (1975): Megestrol acetate for treat-

ment of advanced carcinoma of the prostate. *J. Surg. Oncol., 7,* 9.

24. Miller, G. M. and Hinman, F. (1954): Cortisone treatment in advanced carcinoma of the prostate. *J. Urol., 72,* 485.
25. Mobbs, B. G., Johnson, I. E. and Connolly, J. G. (1975): In vitro assay of androgen binding by human prostate. *J. Steroid Biochem., 6,* 453.
26. Walsh, P. C., McLoughlin, M. G., Menon, M. and Taninis, C. (1976): Measurement of androgen receptors in human prostatic tissue: Methodological considerations. In: *Prostatic Disease,* p. 159. Editors: H. Marberger, H. Haschek, H. K. A. Schirmer, J. A. C. Colston and E. Witkin. A. R. Liss, New York.
27. Menon, M., Taninis, C. E., McLoughlin, M. G., Lippman, M. E. and Walsh, P. C. (1977): The measurement of androgen receptors in human prostatic tissue utilizing sucrose density gradient centrifugation and a protamine precipitation assay. *J. Urol., 117,* 309.
28. Ekman, P., Snochowski, M., Dahlberg, E., Bression, D., Högberg, B. and Gustafsson, J.-Å. (1979): Steroid receptor contents in cytosol from 'normal' and hyperplastic human prostates. *J. Clin. Endocrinol. Metab., 49,* 205.
29. Albert, J., Geller, J., Geller, S. and Lopez, D. (1976): Prostate concentrations of endogenous androgen by radioimmunoassay. *J. Steroid Biochem., 7,* 301.
30. Fang, S. and Liao, S. (1971): Androgen receptors. Steroid- and tissue specific retention of a 17β-hydroxy-5α-androstan-3-one-protein complex by the cell nuclei of ventral prostate. *J. Biol. Chem., 246,* 16.
31. Menon, M., Taninis, C. E., McLoughlin, M. G. and Walsh, P. C. (1977): Androgen receptors in human prostatic tissue: A review. *Cancer Treat. Rep., 61,* 265.
32. Bruchovski, N. and Wilson, J. D. (1968): The conversion of testosterone to 5α-androstan-17β-ol-3-one by rat prostate in vivo and in vitro. *J. Biol. Chem., 243,* 2012.
33. Snochowski, M., Pousette, Å., Ekman, P., Bression, D., Andersson, L., Högberg, B. and Gustafsson, J.-Å. (1977): Characterization and measurement of the androgen receptor in human benign prostatic hyperplasia and prostatic carcinoma. *J. Clin. Endocrinol. Metab., 45,* 920.
34. Bonne, C. and Raynaud, J.-P. (1976): Assay of androgen binding sites by exchange with MT (R 1881). *Steroids, 27,* 497.
35. Menon, M., Taninis, C. E., Hicks, L., Hawkins, E. F., McLoughlin, M. G., and Walsh, P. C. (1978): Characterization of the binding of a potent synthetic androgen, methyltrienolone, to human tissues. *J. Clin. Invest., 61,* 150.
36. Gustafsson, J.-Å., Ekman, P., Pousette, Å., Snochowski, M. and Högberg, B. (1978): Demonstration of a progestin receptor in human benign prostatic hyperplasia and prostatic carcinoma. *Invest. Urol., 15,* 361.
37. Ekman, P., Snochowski, M., Zetterberg, A., Högberg, B. and Gustafsson, J.-Å. (1979): Steroid receptor content in human prostatic carcinoma and response to endocrine therapy. *Cancer, 44,* 1173.
38. Veenema, R. K. (1953): A simplified prostatic perineal biopsy punch. *J. Urol., 69,* 320.
39. Raynaud, J.-P., Bouton, M. M., Ballet-Bourquin, D., Philibert, D., Tournemine, C. and Azadien-Boulanger, G. (1973): Comparative study of estrogen action. *Mol. Pharmacol., 9,* 520.
40. Philibert, D. and Raynaud, J.-P. (1973): Progesterone binding in the immature mouse and rat uterus. *Steroids, 22,* 89.
41. Baxter, J. D. and Tomkins, G. M. (1970): The relationship between glucocorticoid binding and tyrosine aminotransferase induction in hepatoma tissue culture cells. *Proc. Natl. Acad. Sci. U.S.A., 65,* 709.
42. Scatchard, G. (1949): The attraction of proteins for small molecules and ions. *Ann. N.Y. Acad. Sci., 41,* 660.
43. Chamness, G. C. and McGuire, W. L. (1975): Scatchard plots: Common errors in correction and interpretation. *Steroids, 26,* 538.
44. Jönsson, G. (1971): Treatment of prostatic carcinoma with polyestradiol phosphate combined with ethinylestradiol. *Scand. J. Urol. Nephrol., 5,* 97.

45. Jönsson, G., Olsson, A. M., Luttrop, W., Cekan, Z., Purvis, K. and Diczfalusy, E. (1975): Treatment of prostatic carcinoma with various types of estrogen derivatives. *Vitam. Horm. (N.Y.), 33,* 351.
46. Wallace, D. M., Chisholm, G. D. and Hendry, W. F. (1975): TNM Classification for urological tumours (U.I.C.C.)-1974. *Br. J. Urol., 47,* 1.
47. Fergusson, J. D. and Franks, L. M. (1953): The response of prostatic carcinoma to oestrogen treatment. *Br. J. Surg., 40,* 422.
48. Shain, S. A. and Boesel, R. W. (1978): Androgen receptor of the normal and hyperplastic canine prostate. *J. Clin. Invest., 61,* 654.
49. Wagner, R. K., Schulze, K. H. and Jungblut, P. W. (1975): Estrogen and androgen receptor in human prostate and prostatic tumor tissue. *Acta Endocrinol. (Copenhagen), Supplement 193,* 52.
50. Hawkins, E. F., Nijs, M., Brassinne, C. and Tagnon, H. J. (1975): Steroid receptors in the human prostate. I. Estradiol-17β-binding in benign prostatic hypertrophy. *Steroids, 26,* 458.
51. Bashirelahi, N., O'Toole, J. H. and Young, J. D. (1976): A specific 17β-estradiol receptor in human benign hypertrophic prostate. *Biochem. Med., 15,* 254.
52. Hawkins, R. A., Hill, A. and Freedman, B. (1975) A simple method for the determination of oestrogen receptor concentration in breast tumours and other tissues. *Clin. Chim. Acta, 64,* 203.
53. Kodama, T., Honda, S. and Shimazaki, J. (1977): Androphilic proteins in cytosols of human benign prostatic hypertrophy. *Endocrinol. Jpn., 24,* 565.
54. Shain, S. A., Boesel, R. W., Lamm, D. L. and Radwin, M. M. (1978): Characterization of unoccupied (R) and occupied (RA) androgen binding components of the hyperplastic human prostate. *Steroids, 31,* 541.
55. Sirett, D. A. N. and Grant, J. K. (1978): Androgen binding in cytosols and nuclei of human benign hyperplastic prostatic tissue. *J. Endocrinol., 77,* 101.
56. Mobbs, B. G., Johnson, I. E., Connolly, J. G. and Clark, A. F. (1978): Androgen receptor assay in human benign and malignant prostatic tumour cytosol using protamine sulphate precipitation. *J. Steroid Biochem., 9,* 289.
57. de Voogt, H. J. and Dingjan, P. (1978): Steroid receptors in human prostatic cancer. *Urol. Res., 6,* 151.
58. Franks, L. M. (1977): Etiology and epidemiology of human prostatic disorders. In: *Urological Pathology: The Prostate,* p. 23. Editor: M. Tannenbaum. Lea & Febiger, Philadelphia.
59. Moore, R. A. (1935): The evolution and involution of the prostate gland. *Am. J. Pathol., 12,* 599.
60. Franks, L. M. (1954): Atrophy and hyperplasia in the prostate proper. *J. Pathol., 68,* 617.
61. Cowan, R. A., Cowan, S. K. and Grant, J. K. (1977): Binding of methyltrienolone (R 1881) to a progesterone receptor-like component of human prostatic cytosol. *J. Endocrinol., 74,* 281.
62. Asselin, J., Labrie, F., Gourdeau, Y., Bonne, C. and Raynaud, J.-P. (1976): Binding of (^{3}H)methyltrienolone in rat prostate and human benign prostatic hypertrophy (BPH). *Steroids, 28,* 449.
63. Zava, T., Landrum, B., Horwitz, K. B. and McGuire, W. L. (1979): Androgen receptor assay with (^{3}H)methyltrienolone (R 1881) in the presence of progesterone receptors. *Endocrinology, 104,* 1007.
64. Milgrom, E., Thi, M. L. and Baulieu, E. E. (1973): Control mechanism of steroid hormone receptors in the reproductive tract. *Acta Endocrinol. (Copenhagen), Supplement 180,* 380.
65. Forsgren, B., Björk, P., Carlström, K., Gustafsson, J.-Å., Pousette, Å. and Högberg, B. (1979): Purification and distribution of a major protein in the rat prostate that binds estramustine, a nitrogen mustard derivative of estradiol-17β. *Proc. Natl. Acad. Sci. U.S.A., 76,* 3149.
66. Jönsson, G. and Högberg, B. (1971): Treatment of advanced prostatic carcinoma with Estracyt®, a preliminary report. *Scand. J. Urol. Nephrol., 5,* 103.

67. Andersson, L., Boman, J., Collste, L., Edsmyr, F., Esposti, P.-L., Gustafson, H., Hed-lund, P. O., Hultgren, L., Kelly, J., Könyves, I. and Leander, G. (1980): Estracyt versus conventional estrogen treatment – a randomized study. *Scand. J. Urol. Nephrol.* (in press).
68. Ballard, P. L., Baxter, J. D., Higgins, S. J., Rousseau, G. G. and Tomkins, G. M. (1974): General presence of glucocorticoid receptors in mammalian tissues. *Endocrinology, 94,* 998.
69. Ekman, P., Snochwoski, M., Dahlberg, E. and Gustafsson, J.-Å. (1979): Steroid receptors in metastatic carcinoma of the human prostate. *Eur. J. Cancer, 15,* 257.

Discussion

N. Bruchovsky (Edmonton, Alberta, Canada): Since receptor testing will increase the response rate from ~ 75% in unselected patients to 86% in receptor-positive cases, the impact of a receptor assay is relatively small. Do you think that the effort of performing such an analysis can be justified on the basis of the slim improvement in response rate?

P. Ekman: From a clinical standpoint, certainly, this is an important question. I think we should not be satisfied until the correlation between the results of receptor assays and response to endocrine therapy approaches 100%. However, I doubt that this goal will be reached until more sophisticated assay methods are available, as I mentioned in my lecture. We still have a long way to go before the assays are ready to be introduced into more widespread clinical practice.

Endocrine therapy has many undesired side effects and all methods providing tools for a more individualized therapeutical approach should be of great value. Moreover, I guess that in the future we will have several new and potent alternatives to endocrine therapy in the treatment of prostatic carcinoma.

G. Concolino (Rome, Italy): Did you ever try progestational treatment in patients relapsing after estramustine phosphate?

P. Ekman: No. At our clinic the progestational anti-androgen cyproterone acetate has only been used in the conservative treatment of BPH.

Androgen receptors and treatment of prostatic cancer

B. G. Mobbs, I. E. Johnson and J. G. Connolly
Department of Surgery, University of Toronto, Toronto, Canada

Introduction

Many of the difficulties encountered in initial attempts to detect and quantitate androgen receptor (AR) in the human prostate, such as tissue contamination with sex hormone-binding globulin (SHBG) [1–4], instability of receptor protein [5] and the possible metabolism of the natural ligand androstanolone (dihydrotestosterone, DHT), have been or are being resolved by modification of techniques. Other problems, such as the histopathological heterogeneity of many surgical specimens, remain and continue to cause difficulties in the interpretation of results. Nevertheless, we have found that when care is taken in the selection of tissue and if the endocrine status of the patient is taken into account, certain relationships emerge between the latter, the concentration of cytosol AR and the apparent hormonal sensitivity of the tumour as assessed by clinical response to therapy.

Using a protamine sulphate precipitation technique, we have assayed 'free' cytosol AR (*i.e.*, AR unoccupied by endogenous androgen) in over 100 human prostate specimens. This assay was validated on a tissue 'mixture' model, using rat ventral prostate (RVP) cytosol, to provide a known amount of AR, mixed with human prostate and diluted human serum [6]. The assay was found to be sensitive and reproducible. When human prostate was assayed alone it was found that the high affinity binding of tritiated androstanolone (^{3}H-DHT) had similar characteristics to that in RVP, including ligand specificity. Using protamine sulphate-precipitated AR, we have also carried out initial experiments to assay total AR in human prostate cytosol using an exchange technique to replace endogenously-bound androgen with radioactive ligand. We have investigated the effect of therapy on both free and total AR in human prostatic cytosol and have examined the relationship of free AR in treated patients and their response to hormonal manipulation wherever a satisfactory assessment was possible.

Conventional therapy for prostatic carcinoma produces its effect by lowering serum androgen levels, either by removal of the source of androgens (by orchiectomy and, sometimes, by adrenal suppression) or by feed-back inhibition of gonadotrophin secretion by pharmacological doses of oestrogen. However, recent knowledge of the mechanism of action of androgens in the target cells suggests other possible modes of therapy. One of these might be the inhibition of 5α-reductase, thus depressing the formation of DHT from testosterone. Oestrogens, progestogens and, possibly, the synthetic antiandrogen cyproterone acetate (SH 714, CA), are known to have this effect [7–10]. However, since in the absence of DHT testosterone itself may bind to receptor and, possibly, stimulate growth [11], a more effective mode of therapy might be to block formation of the androgen-receptor complex by competition by antiandrogens. The ability of some therapeutic agents to compete with DHT for free AR was examined in a few specimens of prostatic carcinoma.

Materials and methods

Chemicals

[1,2-³H]-DHT (³H-DHT) (40–60 Ci/mM) was obtained from New England Nuclear Corp. On arrival it was diluted to 10 μCi/ml in redistilled benzene-ethanol (9 : 1, v/v) and stored at 4°C. An appropriate aliquot was prepared before each experiment by evaporating the solvent under nitrogen and redissolving the ³H-androgen in buffer.

CA was kindly provided by Schering Berlin, and tamoxifen by I.C.I. Americas Inc. Unlabelled steroids, chlorotrianisene (TACE), diethylstilboestrol (DES), deoxyribonucleic acid (DNA) standard (sodium salt from salmon testes), protamine sulphate (Grade 1) and bovine serum albumin (BSA) were obtained from Sigma Chemical Company, MO; Dextran T 70 from Pharmacia, Montreal; charcoal (Norit A) from Matheson, Coleman and Bell. The scintillator used was 5 g diphenyloxazole (PPO) and 0.1 g 1,4-bis [5-phenyloxazolyl)] (POPOP) (Amersham-Searle) per litre of toluene.

Patients and treatment

The patients were all undergoing surgery for benign prostatic hyperplasia (BPH) or prostatic carcinoma. Twenty-six were diagnosed as having BPH and were untreated except for the surgery. Another 14 tumours had been diagnosed by needle biopsy as prostatic carcinoma and had been treated with oestrogen or by orchiectomy but no malignant tissue was detected in the transurethral prostatectomy (TURP) specimen. Twenty-one patients had untreated prostatic carcinoma and the remaining 49 carcinoma patients had undergone some form of endocrine manipulation, either oestrogen treatment, orchiectomy or both. The synthetic oestrogen generally used was DES (3–15 mg per day). Fosfestrol (Honvol) was administered i.v. or orally (250–1,000 mg per day). Chlorotrianisene (12.5–75 mg per day) and poly-estradiol phosphate (Estradurin) were also administered. Patients had been under oestrogen treatment for periods varying from 2 days to more than a year. Specimens were received from 11 patients who had been orchiectomized from 3 days to 4.5 years previously. Eight additional patients who had been orchiectomized from several months to 11 years previously were also on oestrogen treatment, sometimes of very long duration. Two specimens were received from each of 4 patients, with an interval of 4–9 months between biopsies.

Assessment of endocrine status

In order to establish the extent of the effect of hormone manipulation, 10 ml non-heparinized venous blood was taken from some patients at the time of surgery. The serum was spun off and stored at $-17°C$ until assay of serum testosterone concentration (and in some cases the testosterone free index (TFI)) and high affinity ^{3}H-DHT-binding capacity of the serum, which is considered to be equivalent to SHBG concentration [12].

Serum testosterone was assayed at the Department of Biochemistry, Queen's University, Ontario, by courtesy of Dr. A. F. Clark. The TFI was measured using a modification of the equilibrium dialysis method of Forest *et al.* [13]. It is calculated as ng/100 ml by multiplying total plasma testosterone (ng/100 ml) by the unbound fraction (%).

For the measurement of ^{3}H-DHT-binding capacity, serum was diluted 1 : 100 or 1 : 200–500 (in oestrogen treated patients) with 7 nM tris-HCl buffer (pH 7.4), containing 1.5 mM EDTA and glycerol 10% v/v (TEG buffer). One ml aliquots were incubated with an equal volume of 2 nM ^{3}H-DHT ± 200 nM 'cold' DHT in TEG buffer for 2 hours at $0°C$. One ml of TEG containing a suspension of 0.5% charcoal and 0.05% dextran was added to each aliquot. The tubes were vortexed, allowed to stand in an ice-bath for 15 minutes and centrifuged at 15,000 g for 10 minutes. The supernatant was removed and recentrifuged to remove the charcoal completely. Bound ^{3}H-DHT was extracted with methylene chloride which was evaporated in counting vials. Scintillator was added and radioactivity was counted.

Assessment of response to therapy

Collaborating urologists were asked to provide relevant facts on the treatment and response of patients both before and after the operation from which the prostatic specimens were obtained. Whenever possible data pertaining to objective evidence of the degree of hormonal sensitivity of the tumour were noted, e.g. changes in prostatic size, serum acid phosphatase values, changes in intravenous pyelogram and changes in metastatic picture as provided by bone scans and X-rays. Changes in bone pain and the level of the patients' activity were also recorded but evaluation of response was not based on these alone.

Handling of tissue

The majority of the operations performed were transurethral resections, but tissue was also obtained from retropubic prostatectomy or open biopsy in a few cases. Multiple needle biopsies were obtained in one case. Metastatic tissue was obtained in 2 cases from involved neck and inguinal lymph nodes. Immediately after removal the tissue was placed in a glass vial refrigerated on ice until transfer, in ice, to the laboratory (usually within half an hour). All tissue handling and assay procedures were carried out at $0–4°C$ with precooled equipment, glassware and buffer solutions unless otherwise stated. Prostate chips from transurethral resections were carefully trimmed of damaged portions and rinsed briefly in TEG buffer. Excess buffer was removed with Kimwipes, and representative portions were fixed for histological examination to ensure that the specimen for assay was representative of the tumour. The remaining tissue was either assayed immediately or refrigerated overnight.

The proportion of malignant tissue present in the carcinoma specimen was estimated by a pathologist from the histological specimen prepared in the pathology department: this usually represented a larger portion of the total tumour than the specimen sent for assay. The proportion of tissue which was malignant varied very widely. Occasionally, a specimen diagnosed as carcinoma contained no malignant tissue in the prostatectomy specimen. Carcinomas were also variable in their degree of differentiation and some also contained areas of fibromuscular and glandular hyperplasia.

Assay of androgen receptor

(a) Free sites.   Prostatic tissue was homogenized (approximately 100 mg/ml TEG buffer) using a Potter-Elvejhem type homogenizer at approximately 800 revolutions per minute (rpm) in an ice-bath in 15 second bursts, with 45 second cooling intervals. If enough material was available, an aliquot of the homogenate was removed for DNA determination by the method of Dische [14]. The remainder of the homogenate was spun at 12,000 g for 10 minutes to yield a pellet and a crude supernatant. For small samples the pellet was used for DNA determination. An aliquot of the crude supernatant was removed for assay of the approximate protein concentration by the method of Layne [15]. The remainder was divided into a number of aliquots depending upon the number of experimental conditions to be investigated. These aliquots were transferred to polyallomer tubes and an equal volume of TEG buffer containing 20 nM ^{3}H-DHT was added. For routine assay unlabelled DHT was added to some aliquots at 1 or 4 μM (= M $\times$ 10^{-6}) in order to correct for low affinity binding. For ligand specificity studies competing compounds were added at concentrations varying from 1$-$1,000 times that of ^{3}H-DHT. Blanks using buffer instead of cytosol were run concurrently. Cytosol was then separated from each aliquot by centrifuging at 105,000 g for 1 hour. The supernatant cytosol was then transferred to glass tubes and allowed to stand on ice for the remainder of the 2 hour incubation period. If accurate estimation of protein concentration in the cytosol was needed the method of Lowry [16] was used at this stage.

Pyrex tubes (10 $\times$ 75 mm) for protamine precipitation were prepared as described by Chamness *et al.* [17]. They were etched with chromic acid, washed and incubated for 10 minutes at 30°C with a solution of BSA (1 mg/ml of TE buffer (7 mM tris + 0.1 mM EDTA), pH 7.4). They were then rinsed with ice-cold TE buffer. 0.5 ml aliquots of incubated cytosol were transferred to the prepared tubes and protamine sulphate in an equal quantity of TE buffer was added so that the final concentration of protamine sulphate was 0.05% w/v. The tubes were vortexed and allowed to stand in ice for 10 minutes. They were then spun at 3,000 g for 10 minutes. The supernatants were discarded and the precipitates washed very thoroughly (at least 6 times) with tris buffer. The washed precipitates were extracted with 1.5 ml methylene chloride overnight at 0$-$4°C. The solvent was quantitatively transferred to counting vials and evaporated. Scintillation fluid was added and counting was carried out in a Packard liquid spectrometer, Model 3375. High-affinity binding of ^{3}H-DHT was calculated by subtracting low-affinity binding (in the presence of competitor) from total binding (in the absence of competitor). Binding was related to wet weight of tissue and to

DNA concentration of the tissue in order to correct for variations in cellularity between specimens.

(b) *Total sites.* Total site assay was based on the method of Davies *et al.* [18]. Our recent assays, including all the total site assays, have been carried out using tissue homogenized with a Polytron P-10 homogenizer (Brinkman Instruments, Inc.), setting 3.5, for 2×10 second bursts, with a cooling interval of 50 seconds. The homogenate concentration was approximately 85 mg/ml TEG buffer, resulting in a protein concentration of approximately 1.8 mg/ml of cytosol. Assay was carried out on replicate aliquots of 0.2–0.5 ml. Some aliquots were pipetted into prepared glass tubes for free site assay as already described. Others were transferred to 12×75 mm polystyrene tubes. AR was precipitated by protamine sulphate as for the free site assay and thoroughly washed with tris buffer. For exchange, the precipitate was dispersed using a rubber policeman or, more recently, by sonication, into 1 ml TE buffer containing 25 nM ^{3}H-DHT $\pm$ 2.5 μM 'cold' DHT, and incubated at 15°C overnight. The exchange medium was then removed after centrifugation at 800 g for 5 minutes and the precipitate washed 5 times with 2 ml tris buffer (pH 7.4) containing 1% Tween 80. The tubes were centrifuged between washings and the supernatant removed by aspiration. Radioactivity bound to the precipitate was extracted into ethanol and counted. Using 12 aliquots, six of which contained excess 'cold' DHT to permit correction for low affinity binding, the average coefficient of variation was $14.5 \pm 7.7\%$ (standard deviation), calculated from twelve experiments.

Results

Endocrine status in untreated and treated patients

Total serum testosterone, TFI values and the high affinity ^{3}H-DHT-binding capacity of the serum of patients from whom blood was obtained are listed in Table I. The effects of treatment on endocrine status were usually those expected. The range of total serum testosterone values in untreated patients extended somewhat beyond the normal range (300–1,000 ng/100 ml),

Table I Serum testosterone levels and high affinity ^{3}H-DHT-binding capacities of serum (SHBG concentrations) (means and ranges) in untreated and treated patients.

| Treatment | Testosterone (ng/100 ml) | | ^{3}H-DHT binding capacity (μg/100 ml) |
	Total	TFI	
None	427 (204–1,170) n = 28	33.95 (15.8–88.9) n = 15	0.891 (0.270–3.772) n = 45
Oestrogen	119 (undetectable- 357) n = 34	3.1 (0.6–8.8) n = 16	3.842 (1.56–8.88) n = 37
Orchiectomy	101 (8–684) n = 14	2.3 (0.6–9.8) n = 6	1.369 (0.33–1.70) n = 12
Oestrogen + Orchiectomy	66 (6–178) n = 7	0.8 (0.1–1.8) n = 5	5.537 (3.260–8.84) n = 7

n = number of patients.

and the TFI values in four patients were lower than is considered normal (24.6—93.6 ng/100 ml). This may have been related to the advanced age of the patients. The ^{3}H-DHT-binding capacity of the serum of one patient was unexpectedly high, possibly due to a thyroid problem [19]. The TFI values in all treated patients in whom this was measured were below normal, as was the total serum testosterone, except in 3 oestrogen-treated and one orchiectomized patient. As expected, the ^{3}H-DHT-binding capacity of the serum in all oestrogen-treated patients was above normal, except in one patient whose serum testosterone was also normal. Orchiectomy combined with oestrogen treatment resulted in the lowest mean values of serum testosterone and of TFI and the highest mean value of ^{3}H-DHT-binding capacity observed. However, the ranges of all parameters in all the treated groups overlapped.

Androgen receptor concentration and therapy

(a) Free site assay. The results of the free site assay in the prostatic tissue from the patients in the treatment groups are presented in Table II. In figure 1 the free AR concentration in each specimen, expressed as fM $(= M \times 10^{-15})/$ mg tissue, is plotted against the serum testosterone value in the patient. It is clear that the free androgen receptor concentration in prostatic cytosol from patients whose serum testosterone values were in the normal range was low, i.e. < 0.5 fM/mg tissue. The mean and range of the AR values in these patients was similar whether the prostatic tissue was benign or malignant and whether it was obtained by TURP or open biopsy. The mean value was equivalent to approximately 250 sites per cell, assuming the DNA content per cell to be 7 pg $(= g \times 10^{-12})$ [20]. This estimated number of free sites per cell may be an overestimate for some carcinomas, as Frederiksen *et al.* have observed mixed populations of cells with diploid and hyperdiploid amounts of DNA in some carcinoma specimens [21]. Tissue from patients whose serum testosterone values were lowered by treatment showed a much wider range of AR values. About one quarter of these patients had AR

Table II   *Concentration of 'free' androgen receptor in prostatic cytosols in untreated and treated patients with BPH and prostatic carcinoma.*

Diagnosis and treatment (no. of specimens)	Protamine sulphate-precipitated high-affinity ^{3}H-DHT binding (mean and range)	
	fM/mg tissue	fM/mg DNA
BPH, untreated (22)	0.21 (0—0.64)	60 (0—110)
Carcinoma, untreated (21)	0.24 (0—0.53)	61 (0—190)
Non malignant tissue, oestrogen-treated (12)	0.56 (0.12—1.35)	72 (20—200)
Carcinoma, orchiectomy (14)*	0.89 (0.14—6.74)	191 (40—1,400)
Carcinoma, oestrogen-treated (33)*	1.07 (0.11—11.72)	222 (20—1,670)
Carcinoma, oestrogen-treated + orchiectomy (8)	1.05 (0.28—3.56)	224 (40—660)

* Three patients in the oestrogen-treated group, and one patient in the orchiectomized group did not have serum testosterone levels < 300 ng/100 ml. The prostatic cytosol in each of these patients had a very low binding capacity.

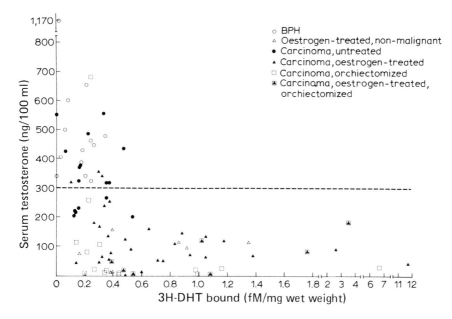

Fig. 1. High affinity binding of ³H-DHT by human prostatic cytosols plotted against serum testosterone values. The horizontal dotted line respresents the lower limit of the normal range of serum testosterone values (300 ng/100 ml).

values > 1 fM/mg tissue, the maximum concentration being equivalent to approximately 7,000 sites per cell (assuming the cells to be diploid). However, only one of the specimens in which no malignant tissue was observed had an AR value > 1 fM/mg. In patients whose serum testosterone levels were < 200 ng/100 ml the AR values did not appear to be related to the serum testosterone levels or to the length or type of treatment.

In figure 2, the AR concentration in the prostatic cytosol of each treated patient is plotted against the high-affinity ³H-DHT-binding capacity (SHBG concentration) of his serum. It is clear that there is no relationship between the SHBG content of the serum and the amount of ³H-DHT bound with high affinity in the protamine sulphate precipitate, at least in patients whose serum bound < 5 µg ³H-DHT/100 ml. In patients with SHBG levels greater than 5 µg/100 ml the data suggest that there is a possibility that SHBG present in the cytosol may be contributing a small amount of high-affinity ³H-DHT-binding to the precipitate. However, the number of patients with such elevated SHBG levels is small and more data are needed to confirm this. In any case, these results are in marked contrast to the strong correlation observed between the ³H-DHT-binding capacity of the serum and the total high-affinity ³H-DHT-binding capacity of prostatic cytosol as measured by the DCC method [22 and our unpublished results].

Free site assays were carried out on two biopsies from each of 4 patients with an interval of several months between biopsies. The assay results on these patients are presented in Table III. All of them had had oestrogen treatment before the first resection. After this, two were orchiectomized and the other two were changed to a different form of oestrogen treatment. However, regrowth of the prostate occurred necessitating a further resection. In 2 of the patients the AR concentrations were low in both biopsies despite

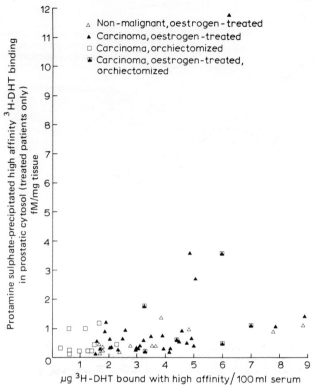

Fig. 2. High affinity binding of ³H-DHT precipitated from human prostatic cytosol by protamine sulphate plotted against SHBG concentration in the serum of each patient.

Table III   Androgen receptor concentration in first and subsequent prostatic carcinoma specimens.

Patient	Biopsy number	Treatment before biopsy	Serum testosterone (ng/100 ml)	High affinity ³H-DHT bound in protamine precipitate		Interval between biopsies (months)
				fM/mg tissue	fM/mg DNA	
A.H.	1.	DES 5 mg t.i.d. for 3 days	139	0.36	90	
	2.	♋ 9 months	10	0.43	100	9
E.L.	1.	DES 2 mg t.i.d. for 6 days	239	0.34	150	
	2.	♋ 6 months	11	0.20	50	6
C.H.	1.	DES (intermittent)	N.D.	1.56	240	
	2.	Polyestradiol phosphate 9 months	N.D.	0.46	130	9
M.B.	1.	Chlorotrianisene 12.5 mg t.i.d. for 6 days	65	0.37	70	
	2.	5-FU for 2 weeks DES 1 mg. t.i.d. for 1 month	108	0.84	220	4

N.D. = Not determined; ♋ = orchiectomized.

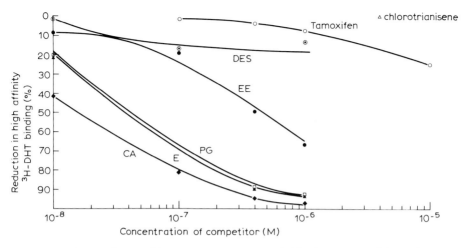

Fig. 3. Ligand specificity of human prostate cytosol AR demonstrated by reduction in high-affinity binding of ^3H-DHT precipitated by protamine sulphate. Competitors were used at concentrations 1–1,000 times the concentration of ^3H-DHT (10 nM).

serum testosterone levels below normal. The value in one patient (C.H.) was lower after polyestradiol phosphate treatment than after DES, possibly due to competition for AR binding sites by the estradiol (see later). The AR value for the fourth patient (M.B.) was higher in the second biopsy (after DES treatment) than in the first biopsy (after chlorotrianisene), although on both occasions his serum testosterone level was well below normal.

Effect of possible therapeutic agents on binding of ^3H-DHT to free receptor sites. ^3H-DHT-binding competition curves for some agents used, or considered for use, in the therapy of prostatic carcinoma are shown in figure 3. The synthetic oestrogens most frequently used (DES and chlorotrianisene) showed no ability to compete with ^3H-DHT for high-affinity binding sites. There has been some interest in the use of ethinylestradiol and the anti-oestrogen tamoxifen for the treatment of prostatic carcinoma. The latter showed no ability to compete with DHT for androgen receptor. Ethinylestradiol was slightly more effective, but much less effective than estradiol or progesterone. Cyproterone acetate was a more effective inhibitor than either estradiol or progesterone.

(b) Total site assay. Preliminary results using the total AR assay are presented in Table IV, expressed as fM/mg DNA. The control tissue was an inguinal node which was replaced by squamous cell carcinoma of unknown origin in a patient who had been orchiectomized for prostatic carcinoma 6 months previously. Assay of free and total sites was carried out on 8 BPH specimens. As expected from the assay results already described, free site concentration was low, the mean value being only about twice that in the control tissue. Total site concentration ranged from about twice to fifteen times that in the control tissue and 86–99% of the sites were measurable only after exchange. The results in 2 untreated carcinoma specimens were similar to those in the BPH specimens as regards total sites although free site concentrations were slightly higher. To date, only 3 specimens have been assayed from 2 treated patients, one of whom had been orchiectomized and

Table IV

Tissue	Treatment	AR sites (fM/mg DNA)		
		Total	Free	% Occupied
Control	Orchiectomy 6 months earlier	136	25	82
BPH (8)	None	1,000 (221–2,094)	58 (9–106)	92 (86–99)
Carcinoma	None	971	149	85
Carcinoma	None	1,593	144	91
Non-malignant	Orchiectomy 6 days earlier	302	108	64
Non-malignant	Orchiectomy 3 weeks earlier	215	84	61
Non-malignant	DES for 1 year	307	157	49

the other treated with DES (1 mg t.i.d.). No malignant tissue was detected
in any of these specimens. The total site concentration was at the low end
of the range found in the BPH specimens but a greater proportion of sites
was detectable before exchange. As yet we have no data on the serum
testosterone levels in these patients.

Correlation between AR concentration and response to therapy. In view
of the wide range of free AR values observed after treatment in patients
whose serum testosterone levels were below 200 mg/100 ml it was of interest
to investigate a possible relationship between the AR concentration and the
response of the patient to endocrine manipulative therapy. As yet we do
not have sufficient data from the total AR assay to examine this question in
untreated patients. In examining a possible correlation in the treated patients
we restricted ourselves to patients whose tumours were estimated to contain
> 60% malignant tissue and for whom objective information concerning
response was available. To date, these conditions have been satisfied for
19 patients. Some of these were in relapse after one or more courses of endocrine treatment while others had undergone a brief course of hormonal
manipulation before operation and their response to continued treatment
was evaluated postoperatively. The data on these patients are presented in
figure 4. When AR concentrations were expressed as fM/mg tissue the
patients fell into 3 groups. Those whose prostatic cytosol contained < 0.4
fM/mg were all in relapse at the time of operation or did not respond to
treatment afterwards. The 7 patients whose AR concentration was 0.4–1.2
fM/mg all showed some degree of response to hormonal treatment. Three of
these showed a mixed response, *i.e.*, one or more parameters indicated a
positive response, while another or others indicated progression of disease.
In the third group (AR > 1.3 fM/mg) one patient whose free prostatic cytosol AR concentration was 3.6 fM/mg experienced remission but the remaining 5 patients were in relapse at the time of operation or failed to respond
to treatment postoperatively. When the AR concentrations were expressed
per unit of DNA a similar pattern emerged, although there was some overlap
between the second and third groups of patients.

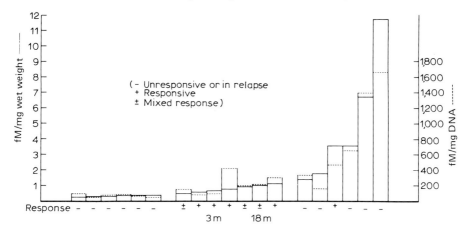

Fig. 4. Relationship between concentration of AR in human prostatic cytosols and response to hormonal manipulation in patients with prostatic carcinoma. The proportion of malignant tissue in each of these tumours was > 60%, and all patients had undergone hormonal manipulation resulting in low serum testosterone values at the time of operation.

Discussion

Effects of therapy on AR concentration

The consistently low free AR values observed in prostatic tissue from untreated patients supported the finding of Rosen *et al.*, that 90% of the AR sites in BPH cytosol were occupied by endogenous androgen [2]. This is confirmed by our results using the total cytosol AR assay, although it should be stressed that those results are very preliminary and are presented tentatively. Nevertheless, the mean value for total cytosol AR when expressed per mg wet weight of tissue (3.6 fM/mg) is close to that observed by Rosen *et al.* using radioimmunoassay of DHT in the 8S receptor peak after sucrose density gradient centrifugation (2.6 fM/mg). In prostatic tissue from some treated carcinoma patients the free site concentration was much higher, presumably because of the 'emptying' of sites formerly occupied by endogenous androgen and/or release of sites from the nucleus into the cytosol. However, in others the concentration of sites was not raised, and from the data so far collected it appears that these tumours were not sensitive to endocrine therapy. In these cases lack of a significant concentration of AR sites may result from selective loss of hormonally sensitive cells due to androgen deprivation during treatment, leaving a population of autonomous cells which did not require androgen stimulation for growth.

Two biopsies were taken from each of 4 oestrogen-treated patients, with an interval of 4–9 months between biopsies. The results from 2 of these patients, both of whom had a high proportion of malignant tissue in both biopsies, are of particular interest (Table III). After the first biopsy, which showed a moderately high concentration of AR, one patient (C.H.) was transferred from DES treatment, which he found difficult to tolerate, to monthly i.m. injections of polyestradiol phosphate. After 9 months a second biopsy showed a reduction in AR concentration to approximately 50% of the former value. This may have been due to competition for AR sites by the estradiol released from the depot of polyestradiol phosphate. Three weeks later this patient underwent bilateral orchiectomy, after which his acid phosphatase levels returned to normal and kidney obstruction disappeared. He remained in remission for more than 15 months. The first biopsy from patient M.B. (after chlorotrianisene therapy) contained a low concentration of AR sites. He was treated with fluorouracil (5-FU) for 2 weeks before being placed on DES for 1 month, when a second biopsy was taken. During this treatment his condition deteriorated but the second biopsy had a higher concentration of AR sites than the first, although his serum testosterone level was higher. One could speculate that during the period of chemotherapy, when serum testosterone levels presumably returned to normal, there was regrowth of a hormone-sensitive cell population containing a higher concentration of AR than in the first biopsy. Prednisone was then added to the DES treatment, serum acid phosphatase fell to normal, leg oedema which was thought to be due to obstruction subsided and the patient was able to return to full-time work. This improvement lasted for 9 months. The biopsies obtained from the other 2 patients showed less malignant involvement. In patient E.L. orchiectomy appeared to result in a decreased site concentration and the patient's disease progressed. In the other (A.H.) a lower serum testosterone level at the time of the second biopsy was associated with a slightly higher concentration of free sites than in the first biopsy. Although orchiectomy resulted in a drop of serum acid phosphatase to a near normal value this patient developed progressive disease after 7 months.

The results from the total site assay suggest that there may have been some loss of AR sites in the tissue from the treated patients in comparison with that of the untreated patients. Treatment appeared to have 'emptied' 40–50% of the remaining sites. The question remains as to the nature of the remaining 50% of the sites (and the *in vivo* ligand) in these specimens. It is tempting to speculate that these sites may have been filled with androgens of adrenal origin [23, 24] which may have been metabolized to testosterone and DHT, either peripherally [25], contributing to residual serum testosterone values, or locally in the prostate itself [26–28]. Many more data are needed in order to investigate this possibility further.

The competition studies carried out with the free site assay confirm that competition for androgen-binding sites is not an element in the therapeutic action of the commonly used synthetic oestrogens. Investigation of the ability to compete with DHT for AR *in vitro* may however be a useful preliminary screening technique for new antiandrogens, provided it is combined with the investigation of possible metabolism of the agent and the induction of side effects *in vivo*.

Does AR concentration relate to responsiveness of prostatic carcinoma to endocrine therapy?

The relationship between AR concentration and response to treatment is presented in Figure 4. This does not include results from patients in whom 2 biopsies were obtained, which have already been discussed. All patients whose tumours contained a free cytosol AR concentration of < 0.4 fM/mg and 90 fM/mg DNA were either in relapse at the time of biopsy or did not respond to subsequent endocrine manipulation. Thus a certain 'threshold' concentration of AR appears to be a requisite for response to hormonal manipulation. It may be of interest to note that the apparent 'threshold' concentration of free cytosol AR in prostatic carcinomas from treated (androgen-deprived) men (0.4 fM/mg tissue, 80–90 fM/mg DNA) is approximately half that used in this laboratory as the threshold concentration of free cytosol oestrogen receptor required for hormonal sensitivity of breast carcinoma in post-menopausal (oestrogen deprived) women (0.8 fM/mg tissue, 200 fM/mg DNA). The most definite responses to endocrine manipulation occurred in patients whose prostatic cytosol contained free AR at concentrations of 0.6–3.6 fM/mg, 80–475 fM/mg DNA. The tumours with the highest concentrations of AR did not appear to be sensitive to hormonal manipulation: possibly this receptor protein is an abnormal one or is an irrelevant product, not linked to processes which control androgen sensitivity. Possibly, as in breast carcinoma, a significant concentration of hormone receptor is a necessary condition for hormonal sensitivity but does not guarantee it.

On the evidence presented here we believe that it is possible to obtain an indication of the likely response of prostatic carcinoma patients to treatment by hormonal manipulation from the result of a free cytosol AR assay, provided that the specimen assayed contains a high proportion of malignant tissue and that the serum testosterone levels are low. Further work on an exchange assay should make possible investigation of a possible correlation of total AR and response in patients untreated before biopsy.

Acknowledgements

This investigation is supported by Grant Number 251 from the Ontario Cancer Treatment and Research Foundation. We greatly appreciate the collaboration of urologists and operating room staff in several Toronto hospitals and of pathologists Dr F. Sims and Dr S. Carlyle. Serum testosterone assays were kindly carried out in the laboratories of Dr A. F. Clark, Department of Biochemistry, Queen's University, Kingston, Ontario. Thanks are also due to Dr M. Lippman, N.I.H., Bethesda, for his advice in setting up the free site assay. Conscientious technical assistance was provided by Mrs S. Parnell.

References

1. Steins, P., Krieg, M., Hollman, H. J. and Voigt, K. D. (1974): *In vitro* studies of testosterone and 5α-dihydrotestosterone binding in benign prostatic hypertrophy. *Acta endocrinol. (Copenhagen), 75*, 773.
2. Rosen, V., Jung, I., Baulieu, E. E. and Robel, P. (1975): Androgen-binding proteins in human benign prostatic hypertrophy. *J. Clin. Endocrinol. Metab., 41*, 761.
3. Mobbs, B. G., Johnson, I. E. and Connolly, J. G. (1975): *In vitro* assay of androgen-binding by human prostate. *J. Steroid Biochem., 6*, 453.
4. Cowan, R. A., Cowan, S. K., Giles, C. A. and Grant, J. K. (1976): Prostatic distribution of sex hormone-binding globulin and cortisol-binding globulin in benign prostatic hyperplasia. *J. Endocrinol., 71*, 121.
5. Castaneda, E. and Liao, S. (1975): The use of anti-steroid antibodies in the characterization of steroid receptors. *J. Biol. Chem., 250*, 883.
6. Mobbs, B. G., Johnson, I. E., Connolly, J. G. and Clark, A. F. (1978): Androgen receptor assay in human benign and malignant prostatic tumour cytosol using protamine sulphate precipitation. *J. Steroid Biochem., 9*, 289.
7. Shimazaki, J., Kurihara, H., Ito, Y. and Shida, K. (1965): Testosterone metabolism in prostate: formation of androstan-17β-ol-3-one and androst-4-ene-3,17-dione, and inhibitory effect of natural and synthetic estrogens. *Gunma J. Med. Sci., 14*, 313.

8. Altwein, J. E., Rubin, A., Klose, K., Knapstein, P. and Orestano, F. (1974): Kinetik der 5-alpha-Reduktase in Prostatadenom in Gegenwart von Oestradiol, Diäthylstilböstrol, Progesteron und Gestonoron-Capronat (Depostat). *Urologe Ausg, A, 13,* 41.

9. Jenkins, J. S. and McCaffery, V. M. (1974): Effect of oestradiol-17β and progesterone estradiol-binding globulin activity in human plasma. *J. Clin. Endocrinol. 63,* 517.

10. Tan, S. Y., Antonipillai, I. and Murphy, B. E. P. (1974): Inhibition of testosterone metabolism in the human prostate. *J. Clin Endocrinol. Metab., 39,* 936.

11. Krieg, M. and Voigt, K. D. (1977): Biochemical substrate of androgenic actions at a cellular level in prostate, bulbocavernosus/levator ani and in skeletal muscle. *Acta Endocrinol., Supp. 214,* 43.

12. Rosner, W. (1972): A simplified method for the quantitative determination of testosterone-estradiol-binding globulin activity in human plasma. *J. Clin. Endocrinol. Metab., 34,* 983.

13. Forest, M. G., Rivarola, M. A. and Migeon C. J. (1968): Percentage binding of testosterone, androstenedione and dihydroisoandrosterone in human plasma. *Steroids, 12,* 323.

14. Dische, Z. (1955): Color reactions of nucleic acid components. In: *The Nucleic Acids,* 1st ed., Vol. I. Editors: S. P. Chargaff and J. N. Davidson. Academic Press, New York.

15. Layne, E. (1957): Spectrometric and turbimetric methods for measuring proteins. In: *Methods in Enzymology,* Vol. III. Editors: S. P. Colowick and N. O. Kaplan. Academic Press, New York.

16. Lowry, O. H., Rosenbrough, N. J., Farr, A. L. and Randall, R. J. (1951): Protein measurement with the Folin phenol reagent. *J. Biol. Chem., 193,* 265.

17. Chamness, G. C., Huff, K. and McGuire, W. L. (1975): Protamine-precipitated estrogen receptor: a solid-phase ligand exchange assay. *Steroids, 25,* 627.

18. Davies, P., Thomas, P. and Griffiths, K. (1977): Measurement of free and occupied cytoplasmic and nuclear androgen receptor sites in rat ventral prostate gland. *J. Endocrinol., 74,* 393.

19. Tulchinsky, D. and Chopra, I. J. (1973): Competitive ligand-binding assay for measurement of sex hormone-binding globulin (SHBG). *J. Clin. Endocrinol. Metab., 37,* 873.

20. Vendrely, R. (1955): The deoxyribonucleic acid content of the nucleus. In: *The Nucleic Acids,* 1st ed., Vol. II, p. 166. Editors: S. P. Chargaff and J. N. Davidson, Academic Press, New York.

21. Frederiksen, P., Thommesen, P., Kjaer, T. B. and Bichel, P. (1978): Flow cytometric DNA analysis in fine needle aspiration biopsies from patients with prostatic lesions. Diagnostic value and relation to clinical stages. *Acta pathol. Microbiol. Scand. Sect. A, 86,* 461.

22. Mobbs, B. G., Johnson, I. E., Connolly, J. G. and Clark, A. F. (1977): Evaluation of the use of cyproterone acetate competition to distinguish between high-affinity binding of [³H]-dihydrotestosterone to human prostate cytosol receptors and to sex hormone binding globulin. *J. Steroid Biochem., 8,* 943.

23. Robinson, M. R. G. and Thomas, B. S. (1971): Effect of hormonal therapy on plasma testosterone levels in prostatic carcinoma. *Br. Med. J., 4,* 391.

24. Sciarra, F., Sorcini, G., di Silverio, F. and Gagliardi, V. (1978): Plasma testosterone and androstenedione after orchiectomy in prostatic adrenocarcinoma. *Clin. Endocrinol. (Oxford), 2,* 101.

25. Longcope, C., Pratt, J. H., Schneider, S. H. and Fineberg, S. E. (1976): The *in vivo* metabolism of androgens by muscle and adipose tissue of normal men. *Steroids, 28,* 521.

26. Collins, W. P., Koullapis, E. N., Bridges, C. E. and Sommerville, I. F. (1970): Studies on steroid metabolism in human prostatic tissue. *J. Steroid Biochem., 1,* 195.

27. di Silverio, F., Gagliardi, V., Sorcini, G. and Sciarra, F. (1976): Biosynthesis and metabolism of androgenic hormones in cancer of the prostate. *Invest. Urol., 13,* 286.

28. Harper, M. E., Pike, A., Peeling, W. B. and Griffiths, K. (1974): Steroids of adrenal origin metabolized by human prostatic tissue both *in vivo* and *in vitro. J. Endocrinol., 60,* 117.

Discussion

M. Krieg (Hamburg, FRG): What type of carcinoma, in terms of highly differentiated or poorly differentiated carcinoma, did the samples with high receptor concentration show?

B. G. Mobbs: Three of the four carcinomas with the highest concentrations of receptor were poorly differentiated.

Androgen, oestrogen and progestogen and their distribution in epithelial and stromal cells of human prostate

N. Bashirelahi, J. D. Young, Jr., S. M. Sidh and H. Sanefuji
Department of Biochemistry, School of Dentistry and the Departments of Surgery (Division of Urology) and Pathology, School of Medicine, University of Maryland, Baltimore, Maryland, U.S.A.

Introduction

Function and growth of human prostate may be hormonally regulated by androgen, oestrogen, and progestogen. Various investigators have established the presence of cytoplasmic receptors for androstanolone [1–4], estradiol [5–16], and progesterone [17–20] in the human prostate. It is well established that the growth and function of the prostate and seminal vesicle are, in part, dependent on androgenic stimulus. Various investigators have concluded that oestrogens in a variety of species are capable of producing squamous metaplasia of epithelium and growth of the fibromuscular stroma in male sex accessory organs [21–23].

The presence of oestrogen receptors in the guinea pig prostate and in the separated epithelium and muscle of guinea pig seminal vesicles has been established [23, 24]. Furthermore, the muscle of guinea pig seminal vesicles possesses the highest level of cytosolic estradiol binding, indicating that the receptor may be primarily associated with the muscular portion of the glands. It is interesting to note that the fibromuscular portions of young, sexually mature rat seminal vesicles were selectively stimulated to grow after oestrogen treatment of castrated adrenalectomized rats [23, 25]. On the other hand, Lasnitzki [26] and Tesar and Scott [27] reported that the main effect of androgen on rat prostate is confined to the epithelial structures which become hypertrophied and functionally active. Asselin *et al.* [17] using ^{3}H-R5020 (R5020 = promegestone), a synthetic progestogen which binds to the progesterone receptor in human endometrium and myometrium (but not to corticosteroid-binding globulin (CGB)), were able to demonstrate that it binds to benign prostatic hypertrophic (BPH) tissue. On this basis they suggested the presence of progestogen-binding components or an atypical androgen receptor in human BPH cytosol. Dube *et al.* [18] have also suggested the presence of a progesterone receptor-like component in the cytosols of human benign hyperplastic prostate.

Menon *et al.* [20] compared the binding affinity of ^{3}H-R1881 (R1881 =

metribolone) and ^{3}H-R5020 by Scatchard analysis of the cytosol of human BPH, seminal vesicle, and epididymis. They detected the presence of specific high affinity sites for ^{3}H-R5020. However, the affinity for R5020 was lower than the affinity observed for R1881. Recently, Gustafsson *et al.* [19] identified a progestogen receptor in cytosol from human BPH and carcinomatous prostatic tissue using ^{3}H-R5020. They reported that the ^{3}H-R5020 receptor complex had a sedimentation coefficient of approximately 4S.

It is known that alteration in the hormonal environment causes a favourable response in hormone-dependent neoplasms such as those of the breast and prostate. However, the quality and duration of response is unpredictable. The role of oestrogen receptors in human mammary cancer as a useful marker of hormone sensitivity or resistance has been well established. Oestrogen receptor-positive breast tumours have a 55 to 60% response rate to endocrine treatment but in oestrogen receptor-negative tumours the response is only 10% [28].

The significance of oestrogen and progestogen receptor protein(s) as markers to predict the response of prostatic carcinoma to hormonal treatment remains to be established. In two separate studies conducted in our laboratory we were able to demonstrate the presence of a specific estradiol-binding protein or proteins in extents ranging from 1.4 to 126.0 fM (= M $\times$ 10^{-15})/mg protein in 33 of the 50 patients with metastatic carcinoma of the prostate [29, 30]. In these studies most patients who demonstrated the presence of a significant amount of estradiol-binding protein responded favourably to hormonal manipulation; on the other hand, patients who demonstrated low levels of oestrogen receptors and high levels of androgen-binding protein became resistant to endocrine treatment after an initial brief favourable response.

In the present study, we have measured estradiol-, androstanolone- and progesterone-binding protein(s) in epithelial and stromal cells of normal, BPH, and carcinomatous human prostates. Evidence will be presented in favour of a possible correlation between estradiol, progesterone and androstanolone receptors and hormonal treatment of prostatic carcinoma and benign hyperplasia. We will also present data to demonstrate the presence of a cytoplasmic progesterone receptor with a sedimentation coefficient of approximately 4S and 8S in both epithelial and stromal cells of human benign hyperplastic prostate.

Experimental procedures

Fresh human prostatic tissue was obtained by transurethral resection from patients with metastatic prostatic carcinoma or following retropubic operation at the University of Maryland, Maryland General and Veterans' Administration Hospitals. Prostatic chips were frozen immediately in liquid nitrogen and stored at $-70°$C in a deep freeze. In experiments using epithelial and stromal cells, the tissue was placed in saline and in an ice bath immediately after open prostatectomy. A trained surgical pathologist dissected the tissue into epithelial and stromal tissue under a dissecting microscope in a walk-in cold room (temperature 0–4°C). Prostatic specimens were frozen immediately in liquid nitrogen and stored at $-70°$C in a deep freeze. It should be mentioned that histological examination of these tissues revealed that stroma is almost free of epithelial cells while epithelial tissue contains some stromal cells. Frozen prostate tissue was pulverized and allowed to thaw in the presence of three volumes of trometamol-edetic acid (tris-EDTA) buffer (10 mM tris, 1.5 mM EDTA, 0.5 mM dithioerythritol). Pulverized and thawed tissue was homogenized with a Polytron PT 10–35 homogenizer with PT 10 probe (Brinkman Instrument Inc., Westbury, New York). The homogenate was then centrifuged at 100,000 g for 1 hour in a Beckman type 50.1 rotor. After centrifugation, the protein concentration in the super-natant (cytosol) was measured according to the method of Lowry et al. [31] using bovine serum albumin as standard.

The cytosol was incubated with ^{3}H-estradiol ((1,2,6,7-^{3}H)-estradiol), ^{3}H-R1881 (^{3}H-metribolone) or ^{3}H-R5020 (^{3}H-promegestone) in the presence or absence of 100-fold excess unlabelled competing steroids (diethylstil-boestrol (DES), androstanolone or progesterone) for 16 to 24 hours at 0–4°C. In order to differentiate the specific estradiol receptor protein from other binding proteins, excesses of both nonlabelled androstanolone and diethylstilboestrol (1×10^{-6}M) were also used.

Charcoal-dextran assays for bound steroid were performed as described by Miller et al. [32] with minor modifications. Briefly, 0.5 ml samples were incubated for 30 minutes with 0.5 ml of 2.5% charcoal, 0.25% Dextran T-40, and 2% ovalbumin in 10% (v/v) glycerol. After centrifugation for 20 minutes at 2,500 g aliquots of the supernatant fluid were taken for glycerol density gradient centrifugation and determination of radioactivity according to the method of Patterson and Greene [33] using triton X-100 and toluene.

Linear 10–30% (w/v) glycerol density gradients (5 ml volume) in cellulose nitrate tubes were prepared in TED buffer (10 mM tris, 1.5 mM EDTA, 0.5 mM dithioerythritol) using a gradient former of local manufacture and a peristaltic pump (Technicon Instrument Corporation, Tarrytown, New York). The linearity of the gradients was checked periodically by the use of a Bausch and Lomb refractometer.

Three-tenths ml of labelled unfractionated or fractionated prostate cytosol was layered on to the gradients. The sedimentation coefficients of the ^{3}H-steroid labelled binding proteins were estimated by comparison with the rate of migration of ^{14}C-protein markers added to a parallel marker tube. The parallel marker tube was prepared by layering 0.4 ml of corresponding buffer, containing 10 μl of both ^{14}C-ovalbumim and ^{14}C-gamma globulin (1,800 disintegrations per minute (DPM) per 10 μl of each ^{14}C-protein), on a separate glycerol density gradient. Gradients were centrifuged at 149,000 g for 16 hours using a Beckman SW50.1 swinging bucket rotor in a Sorvall OTD-2 ultracentrifuge. Fractions were collected by inserting a thin steel tube from the top to the bottom of the gradient and removing the glycerol density gradient with a Technicon peristaltic pump. Three drop (0.2 ml) fractions were collected directly into liquid scintillation vials. Four ml of scintillation cocktail was added to each vial and the radioactivity was measured.

For Scatchard analysis cytosol was incubated with steroid solutions con-taining radioactive steroid at concentrations ranging from 4×10^{-11}M to 2×10^{-9}M for 16–24 hours at 0-4°C. At the end of the incubation period, total radioactivity was measured using 10 μl samples. Free steroid was then extracted by the addition of 125 μl of a dextran-coated charcoal suspension (1.25 g of Norit A and 0.625 g Dextran T-40 per 100 ml TED buffer). The charcoal-cytosol mixture was incubated for 20 minutes at 0-4°C and the charcoal was then sedimented by centrifugation at 3,000 g for 20 minutes. The radioactivity in the supernatant was then measured using 100 μl samples.

The plots were corrected for nonsaturable binding as described by Chamness and McGuire [34].

Results

The initial series of experiments were carried out to characterize the binding of ^{3}H-R5020 in cytosol prepared from specimens of stroma of benign prostatic hyperplasia (Figure 1). A distinct peak of bound ^{3}H-R5020 was resolved from ^{14}C-gamma globulin and was characterized by a sedimentation coefficient of $\sim$ 8S. Binding of ^{3}H-R5020 in the 8S region was displaced completely by a 100-fold excess of unlabelled R5020 or progesterone. However, binding of ^{3}H-R5020 in the 4S region was partially reduced by a 100-fold excess of progesterone or R5020. When the binding of ^{3}H-R5020 in the presence of a 100-fold excess of unlabelled DES, progesterone and R5020 was measured displacement of the 8S region binding could be demonstrated only by progesterone and R5020 but not by DES.

In order to demonstrate that binding in the 8S region is not due to the presence of CBG, binding of ^{3}H-R5020 was compared in the presence of a 100-fold excess of unlabelled hydrocortisone or of progesterone. The results, shown in figure 2, demonstrate that progesterone, not hydrocortisone, competes for binding in the 8S region. Because ^{3}H-R1881 binds to both androgen and progestogen receptors, the specificity of binding of ^{3}H-R5020 was investigated further. It can be seen that R1881 was as effective as R5020 and progesterone in displacing ^{3}H-R5020 binding in the 8S region.

Typical saturation curves for the binding of ^{3}H-R5020 in cytosol prepared from stromal and epithelial cells of BPH specimens are shown in figures 3 and 4. Specific binding was saturable at low steroid concentrations (5 $\times$ 10^{-13}M), indicating a limited number of binding sites. The data shown in figures 5 and 6 were analysed according to the method of Scatchard and corrected for non-specific binding by the method of Chamness and McGuire [34]. Data from figure 3 indicate a corrected dissociation constant of 1.5 $\times$ 10^{-10}M (1.2 $\times$ 10^{-10}M uncorrected). The number of apparent binding sites was 7 $\times$ 10^{-15}M/mg protein (15 $\times$ 10^{-15}M/mg for uncorrected). Data in figure 4 indicate a corrected dissociation constant of 2.1 $\times$ 10^{-10}M (4.2 $\times$ 10^{-10}M uncorrected). The number of apparent binding sites was 15 $\times$ 10^{-15}M/mg protein (59 $\times$ 10^{-15}M/mg protein uncorrected).

In order to investigate steroid specificity of the R5020-binding protein, cytosols prepared from stromal and epithelial cells were incubated with 1 nM (= M $\times$ 10^{-9}) ^{3}H-R5020 in the absence or presence of a 10-, 100- and 1,000-fold excess of nonradioactive steroids. Nonspecific binding, defined as that binding not displaced by the addition of either a 100- or 1,000-fold excess of nonradioactive R5020 or progesterone, was subtracted in all instances. R5020 and progesterone were equally potent in competing for specific binding of ^{3}H-R5020 by the receptor present in the cytosol of human BPH specimens. Steroids such as estradiol and hydrocortisone and synthetic oestrogen (DES) were ineffective in inhibiting binding (Figure 5). Triamcinolone acetonide, which blocks binding to the progesterone receptors [35], was effective but not as effective as progesterone and R5020 in low concentrations. Androstanolone showed approximately 50% inhibition only at 1,000-fold excess concentration.

In the next series of experiments, the specificity of the binding of ^{3}H-progesterone was assessed in cytosol from stromal and epithelial cells of

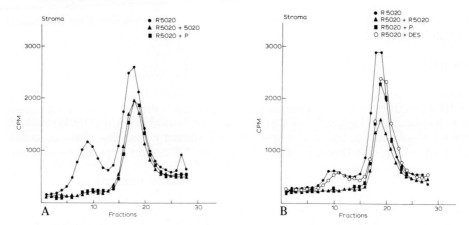

Fig. 1. Glycerol density gradient centrifugation of prostatic cytosol (stromal cells) after incubation with ³H-R5020. (A) Aliquots of cytosol were incubated for 20 hours at 0°C with 1 × 10⁻⁸M ³H-R5020 without (●——●) or with 100-fold excess unlabelled R5020 (▲——▲) or progesterone (■——■). (B) Aliquots of cytosol were incubated for 20 hours at 0°C with 1 × 10⁻⁸M ³H-R5020 in the absence (●——●) or presence of 100-fold excess unlabelled R5020 (▲——▲), progesterone (■——■) or DES (○——○). Free steroids were removed by dextran-coated charcoal treatment at 0-4°C. Aliquots of 0.3 ml were placed on 10–30% glycerol gradients, and the tubes were centrifuged at 149,000 g for 16 hours. Two hundred microlitre fractions were collected and assayed for radioactivity.

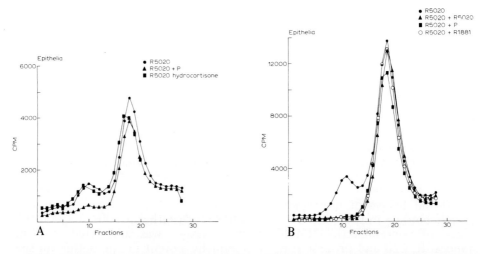

Fig. 2. Glycerol density gradient centrifugation of prostatic cytosol (epithelial cells) after incubation with ³H-R5020. (A) Aliquots of cytosol were incubated for 20 hours at 0°C with 1 × 10⁻⁸M ³H-R5020 in the absence (●——●) or presence of 100-fold excess un-labelled progesterone (▲——▲) or hydrocortisone (■——■). (B) Aliquots of cytosol were incubated for 20 hours at 0°C with 1 × 10⁻⁸M ³H-R5020 without (●——●) or with 100-fold excess unlabelled R5020 (▲——▲), progesterone (■——■) or R1881 (○——○). Free steroids were removed by dextran-coated charcoal treatment at 0-4°C. Aliquots of 0.3 ml were placed on 10–30% glycerol gradients, and the tubes were centrifuged at 149,000 g for 16 hours. Two hundred microlitre fractions were collected and assayed for radioactivity.

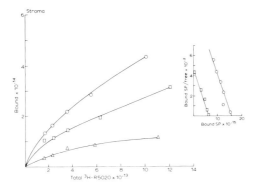

Fig. 3. Binding as a function of increasing concentration of R5020. Cytosol (from stromal tissue) was incubated for 20 hours at 0°C with 4 × 10⁻¹¹ to 2 × 10⁻⁹M ³H-R5020 in the absence or presence of a 100-fold excess of unlabelled progesterone and analysed by dextran-coated charcoal technique. Scatchard analysis of binding, data for which was corrected for non-specific binding according to the method of Chamness and McGuire [34]. The linear regression of bound:free R5020 vs. fM R5020 bound/mg cytosol protein yielded intercepts on the abcissa (binding site concentration) of 7 (15 for uncorrected). Dissociation constants estimated from the slopes of the regression equations were 1.5 × 10⁻¹⁰M (1.2 × 10⁻¹⁰M for uncorrected).

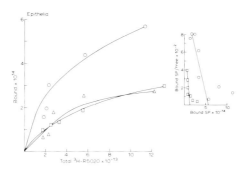

Fig. 4. Binding as a function of increasing concentration of R5020. Cytosol (from epithelial tissue) was incubated for 20 hours at 0°C with 4 × 10⁻¹¹ to 2 × 10⁻⁹M ³H-R5020 in the absence or presence of a 100-fold excess of unlabelled progesterone and analysed by dextran-coated charcoal technique. Scatchard analysis of binding, data for which was corrected for non-specific binding according to the method of Chamness and McGuire [34]. The linear regression of bound:free R5020 vs. fM R5020 bound/mg cytosol protein yielded intercepts on the abcissa (binding site concentration) of 15 (59 for uncorrected). Dissociation constants, estimated from the slopes of the regression equation, were 2.1 × 10⁻¹⁰M (4.2 × 10⁻¹⁰M for uncorrected).

human prostate. In these experiments cytosol from stromal and epithelial cells was incubated with 1 nM ³H-progesterone in the absence or presence of 10-, 100-, and 1,000-fold excesses of nonradioactive R5020, progesterone or hydrocortisone. These experiments were intended initially to demonstrate whether ³H-progesterone binds to the same protein as R5020 and secondly to investigate the specificity of progesterone-binding protein. Figure 6 shows that ³H-progesterone can compete equally with progesterone, R5020 and, to a lesser extent, triamcinolone acetonide but not with hydrocortisone.

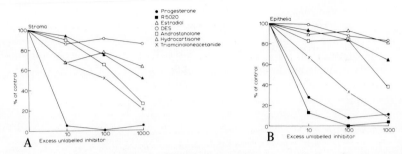

Fig. 5. *Steroid specificity of* [3]*H-R5020-binding by prostatic cytosol prepared (A) from stromal and (B) from epithelial cells. Aliquots of prostatic cytosol were incubated with 1.0 nM* [3]*H-R5020 in the absence or in the presence of 10-, 100- and 1,000-fold excess nonradioactive competing-steroid for 20 hours at 0°C. Nonspecific binding (binding not displaced by the addition of 1,000-fold excess R5020 or progesterone) was subtracted in all instances. Free steroids were removed by dextran-coated charcoal treatment at 0-4°C for 20 minutes. Dublicate aliquots of 100 μl of the supernatant were assayed for radioactivity.*

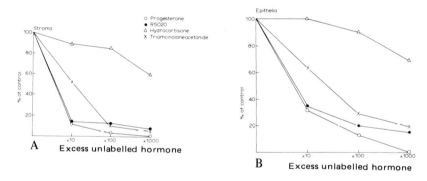

Fig. 6. *Steroid specificity of* [3]*H-progesterone-binding by prostatic cytosol prepared (A) from stromal and (B) from epithelial cells. Aliquots of prostatic cytosol were incubated with 1.0 nM* [3]*H-progesterone in the absence or presence of 10-, 100-, and 1,000-fold excess nonradioactive competing steroid for 20 hours at 0°C. Nonspecific binding (binding not displaced by addition of 1,000-fold excess R5020 or progesterone) was subtracted in all instances. Free steroids were removed by dextran-coated charcoal treatment at 0-4°C for 20 minutes. Duplicate aliquots of 100 μl of the supernatant were assayed for radioactivity.*

It should be mentioned that the results of experiments with ^{3}H-progesterone are not as consistent as the results of experiments with ^{3}H-R5020. The problem may be due to the fact that ^{3}H-progesterone is metabolized readily or that the receptor is more heat sensitive than androgen and oestrogen receptors under our experimental conditions.

In the next series of experiments, we have measured the concentration of oestrogen, androgen, and progesterone receptors in normal, BPH, and carcinomatous prostates.

Table I is a tabulation of the oestrogen receptor concentration (fM/mg protein) in immediate autopsy (normal prostate). It can be seen from this very small sample of true normal human prostates that there are measurable amounts of oestrogen receptor in both stromal and epithelial cells.

Table II shows androgen receptor concentrations in the same group of individuals with normal prostates. It can be seen that androgen receptor is present in both stromal and epithelial cells. It is possible that the concentration of free receptor is not very large due to the high concentration of circulating androgen. Table III records oestrogen receptor concentrations in the prostatic cytosols of 29 BPH patients of age ranging from 56 to 83

Table I Oestrogen receptor concentration (fM/mg protein). Immediate autopsy (normal prostate).

Patient no.	Age	Specific binding (100-fold excess estradiol)		Specific binding (100-fold excess DES)	
		Epithelium	Stroma	Epithelium	Stroma
1.	20	5.4	52.4	6.1	26.7
2.	28	7.8	14.0	0	0
3.	30	–	–	–	74.0
4.	33	*14.3	*9.8	*4.2	*20.3
5.	48	–	–	15.9	3.8
6.	58	2.4	0	1.6	0

Cytosols were prepared from epithelial and stromal tissue or from whole tissue (not dissected) human prostate and incubated with 1×10^{-8}M ^{3}H-estradiol (91.8 Ci/mM) for 18–24 hours at 2-4°C. The reaction was stopped by addition of an equal volume of dextran-coated charcoal followed by a twenty minute incubation at 0°C. The suspension was then centrifuged for twenty minutes at 3,079 g in a refrigerated centrifuge. The radioactivity in the supernatant was measured. Specific binding was determined by the difference between values obtained in the absence or presence of a 100-fold excess unlabelled steroid. Asterisks indicate the presence of 1×10^{-6}M unlabelled androstanolone in the incubation medium to saturate SHBG.

Table II Androgen receptor concentration (fM/mg protein). Immediate autopsy (normal prostate).

Patient no.	Age	Specific binding (100-fold excess R1881)		Specific binding (100-fold excess androstanolone)	
		Epithelium	Stroma	Epithelium	Stroma
1.	20	24.3	15.5	18.6	7.3
2.	28	12.0	14.0	–	–
3.	30	0.0	0.0	–	–
4.	33	6.9	14.3	7.0	13.0
5.	48	51.2	50.0	–	–
6.	58	6.7	15.4	14.8	7.0

Cytosol from fresh and frozen human prostate was prepared and incubated with 1×10^{-8}M (^{3}H-R1881) (87.0 Ci/mM) in the presence or absence of a 100-fold excess unlabelled hormone. The free steroid was removed by dextran-coated charcoal treatment for 20 minutes at 0-4°C. The suspension was centrifuged for 20 minutes at 2,500 g under refrigeration and the radioactivity in the supernatant was measured. Specific binding was determined by subtracting nonspecific binding (in the presence of a 100-fold excess of unlabelled steroid) from total binding in the absence of unlabelled steroid.

years. On the basis of these results, there may be more oestrogen receptors in the samples of stromal cells than in those of epithelial cells. Table IV lists androgen receptor concentrations in prostatic cytosols of the same 29 patients with BPH. It can be seen that both stromal and epithelial cells contain androgen receptors but there may be more androgen receptor in epithelial than in stromal cells. Table V shows progesterone receptor concentrations (as measured with ^{3}H-R5020) in prostatic cytosols of 12 BPH patients with ages ranging from 61 to 76 years. It can be seen that, as with oestrogen and androgen receptors, there is a progesterone receptor in both epithelial and stromal cells. However, as with oestrogen receptor, there may be more progesterone receptor in stromal than in epithelial cells.

Twelve patients with metastatic carcinoma of the prostate were analysed for estradiol, androstanolone and progesterone receptor proteins. In all but one patient receptor protein assays were performed prior to hormonal manipulation with either DES, 1–3 mg orally/day, or bilateral orchiectomy or

Table III   Oestrogen receptor concentration (fM/mg protein) in patients with benign prostatic hypertrophy.

Patient no.	Age	Specific binding (100-fold excess R1881)			Specific binding (100-fold excess androstanolone)		
		Epithelium	Stroma	Whole	Epithelium	Stroma	Whole
1.	56	—	—	—	*3.9	*19.0	—
2.	58	*9.8	*26.6	—	0	0	—
3.	61	—	—	—	*9.2	*16.0	*7.1
4.	63	*16.1	*25.0	—	13.7	25.1	—
5.	63	0	0	—	0	0	—
6.	64	*1.7	*12.6	—	*0	*3.2	—
7.	64	—	—	—	0	9.1	—
8.	66	—	—	—	*4.0	*35.0	*18.9
9.	68	*0	*0	—	*5.3	*0	—
10.	68	7.4	—	—	10.1	0	—
11.	68	—	—	—	1.3	7.0	—
12.	68	—	—	—	*42.3	—	—
13.	69	—	—	—	*5.0	*57.0	*1.0
14.	70	—	—	—	*29.3	*6.1	*18.9
15.	70	—	—	—	*5.0	*5.0	*26.0
16.	71	—	—	—	*0	*0	*3.0
17.	72	*8.4	*15.0	—	—	—	—
18.	72	0	5.0	—	2.2	3.8	—
19.	72	*0	*21.7	—	*0	*7.4	—
20.	73	*10.6	*20.2	—	*5.0	*10.2	—
21.	73	—	—	—	*0	*75.8	*26.4
22.	74	—	—	—	*4.0	*1.1	—
23.	75	—	*18.3	—	—	*3.4	—
24.	75	7.3	7.4	—	0	0	—
25.	76	—	*69.1	—	—	*27.6	—
26.	76	—	—	—	*14.9	*3.3	—
27.	82	—	—	—	*0	*111.8	*35.4
28.	82	6.9	15.9	—	13.0	11.7	—
29.	83	8.2	—	—	0	31.3	—

Experimental conditions were as described for Table II.

both. The patients were followed for a minimum of 6 months and were classified into three groups, depending upon the response to endocrine therapy. In Group I there were 5 patients, who showed both subjective and objective regression of disease. Group II consisted of 2 patients, who showed some subjective regression of symptoms but no objective regression or progression of the disease. Group III included another 5 patients, whose disease progressed both subjectively and objectively.

Table VI shows the oestrogen, androgen, and progesterone receptor protein concentrations for Group I patients. Binding sites for estradiol were measurable in 4 patients and ranged from 8.6 to 87.2 fM/mg protein. Patient E.I., marked with an asterisk, responded remarkably well to DES therapy with relief of pain, regression of growth locally and stabilization of metastasis for about 3 years before developing recurrent symptoms requiring transurethral resection of the prostate. The receptor protein analysis, at this time, showed very high (87.2 fM/mg protein) estradiol binding sites.

Table IV   Androgen receptor concentration (fM/mg protein). Patients with benign prostatic hypertrophy.

Patient no.	Age	Specific binding (100-fold excess R1881)			Specific binding (100-fold excess androstanolone)		
		Epithelium	Stroma	Whole	Epithelium	Stroma	Whole
1.	56	97.6	101.4	—	52.8	15.0	—
2.	58	167.7	91.1	—	110.0	49.0	—
3.	61	—	—	—	33.8	27.1	39.6
4.	63	*140.3	*92.5	—	*63.5	*57.3	—
5.	63	19.0	—	—	—	—	—
6.	64	32.1	29.8	—	19.8	10.0	—
7.	64	27.1	14.9	—	19.4	0	—
8.	66	—	—	—	1.0	23.2	43.2
9.	68	0	0	—	0.1	0	—
10.	68	10.0	0	—	—	—	—
11.	68	84.0	90.0	—	44.0	42.0	—
12.	68	—	—	—	106.1	—	—
13.	69	—	—	—	63.0	0.0	0.0
14.	70	66.7	119.7	103.9	95.8	101.6	59.4
15.	70	—	—	—	7.0	3.0	12.0
16.	71	—	—	—	5.0	0	0
17.	72	124.9	74.1	—	52.0	2.0	—
18.	72	0	0	—	—	—	—
19.	72	10.6	130.3	—	0	67.7	—
20.	73	113.5	51.1	—	57.7	29.2	—
21.	73	—	—	—	26.6	82.9	24.0
22.	74	71.1	106.0	—	34.1	30.0	—
23.	75	—	—	—	6.0	—	—
24.	75	0	0	—	—	—	—
25.	76	—	—	—	32.5	—	—
26.	76	—	—	—	110.6	92.3	—
27.	82	—	—	—	115.4	130.7	90.3
28.	82	0	—	—	—	—	—
29.	83	0	0	—	—	—	—

Experimental conditions were as described for Table II.

Table V   Progesterone receptor concentration (fM/mg protein). Patients with benign prostatic hypertrophy.

Patient no.	Age	Specific binding (100-fold excess R5020)			Specific binding (100-fold excess progesterone)		
		Epithelium	Stroma	Whole	Epithelium	Stroma	Whole
1.	61	56.1	0	64.5	95.6	0	9.1
2.	64	23.4	11.0	–	24.0	21.9	–
3.	66	0	18.8	47.7	34.2	73.0	11.5
4.	68	0	30.6	–	0	57.5	–
5.	69	88.0	29.0	24.0	87.0	32.0	40.0
6.	70	21.4	72.9	34.7	38.1	68.4	68.9
7.	70	15.0	9.0	8.0	11.0	45.0	13.0
8.	71	28.0	10.0	37.0	37.0	36.0	34.0
9.	72	1.6	190.7	–	26.8	163.0	–
10.	73	0	0.4	–	0.1	0.7	–
11.	75	0	21.1	–	0.5	22.7	–
12.	76	36.1	9.3	–	51.5	54.7	–

Cytosol from fresh and frozen human prostate was prepared and incubated with 1×10^{-8}M $(6,7\text{-}^3\text{H})$-R5020 (87.0 Ci/mM) in the presence of a 100-fold excess of unlabelled hormone. Free steroid was removed with dextran-coated charcoal for 20 minutes at $0\text{-}4^\circ\text{C}$. The suspension was centrifuged for 20 minutes at 2,500 g in a refrigerated centrifuge, and the radioactivity in the supernatant was measured. Specific binding was determined by the difference between values obtained in the absence and in the presence of a 100-fold excess of unlabelled hormone.

Table VI   Oestrogen, androgen and progesterone receptors (fM/mg protein) in hormone sensitive patients (Group I).

Patient no.	Specific binding (^{3}H-estradiol) (100-fold excess DES)	Specific binding (^{3}H-R1881) (100-fold excess androstanolone)	Specific binding (^{3}H-R5020) (100-fold excess progesterone)
1. D.J.	57.6	26.0	–
2. L.B.	20.5	28.2	11.5
3. L.H.	8.6	35.0	18.8
4. E.I.*	87.2	–	–
5. A.B.**	0.0	0.0	10.0

* Treated with DES (3 mg/day) for 3 years prior to receptor protein assay.
** Treated with DES (3 mg/day) for 8 months prior to receptor protein assay.
Cytosol from fresh and frozen human prostate was prepared and incubated with 1×10^{-8} M ^{3}H-estradiol (91.8 Ci/mM), 1×10^{-8} M ^{3}H-R1881 (87.0 Ci/mM) or 1×10^{-8} M ^{3}H-R5020 (87.0 Ci/mM), in the presence or absence of a 100-fold excess of unlabelled hormone. The free steroid was removed with dextran-coated charcoal treatment for 20 minutes at $0\text{-}4^\circ\text{C}$. The suspension was centrifuged for 20 minutes at 2,500 g in a refrigerated centrifuge and the radioactivity in the supernatant was measured. Specific binding was determined by the difference between values obtained in the absence or presence of a 100-fold excess of unlabelled hormone.

Table VII Oestrogen, androgen and progesterone receptors (fM/mg protein) in patients with no regression/progresssion on hormone (Group II).

Patient no.	Specific binding (^{3}H-estradiol) (100-fold excess estradiol)*	Specific binding (^{3}H-estradiol) (100-fold excess DES)	Specific binding (^{3}H-R1881) (100-fold excess androstanolone)	Specific binding (^{3}H-R1881) (100-fold excess progesterone)
1. M.J.	0.0	0.0	52.8	–
2. S.L.	6.6	0.0	15.2	12.0

Experimental conditions were as described for Table VI. Asterisk indicates presence of unlabelled androstanolone in incubation medium to saturate SHBG.

Both patients in Group II showed significantly higher androstanolone binding than estradiol binding, which was not measurable in the presence of excess DES (Table VII). All patients in Group III also showed significantly higher androstanolone-binding concentrations than estradiol-binding protein concentrations (Table VIII).

When one considers the results obtained for androstanolone receptor protein in columns three and four of Tables VII and VIII, it is interesting to note that when progesterone was substituted for androstanolone as a competing steroid values for androstanolone-binding sites were lower. This indicates that R1881 binds to some other proteins (such as progesterone-binding protein) besides androstanolone receptor. Thus the values shown in column three are representative of a specific androstanolone receptor protein. At the same time one can also extrapolate the concentration of progesterone receptor protein as shown in column four.

Table VIII Oestrogen, androgen and progestogen receptors (fM/mg protein) in patients resistant to hormone (Group III).

Patient no.	Specific binding (^{3}H-estradiol) (100-fold excess estradiol)***	Specific binding (^{3}H-estradiol) (100-fold excess excess DES)	Specific binding (^{3}H-R1881) (100-fold excess androstanolone)	Specific binding (^{3}H-R1881) (100-fold excess progesterone)
1. E.H.*	0.2	5.6	131.4	89.4
2. L.L.	9.7	3.8	24.3	6.4
3. A.C.**	0.0	0.0	65.2	30.5
4. J.B.	–	4.8	27.1	–
5. R.J.	–	0.0	47.0	21.0+

* Bil. hydro-uretero nephrosis and paraplegia secondary to pathological fracture T12, L1.
** Died 1 year after diagnosis (urinary obstruction and sepsis).
*** Indicates presence of unlabelled androstanolone in incubation medium to saturate SHBG.
+ Progesterone receptor was measured by using ^{3}H-R5020 competed with unlabelled progesterone.
Experimental conditions were as described for Table VI.

Discussion

Progestational agents like cyproterone acetate have been used in benign prostatic hyperplasia as well as prostatic carcinoma with some success [36–38]. Cytosol extracts prepared from BPH contain a specific progesterone receptor that is completely destroyed by heating to 50°C for 15 minutes (results are not presented in this report). On glycerol density gradient centrifugation, the receptor sediments in the 8S and 4S regions (mostly in 8S). This binding protein has the characteristics of a true receptor: steroid specificity, heat lability, protein nature (results are not presented in this report), 8S sedimentation coefficient and saturability and high affinity binding.

Oestrogen is known to regulate the activity of progesterone receptor in several target tissues [39–41] and the presence of the cytosol receptor characterized here in human prostate, especially in stromal tissue of human prostate may indicate that oestrogen has a primary role in modulating the growth and function of this organ and is in complete agreement with our previous findings concerning the presence of oestrogen receptor in the human prostate. Thus the presence of both progesterone and estradiol receptors in the human prostate may prove to be of considerable importance in elucidating the mechanism of BPH.

It is generally believed that favourable response to oestrogen therapy in hormone sensitive prostatic carcinoma is mediated primarily via suppression of the hypothalamo-hypophyseal axis, thus reducing the circulating androgens. In addition, Mangan *et al.* [42] have proposed a direct action of oestrogen on prostatic carcinoma. If one supposes that the indirect and direct actions of oestrogen in prostatic carcinoma are brought about by reduction in androgen level and the presence of androgen receptors respectively, then tumours from patients responding to endocrine ablative therapy should contain a significant concentration of androgen receptors. Wagner [15] compared receptor pattern with response to endocrine treatment in 11 patients with prostatic carcinoma but failed to show any correlation between androgen (and oestrogen) receptor content and tumour response to endocrine treatment. Only 3 of the 5 patients whose tumours regressed demonstrated measurable androgen receptors.

The results reported in the present study were obtained by using transurethral resection (TUR) specimens. The following points should be made:
 a) the prostatic chips used for receptor assay were of large size,
 b) the charred sections were removed,
 c) pathological diagnoses were made in random fashion on these chips.

In spite of all these precautions there are serious reservations concerning the use of TUR samples but, since radical prostatectomy is not carried out routinely in carcinoma of the prostate, the only other option is the use of needle biopsy samples. However, at the present time, experimental limitations do not allow receptor measurements on needle biopsies. Until that time, we are restricted to the use of TUR specimens.

All 7 patients (of Groups II and III combined) who failed to show objective response to hormonal manipulation as judged by increase in size of primary lesion, elevation of serum acid phosphatase, appearance of lower ureteral obstruction, or new metastatic lesions on bone scan demonstrated significantly high levels of androstanolone receptor protein(s) compared with the level of estradiol receptor protein(s). These results are in agreement with the report of Wagner [15] quoted above. Several other investigators have reported significantly high amounts of assayable androstanolone receptor sites in patients with poorly differentiated tumours and progressive metastatic disease [12, 43].

The presence of a specific estradiol receptor protein in prostatic carcinoma has come to light only recently [7, 8, 9, 14]. We were able to demonstrate it in significant quantity (> 3.5 fM/mg protein) in 8 of the 10 patients in this study. In 4 (50%), the receptor content exceeded 25 fM/mg cytosol protein (Tables VI, VII, VIII).

It is interesting to note that the 4 patients of Group I who responded to endocrine treatment (as judged by decrease in size of primary lesion, relief of pain in metastatic site, stabilization of acid phosphatase and bone metastasis) demonstrated significantly higher oestrogen receptor contents (8.6 to 87.2 fM/mg protein) as compared with the 7 patients of Group II and III combined who failed to respond objectively to such treatment. In 4 of these 7 patients, oestrogen receptor protein was not present in measurable quantity when assays were carried out with DES as a competing steroid and in the other 3 it ranged from 3.8 to 5.6 fM/mg cytosol protein. Based on these preliminary findings, it appears that patients who demonstrate absence or insignificant amounts of oestrogen receptor protein, and/or high androgen receptor content, fail to respond to additive endocrine therapy for any significant length of time. Perhaps they may respond better and more predictably to combination chemotherapy, or other available therapeutic modalities.

We have not treated any of the progesterone receptor-positive patients with progestational agents and are presently unable to predict whether these patients would have responded to such therapy. It would be of interest to investigate whether oestrogen controls the level of progesterone receptor in the human prostate, as is shown to be the case in female reproductive organs.

References

1. Hansson, V., Tveter, K. J., Attramadal, A. C. and Torgenson, O. (1971): Androgenic receptors in human benign nodular prostatic hyperplasia. *Acta Endocrinol. (Copenhagen), 68,* 79–83.
2. Mainwaring, W. I. P. and Milroy, E. J. G. (1973): Characterization of the specific androgen receptors in the human prostate gland. *J. Endocrinol., 57,* 371–374.
3. Davies, P. and Griffiths, K. (1975): Similarities between 5α-dihydrotestosterone receptor complexes from human and rat prostatic tissue: Effect on RNA polymerase activity. *Mol. Cell. Endocrinol., 3,* 143–164.
4. Davies, P. and Griffiths, K. (1974): Further studies on the stimulation of prostatic ribonucleic acid polymerase by the 5α-dihydrotestosterone receptor. *J. Endocrinol., 62,* 385–400.
5. Bashirelahi, N. and Armstrong, E. G. (1975): 17β-Estradiol binding by human prostate. In: *Normal and abnormal growth of the prostate,* Vol. II, p. 632–649. Editor: M. Goland. Thomas, Springfield, Illinois.
6. Hawkins, E. F., Nijs, M., Brassinne, C. and Tagnon, H. J. (1975): Steroid receptors in the human prostate. 1. Estradiol-17β binding in benign prostatic hypertrophy. *Steroids, 26,* 458–469.
7. Hawkins, E. F., Nijs, M. and Brassinne, C. (1976): Steroid receptors in human prostate. 2. Some properties of the estrophilic molecule of benign prostatic hypertrophy. *Biochem. Biophys. Res. Commun., 70,* 854–861.
8. Wagner, R. K., Schulze, K. H. and Jungblut, P. W. (1975): Estrogen and androgen receptor in human prostate and prostatic tumor tissue. *Acta Endocrinol. (Copen-*

hagen), Suppl. 193, Abstract 52.

9. Bashirelahi, N. and Young Jr., J. D. (1976): Specific binding protein for 17β-estradiol in prostate with adenocarcinoma. Urology, 8, 553–558.

10. Bashirelahi, N., O'Toole, J. H. and Young, J. D. (1976): A specific 17β-estradiol receptor in human benign hypertrophic prostate. Biochem. Med. 15, 254–261.

11. Bashirelahi, N., Kneussl, E. S., Vassil, T. C. and Young Jr., J. D. (1979): Measurement and characterization of estrogen receptors in the human prostate. In: Progress in Clinical and Biological Research, Prostate Cancer and Hormone Receptors, Vol. 33, pp. 65–84. Editors: G. P. Murphy and A. A. Sandberg. Alan R. Liss, Inc., New York.

12. Krieg, M., Grobe, I., Voigt, K. D., Altenähr, E. and Klosterhelfen, H. (1978): Human prostatic carcinoma: Significant differences in its androgen binding and metabolism compared to human benign prostatic hypertrophy. Acta Endocrinol. (Copenhagen), 88, 397–407.

13. Pertshuk, L. P., Zava, D. T., Gaetjens, E., Macchia, R. J., Brigati, D. J. and Kim, D. S. (1978): Detection of androgen and estrogen receptors in human prostatic carcinoma and hyperplasia by fluorescence microscopy. Res. Commun. Chem. Pathol. Pharmacol., 22, 427–430.

14. Pertshuk, L. P., Zava, D. T., Tobin, E. H., Brigati, D. T., Gaetjens, E., Macchia, R. J., Wise, G. J., Wax, H. S. and Kim, D. S. (1979): Histochemical detection of steroid hormone receptors in the human prostate. In: Progress in Clinical and Biological Research, Prostate Cancer and Hormone Receptors, Vol. 33, pp. 113–132. Editors: G. P. Murphy and A. A. Sandberg. Alan R. Liss, Inc., New York.

15. Wagner, R. K. (1978): Extracellular and intracellular steroid binding proteins. Properties, discrimination, assay and clinical application. Acta Endocrinol. (Copenhagen), 218 (Suppl. 1), 1–73.

16. Karr, J. P., Wajsman, Z., Madajewicz, S., Kirdani, R. Y., Murphy, G. P. and Sandberg, A. A. (1979): Steroid hormone receptors in the prostate. J. Urol. (in press).

17. Asselin, J., Labrie, F., Gourdeau, Y., Bonne, C. and Raynaud, J. P. (1976): Binding of [³H]methyltrienolone (R1881) in rat prostate and human benign prostatic hypertrophy (BPH). Steroids, 28, 449–459.

18. Dube, J. Y., Chapdelaine, P., Tremblay, R. R., Bonne, C. and Raynaud, J. P. (1976): Comparative binding specifictity of methyltrienolone in human and rat prostate. Horm. Res., 7, 341–347.

19. Gustafsson, J. A., Ekman, P., Pousette, A., Snochowski, M. and Hogberg, B. (1978): Demonstration of a progestin receptor in human benign prostatic hyperplasia and prostatic carcinoma. Invest. Urol., 15, 361–366.

20. Menon, M., Tananis, C. E., Hicks, L., Hawkins, E. F., McLoughlin, M. G. and Walsh, P. C. (1978): Characterization of the binding of a potent synthetic androgen, methyltrienolone to human tissue. J. Clin. Invest., 61, 150–162.

21. Emmens, C. W. and Parkes, A. S. (1947): Effect of exogenous estrogens on the male mammal. Vitam. Horm. (N.Y.), 5, 233–272.

22. Price, D. and Williams-Ashman, H. G. (1961): The accessory reproductive glands of mammals. In: Sex and internal secretions, 3rd ed., p. 366. Editor: W. C. Young. The Williams and Wilkins Co., Baltimore.

23. Mawhinney, M. G. and Belis, J. A. (1975): Androgens and estrogens in prostatic neoplasia. In: Advances in sex hormone research, Vol. II, p. 141–209. Editors: J. A. Thomas and R. L. Singhal. University Park Press, Baltimore.

24. Belis, J. A., Blume, C. D. and Mawhinney, M. G. (1977): Androgen and estrogen binding in guinea pig accessory sex organs. Endocrinology, 101, 726–740.

25. Tisell, L. E. (1971): Growth of the ventral prostate, the dorsolateral prostate, the coagulating glands and the seminal vesicles in castrated and adrenalectomized rats injected with oestradiol and/or cortisone. Acta Endocrinol. (Copenhagen), 68, 485–501.

26. Lasnitzki, I. (1974): The effect of hormones on rat prostatic epithelium in organ culture. In: Normal and abnormal growth of the prostate, Vol. I, p. 29–54. Editor: M. Goland. Thomas, Springfield, Illinois.

27. Tesar, C. and Scott, W. W. (1964): A search for inhibition of prostate stimulations. *Invest. Urol., 1,* 482–498.
28. Osborne, C. K. and McGuire, W. L. (1978): Current use of steroid hormone receptor assays in the treatment of breast cancer. *Surg. Clin. North Am., 58,* 777–788.
29. Sidh, S. M., Young Jr., J. D., Karmi, S. A., Powder, J. R. and Bashirelahi, N. (1979): Adenocarcinoma of prostate: role of 17β-estradiol and 5α-dihydrotestosterone binding proteins. *Urology, 13,* 597–603.
30. Young Jr., J. D., Sidh, S. M. and Bashirelahi, N. (1979): The role of estrogen, androgen and progestogen receptors in the management of carcinoma of the prostate. *Trans. Am. Assoc. Genitourinary Surgeons, 71,* 23–25.
31. Lowry, O. H., Rosebrough, N. J., Fass, A. A. and Randall, R. J. (1951): Protein measurement with the folin phenol reagent. *J. Biol. Chem., 193,* 265–275.
32. Miller, L. K., Diaz, S. C. and Sherman, M. R. (1975): Steroid-receptor quantitation and characterization by electrophoresis in highly cross linked polyacrylamide gels. *Biochemistry, 14,* 4433–4443.
33. Patterson, M. S. and Greene, R. C. (1965): Measurement of low energy beta-emitters in aqueous solution by liquid scintillation counting of emulsions. *Anal. Chem., 37,* 854–874.
34. Chamness, G. C. and McGuire, W. L. (1975): Scatchard Plots: Common errors in correction and interpretation. *Steroids, 26,* 538–542.
35. Zava, D. T., Landrum, B., Horwitz, K. B. and McGuire, W. L. (1978): Measurement of androgen receptor with [^{3}H]methyltrienolone in systems containing both androgen and progesterone receptors. *Clin. Res., 26,* 315A (Abstract).
36. Smith, R. B., Walsh, P. C. and Goodwin, W. E. (1973): Cyproterone acetate in the treatment of the prostate. *J. Urol., 110,* 106–108.
37. Geller, J. and Vazakas, G. (1968): The effect of cyproterone acetate on advanced carcinoma of the prostate. *Surg. Gynecol. Obstet., 27,* 748–758.
38. Popelier, G. (1973): Behandlung des Prostata-Karzinoms mit Gestagen. *Urologe Ausg. A, 12,* 134–139.
39. Baulieu, E. E., Alberga, A., Jung, I., Lebeau, M. C., Mercier-Bodard, C., Milgrom, E., Raynaud, J. P., Raynaud-Jammet, C., Rochefort, H., Truong, H. and Robel, P. (1971): Metabolism and protein binding of sex steroids in target organs: An approach to the mechanism of hormone action. In: *Recent progess in hormone research,* Vol. 27, p. 351–419. Editor: E. B. Astwood. Academic Press, New York.
40. Horwitz, K. B. and McGuire, W. L. (1977): Estrogen and progesterone: Their relationship in hormone-dependent breast cancer. In: *Progesterone receptors in normal and neoplastic tissues,* p. 103–124. Editors: McGuire, W. L., Raynaud, J. P., Baulieu, E. E. Raven Press, New York.
41. Toft, D. O. and O'Malley, B. W. (1972): Target tissue receptors for progesterone, the influence of estrogen treatment. *Endocrinology, 99,* 1041–1045.
42. Mangan, F. R., Neal, G. E. and Williams, D. C. (1976): The effects of diethylstilbestrol and castration on the nucleic acid and protein metabolism of rat prostate gland. *Biochem. J., 104,* 1075–1081.
43. Walsh, P. C., Greco, J. M., Tananis, C. E., Hicks, L. L., McLoughlin, M. G. and Menon, M. (1978): The binding of a potent synthetic androgen methyltrienolone (R1881) to cytosol preparations of human prostatic cancer. *Trans. Am. Assoc. Genitourinary Surgeons, 69,* 78–80.

Discussion

R. Ghanadian (London, U.K.): Have you labelled your progesterone receptor with ^{3}H-progesterone? If not, is it justified to call it progesterone receptor? Your binding is only a binding to R5020 which competes with progesterone. O'Mally and his co-workers have demonstrated progesterone receptor by labelling with ^{3}H-progesterone in chick oviduct, so technically it is possible to demonstrate it.

N. Bashirelahi: Yes, we have used ³H-progesterone as a ligand and it does bind to progesterone receptor protein(s). However, the results are not as consistent as with ³H-R5020.

R. Ghanadian: Have you performed any experiment at temperatures over 0°C?

N. Bashirelahi: All experiments were performed at temperatures 0-4°C.

N. Pfitzenmaier (Heidelberg, FRG): You have shown some investigations concerning oestrogen receptor and dihydrotestosterone receptor in normals. How long after death have you investigated the normal prostates?

N. Bashirelahi: The normal prostates (immediate autopsy) were harvested within 5 hours of cerebral death. During the harvesting the patients were maintained on artificial respiration and infused crystalloid and colloid solutions to keep the systolic blood pressure in the range of 100–120 mm of mercury.

J. Poortman (Utrecht, The Netherlands): Sucrose-gradient profiles show two peaks for R5020: one peak can be abolished by an excess of cold R5020, the second peak can not be abolished. If you change to a DCC-assay, this second peak contributes in your assay as an aspecific amount. So all your DCC-data are too high.

N. Bashirelahi: Results of our experiments with DCC-assay are in complete agreement with our results with sucrose density gradient experiments.

Steroid receptors in metastases of prostatic cancer

F. A. G. Teulings, J. Alexieva-Figusch*, M. S. Henkelman, H. Portengen and
H. A. van Gilse*
*Departments of Biochemistry and *Clinical Endocrinology, Rotterdamsch
Radio-Therapeutisch Instituut, Dr. Daniel den Hoed Kliniek, Rotterdam,
The Netherlands*

Introduction

It is known that non-cancerous as well as cancerous cells are present in prostatic cancer tissues. In studying the presence of hormone receptors using biochemical methods there is doubt whether the receptor originates from malignant cells or not. This problem can be overcome by studying metastatic deposits of prostatic cancer, such as those present in lymph node tissues.

Oestrogen therapy is the standard treatment for advanced prostatic cancer. However, not all cancers respond to oestrogens. The effectiveness of alternative hormonal therapies with medroxyprogesterone acetate (MPA) or cyproterone acetate (CA) is therefore being studied clinically. Although several interactions of these substances with androgen biosynthesis or metabolism, as well as their pharmacological effects [1], are known – and are, in fact, the underlying reasons for the clinical trials – it is not known whether receptors in the cancer cells are of crucial importance for tumour regression. It is of importance, therefore, to know whether or not a particular steroid can bind with high affinity to the receptors in prostatic cancer. It was possible to make some observations in this respect for the androgen receptor present in a lymph node metastasis, using sucrose gradient centrifugation.

Low temperature agar-gel electrophoresis according to Wagner [2] was the method of choice for studying receptors simultaneously. By this method an estimate of the tumour sex hormone-binding globulin (SHBG) content can also be made. During our studies we observed that tumours obtained from patients during oestrogen therapy contain high levels of SHBG. The significance of this observation in oestrogen therapy of prostatic cancer will be discussed.

Materials and methods

Immediately after excision tumour tissues were quickly frozen and kept at

−70°C until analysis. [2,4,6,7-^{3}H]-oestradiol, 90−115 Ci/mmol, [1,2,4,5,6,7-^{3}H]-androstanolone (DHT), 110−150 Ci/mmol, [6,7-^{3}H]-dexamethasone, 35−50 Ci/mmol and (17α-methyl-^{3}H)-promegestone (^{3}H-R5020), 70−87 Ci/mmol were obtained from NEN-Chemicals (Federal Republic of Germany (FRG)). Unlabelled steroids and other chemicals of analytical grade were obtained from Merck (FRG), Serva (FRG) or Sigma (USA).

For analysis, frozen tissue was powdered under liquid nitrogen (Micro-dismembrator, Braun-Melsungen, FRG) and homogenized in TED buffer (10 mM tris, 1.5 mM EDTA, 0.5 mM dithioerythritol, pH 7.5). Cytosol was obtained by ultracentrifugation (Beckman L2-65B, 65 Ti rotor, 100,000 g, 60 minutes, 2°C). Samples were prepared by incubation of cytosol with ^{3}H-steroids for 2 hours at 4°C. Incubation concentrations of ^{3}H ligands were: oestradiol (E) 10 nM, DHT 30 nM, dexamethasone (D) 10 nM and R-5020 10 nM. Samples for correction of non-specific binding were prepared by adding a 200-fold excess of unlabelled diethylstilboestrol (DES) or a 100-fold excess of DHT, D or R-5020, respectively, to a duplicate sample. E and DHT samples were treated after incubation with charcoal-dextran (0.5% w/v charcoal A, 0.05% Dextran T 70 and 0.1% gelatine in TED-buffer) for 90 minutes and R-5020 samples were treated for 15 minutes to reduce albumin binding [3]. Agar-gel electrophoresis was performed on 0.05 ml samples for 90 minutes (21 V/cm, 130 mA, 4°C). After electrophoresis, agar slabs were cut into 9 fractions at the cathodic side and 7 fractions at the anodic side of the origin. The agar fractions were counted for 4 minutes using liquid scintillation counting. Receptor concentrations were expressed in fmol ml cytosol. From protein (Lowry) and albumin (immuno diffusion plates, Behring, FRG) concentrations the tumour-protein concentration was estimated, assuming a plasma-albumin concentration of 60%.

For density gradient centrifugation experiments a linear 5−20% sucrose gradient containing 10% glycerol was prepared in buffer (1.5 mM EDTA, 10 mM tris, 12 mM monothioglycerol and 10% glycerol v/v, pH 7.4). Samples were prepared by incubating cytosol with 10^{-8} M ^{3}H-DHT, with or without an excess of unlabelled competitor, for 2 hours at 4°C. After incubation, samples were treated for 15 minutes with dextran-charcoal. The ultracentrifuge run was made for 16.5 hours (Beckman SW-50 rotor, 50,000 revolutions per minute (rpm), 2°C). Thirty-two fractions of 6 drops were collected.

Results and discussion

Receptors in lymph node metastases

Six lymph node metastases of prostatic cancer were investigated. In comparison with metastatic deposits in 27 postmenopausal breast cancers (Table I) it is striking that the oestrogen and progesterone receptors are present in significantly lower amounts. The dominant receptor in prostatic cancer appears to be the androgen receptor. If steroid hormone receptors are involved in hormonal therapy of prostatic cancer, one should, therefore, look primarily to see if androgen receptors are present. All patients from whom lymph node metastases were obtained were subsequently treated with hormonal therapy (Table II). Patients A and B had high levels of androgen receptor as well as of some of the other receptors. Both patients appeared to respond well to therapy. Patients C and D were treated with MPA. Although significant amounts of androgen receptor were present no objective

Table I Receptor, SHBG and protein concentrations in lymph node deposits.

	Prostate cancer		Breast cancer	
	range	median	range	median
Oestrogen receptor	0– 85	5	0– 770	50
Androgen receptor	0–105	17	0– 150	50
Progesterone receptor	0– 5	0	0–1,480	23
Glucocorticoid receptor	0– 50	0	0– 200	30
Albumin	2– 7	4	2– 10	5
Tumour protein	8– 57	23	2– 56	34
SHBG	0–125	27	0– 145	55

Receptor and SHBG concentrations are expressed in fmol/mg tumour protein. Protein concentrations are expressed in mg/g tissue.

regression was noted in these patients. The response in the patients E and F could not be evaluated, because both patients died within months after starting therapy. Although no conclusions can be drawn from the clinical study the results do not contradict the hypothesis that an androgen receptor needs to be present for effective hormonal therapy of prostatic cancer.

The androgen receptor in alternative hormonal therapy

Not all cancers treated respond to oestrogen therapy. Sometimes a beneficial effect of oestrogen therapy is of short duration only. Some alternative hormonal treatments are the subject of clinical trials, *e.g.* the European Organization for Research on the Treatment of Cancer (EORTC) Urological Group [4] is comparing the effect of CA, MPA and DES in a randomized prospective study in patients with advanced prostatic cancer.

In previous unpublished studies we found that the progestogens megestrol acetate (MA) and MPA have high affinity for progesterone, glucocorticoid and androgen receptors but not for the oestrogen receptor of breast and endometrial cancers. As can be seen from Table III, a 39-fold excess of progesterone or a 27-fold excess of R-5020 suppresses the binding of radio-labelled DHT to the DHT receptor by 50 percent while only a 6-fold excess of MA or a 4-fold excess of MPA is needed. A similar situation was noticed for the dexamethasone receptor.

Although not enough tumour tissue was available to repeat these studies in prostatic cancer, it was possible to perform some competition studies with the androgen receptor present in a lymph node metastasis (patient A, Table II).

By sucrose-glycerol density gradient centrifugation it was shown (Figure 1) that most of the androgen receptor was in the 7–8 S configuration. The amounts of competitors to give about 50 percent suppression of ^{3}H-DHT binding were chosen on the basis of the data in Table III.

MPA, MA, CA and progesterone (PG) suppressed DHT binding in the 7–8 S area. A 100-fold excess of DHT was able to suppress binding completely in the 7–8 S as well as in the 4 S area (not shown in the figure). However, DES, present in a 200-fold excess, was unable to suppress DHT binding.

It can be concluded that MPA, CA and also MA are strong competitors

Table II Receptors in lymph node metastases of prostatic cancer and clinical effect of therapy.

Patient	Therapy	Duration of therapy (months)	Clinical effect	Response objective	Response subjective	AR (fM/mg tumour protein)	ER	PGR	GR
A	Orchiectomy	5 (continuing)	No new metastases	?	+	105	10	5	50
B	Ethinyl-oestradiol	6 (continuing)	Lymph node < Bone <	+	+	40	85	0	0
C	Medroxy-progesterone acetate	3 (continuing)	Slow progression bone	−	pain ↓	25	5	n.d.	n.d.
D	Medroxy-progesterone acetate	1	Lymph node >>	−	−	10	0	0	0
E	Prednisone	2	Not evaluable			0	15	n.d.	n.d.
F	Cyproterone acetate	1	Not evaluable			0	0	n.d.	n.d.

AR = androgen receptor; ER = oestrogen receptor; PGR = progesterone receptor; GR = glucocorticoid receptor; n.d. = not determined, + = remission; − = failure; ? = unknown.

Table III   Relative affinities of progesterone and progestogens for the various receptors.*
Estimated excesses for 50% inhibition of binding.

	E-R	DHT-R	R5020-R	D-R
Progesterone	N.d.	39	n.d.	67
R5020	N.d.	27	n.d.	60
Megestrol acetate	> 100	6	9	9
Medroxyprogesterone acetate	> 100	4	7	4

n.d. = Not determined.
* Mean figures from 3 breast cancers and 1 endometrial cancer.

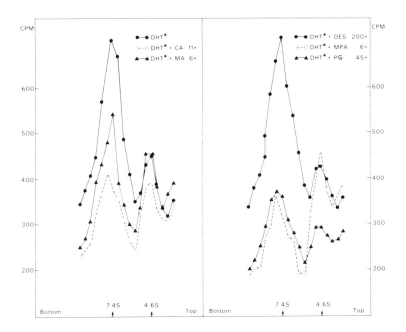

Fig. 1.   Sucrose gradient separation of the 7–8S form of androgen receptor from metastatic prostate cancer tissue. Suppression of DHT binding by CA, MA, DES, PG and MPA also shown.

for the 7–8 S androgen receptor of prostatic cancer. Although there is evidence that these substances also interfere with androgen metabolism, it cannot be excluded that, through competition with DHT for the androgen receptor, a tumour-growth-reducing effect of these substances may be obtained. It has however to be shown in a clinical study whether tumour regression with MPA or CA occurs only in tumours containing a significant amount of androgen receptor.

Tumour-SHBG levels

The presence of SHBG in tumour homogenates has been generally regarded as a contamination of the homogenates with plasma proteins. During the course of a study on androgen receptors in breast and prostatic carcinoma we made some observations on tumour-SHBG levels which could not be explained by assuming plasma contamination to be the only cause of the presence of SHBG.

Low temperature electrophoresis was used to assess the androgen receptor. Separation from SHBG is an important advantage of this method, especially in the case of the androgen receptor. Another advantage, not fully recognized at present, is that an estimate of tumour-SHBG level can be made when the radio-ligand ³H-DHT is used for estimation of the androgen receptor. SHBG, having an affinity for this ligand comparable to that of the androgen receptor, is separated during electrophoresis from the receptors as well as from unbound ligand. Although the estimate cannot be regarded as quantitative, due to dissociation during the procedure, we have performed determinations in a reproducible way and have used the estimated SHBG levels comparatively only.

Separation of SHBG from the androgen receptor is illustrated in figure 2. The tissue was obtained from a patient with cancer of the prostate who had received DES for several years. There is an abundance of SHBG, while the amount of receptor is in the normal range. Very high SHBG levels have been observed in all primary cancers obtained during or directly after finishing oestrogen therapy.

As shown in Table IV the mean tumour-SHBG level in untreated breast cancer tends to be twice that in untreated prostatic tumours. This is in agreement with the observation that plasma SHBG concentrations in men

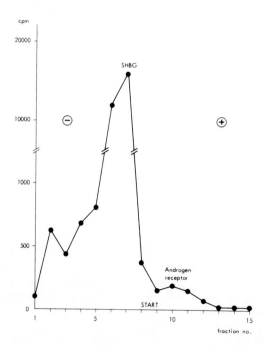

Fig. 2. Agar-gel electrophoresis separation (corrected for non-specific binding) of SHBG and androgen receptor. Tumour tissue obtained from a patient with cancer of the prostate during DES therapy. SHBG fractions 4–8; androgen receptor fractions 9–15.

Table IV SHBG levels in tumour tissues.

fmol/g tissue		Number of patients	Tumour SHBG	
			mean	range
Prostate	BPH	4	1,150	900– 4,500
	Lymph node deposits (no treatment)	6	850	0– 2,800
	Cancer (during oestrogen treatment)	4	22,500	11,200–32,000
Breast (postmenopausal)	Cancer (no treatment)	63	2,600	0–12,900
	Cancer (during oestrogen treatment)	4	23,000	13,000–52,200

are half those in women of comparable age [5]. When comparing the albumin levels of the various groups no important differences are seen. It is unlikely, therefore, that there is a difference in the degree of contamination with plasma proteins during hormonal therapy. From the mean tumour-SHBG levels it can be seen that long-term administration of ethinylestradiol resulted in about an 11-fold increase in tumour-SHBG in the breast cancer patients and, possibly, an even stronger increase during treatment of prostatic cancer with DES. An approximately 5-fold increase of plasma-SHBG during DES administration was reported by Murayama *et al.* [6] for breast cancer and by Houghton *et al.* [7] for cancer of the prostate. Our findings show a much higher increase of SHBG in tumour tissues than was reported for plasma levels, which could mean that SHBG accumulates in tumour tissues. Intracellular presence of SHBG in tumour cells was suggested earlier from experiments of Rosen *et al.* [8] and Steins *et al.* [9]. Our results suggest that administration of oestrogenic substances enhances tumour SHBG levels more strongly than plasma levels. These higher SHBG levels may deprive the cancer cells of DHT. This may explain how tumour regression during oestrogen therapy of prostate cancer occurs, although it still has to be clarified whether the presence of an androgen receptor is crucial to the effectiveness of oestrogen therapy of prostatic cancer.

Acknowledgements

The authors wish to thank W. H. Hirdes, M. C. C. de Jong, Prof. F. H. Schröder and H. P. Vlietstra for providing tumour tissues, J. P. R. van Dalen, D. I. Blonk, R. Menon and A. Talerman for their collaboration in this study, and Mrs. J. Wike for reading the English text.

References

1. Neuman, F. (1978): The physiological action of progesterone and the pharmacological effects of progestogens – a short review. *Postgrad. Med. J., 54,* Supplement 2.
2. Wagner, R. K. (1972): Characterization and assay of steroid hormone receptors and steroid-binding proteins by agar-gel electrophoresis at low temperature. *Hoppe-Seyler's Z. Physiol. Chem., 353,* 1235.
3. Teulings, F. A. G., Blonk-van der Wijst, J., Portengen, H., Henkelman, M. S., Treurniet, R. E. and van Gilse, H. A. (1975): Quantitation of estrogen receptors in human breast cancer by agar gel electrophoresis. *Clin. Chim. Acta, 64,* 27.

4. European Organisation for Research on Treatment of Cancer — Urological Group (1978): Protocol for a randomized prospective study of the treatment of patients with advanced prostatic cancer category T3 and T4 to compare the effect of cyproterone acetate, medroxyprogesterone and stilbestrol. In: *Current Research of the E.O.R.T.C. Cooperative Groups, Project Groups, Clubs, Task Forces and Working Parties*, p. 49. Editor: M. Staquet. E.O.R.T.C., Brussels.
5. Vermeulen, A., Verdonck, L., van der Straten, M. and Orie, R. (1969): Capacity of the testosterone-binding globulin in human plasma and influence of specific binding of testosterone on its metabolic clearance rate. *J. Clin. Endocrinol. Metab., 29,* 1470.
6. Murayama, Y., Utsunomiya, J., Asano, K. and Ogawa, S. (1976): Serum globulin assay of estrogen binding ability during endocrine treatment of postmenopausal advanced breast cancer. *Jpn. J. Surg., 6,* 119.
7. Houghton, A. L., Turner, R. and Cooper, E. H. (1977): Sex hormone binding globulin in carcinoma of the prostate. *Br. J. Urol., 49,* 227.
8. Rosen, V., Jung, I., Baulieu, E. E. and Robel, P. (1975): Androgen binding proteins in human benign prostatic hypertrophy. *J. Clin. Endocrinol. Metab., 41,* 761.
9. Steins, P., Krieg, M., Hollman, H. and Voigt, K. D. (1974): In vitro studies of testosterone and dihydrotestosterone binding in benign prostatic hypertrophy. *Acta Endocrinol. (Copenhagen), 75,* 773.

Discussion

M. Krieg (Hamburg, Federal Republic of Germany): Did you correlate the SHBG concentration in each patient as between tissue and plasma?

F. A. G. Teulings: We observed high SHBG peaks in the agar-gel electrophoresis pattern in a minority of the tumours which we have analysed for receptors. It was found retrospectively that high tumour SHBG levels were associated with tumours obtained from patients receiving oestrogen therapy. By comparing the tumour SHBG determinations in untreated patients with those in oestrogen-treated patients it was found that the levels in the latter were 10–20 times higher. An increase in plasma-SHBG levels during oestrogen treatment is reported in the literature. This increase, however, did not exceed, on average, a factor of 5, as was confirmed during this workshop by Dr. B. Mobbs also.

At present there is no conclusive explanation for the discrepancy between the increases in tumour and plasma-SHBG levels. This has first to be confirmed by quantitative measurements of tumour and plasma levels in patients before and during treatment.

Is there a place for the assay of cytoplasmic steroid receptors in the endocrine treatment of prostatic cancer?

H. J. de Voogt and P. G. Dingjan
Departments of Urology and Pathological Chemistry, University Hospital, Leiden, The Netherlands

Introduction

Our main purpose in undertaking a study of cytoplasmic steroid receptors in human prostatic tissue was to determine their relevance to prognosis of response to endocrine therapy, by analogy with the results obtained in breast cancer. A second, consequential aim was to ascertain if a practical laboratory assay could be developed for routine use. In pursuit of these aims it was decided, after the methodology had been established, to collect data relating to a fairly large number of patients, to allow meaningful statistical analysis.

During the study, in which androstanolone receptor (DHT-R) was first determined, binding of estradiol by prostatic tissue was also noted. This binding had all the characteristics of receptor binding but differed in certain respects from the E2-receptor (E2-R) most often found in oestrogen target tissues such as the uterus or mammae [1]. This receptor has also been described by other authors [2–5]. A third aim, of seeing whether this E2-R might have specific significance in relation to prostatic tissue, therefore arose.

Materials and methods

Between 1975 and 1978 prostatic tissue samples were obtained from 116 patients by way of prostatectomy, trans-urethral resection (TUR) and perineal needle biopsy. Histological investigation revealed that 66 patients had benign prostatic hyperplasia (BPH) and 50 had prostatic cancer. Of these 50, only 47 were available for full evaluation.

The receptor assay method used was the cold agar gel electrophoresis method of Wagner [6], with some slight modifications. This has been described in detail in earlier communications [1, 7] in which the relevant studies on specificity are also recorded.

All carcinoma patients were categorized according to the Tumours-Nodes-Metastases (TNM) system of the UICC (1974). All data were recorded on punched cards for computer analysis.

Each piece of tissue regarded as suitable for receptor assay was cut in half.

One half, selected at random, was given to the pathologist for rough morphometric analysis to determine the amount of carcinomatous/epithelial elements and the quantity of stromal cells present. The other half was then subjected to receptor assay.

Plasma levels of testosterone, estradiol, estrone, hydrocortisone and prolactin were determined in all patients by radioimmunoassay.

The carcinoma patients received endocrine treatment, mainly with diethylstilbestrol (DES), after which response was assessed by the following four criteria:

1. reduction in tumour size (rectal palpation);
2. disappearance of obstructive symptoms;
3. clinical chemical values (acid phosphatase, liver function tests, testosterone values, γ-glutamic acid transaminase; and
4. clinician's evaluation of whether disease had progressed, regressed or remained unaltered.

Statistical analysis in this study mainly involved the Spearman rank correlation and Pearson correlation tests.

Results

Table I shows how four patient-groups were formed. The 15 patients of group 4 were selected from group 2 and treated with DES for 8 months, following which a second assessment, including prostatic biopsy and receptor determinations, was carried out. The values found for DHT- and E2-R binding are given in Table II. The presence or absence of receptor binding is indicated in Table III. The differences in DHT-R binding seen in the BPH group of patients and in the groups suffering from prostatic cancer are significant ($p < 0.05$).

Tables IV and V show the relationship between receptor binding and criteria for response. Reduction of tumour size in group 2 is correlated with increasing DHT-R values and the final clinical evaluation in group 4 cor-

Table I

group 1	66 patients with BPH
group 2	27 patients with prostatic cancer, untreated
group 3	20 patients with prostatic cancer, treated with oestrogens for an average of 38 months
group 4	15 patients from group 2, after 8 months' treatment with oestrogens

Table II   Quantitative binding capacities of DHT-R and E2-R in fmol/mg tissue protein.

Group	N	DHT-R		E2-R	
		median	range	median	range
1	66	8	0– 277	251	0–10,849
2	27	25	0– 206	380	0–15,507
3	20	32	0–1,621	65	0– 1,085
4	15	52	0– 382	113	0– 2,685

N = number of patients.

Table III Presence of DHT-R and E2-R in human prostatic cytosol.

Group	N	DHT-R		E2-R	
		negative* (%)	positive (%)	negative* (%)	positive (%)
1	66	73	27	3	97
2	27	44	56	11	89
3	20	35	65	15	85
4	15	40	60	33	67

* < 20 fmol/mg of tissue protein.

Table IV Spearman rank correlation coefficients between DHT-R and criteria of response to endocrine therapy.

	Group 2			Group 3			Group 4		
	r	N	P	r	N	P	r	N	P
Tumour size	0.42	25	*0.04*	−0.22	20	0.35	−0.43	15	0.10
Patient complaints	0.16	25	0.42	−0.03	20	0.91	−0.31	15	0.25
Laboratory assessments	0.27	25	0.19	−0.17	20	0.47	0.28	15	0.29
Final evaluation	0.003	25	0.99	−0.09	20	0.71	0.13	15	0.62

r = correlation coefficient; a negative correlation means that response is worse when DHT-R increases; N = number of patients or tests done; P = tail probability (when in italics it is ⩽ level of significance $\alpha = 0.05$).

Table V Spearman rank correlations between E2-R and criteria for response to endocrine therapy.

	Group 2			Group 3			Group 4		
	r	N	P	r	N	P	r	N	P
Tumour size	−0.02	25	0.91	0.02	20	0.44	−0.26	15	0.33
Patient complaints	0.07	25	0.72	−0.04	20	0.88	−0.21	15	0.44
Laboratory assessments	−0.27	25	0.18	0.06	20	0.81	−0.49	15	0.065
Final evaluation	0.02	25	0.90	0.28	20	0.21	0.53	15	*0.048*

r = correlation coefficient; a negative correlation means that response is worse when E2-R increases: N = number of patients or tests done; P = tail probability (when in italics it is ⩽ level of significance $\alpha = 0.05$).

relates with high levels of E2-R. No other statistically significant correlations were detected.

In Tables VI, VII and VIII Spearman correlation coefficients between the degree of steroid binding and the amount of cancer tissue (significant negative correlation for E2-R in group 3), tumour grade (no significant correlation) and amount of stromal cells (significant positive correlation for E2-R in group 3) are given.

Table VI Spearman rank correlation coefficients between amount of cancer tissue and binding capacity of steroid hormone receptors.

	DHT-R			E2-R		
	r	N	P	r	N	P
group 2	0.17	27	0.40	−0.28	27	0.16
group 3	0.37	20	0.11	−0.63	20	*0.006*
group 4	0.09	15	0.74	−0.28	15	0.29

r = correlation coefficient; a negative correlation means that response is worse when E2-R increases; N = number of patients or tests done: P = tail probability (when in italics it is ≤ level of significance α = 0.05).

Table VII Spearman rank correlations between tumour grade and binding capacity of steroid hormone receptors.

	DHT-R			E2-R		
	r	N	P	r	N	P
group 2	−0.10	26	0.63	−0.33	26	0.10
group 3	−0.10	19	0.70	−0.33	19	0.16
group 4	−0.03	14	0.92	−0.29	14	0.30

r = correlation coefficient; a negative correlation means that response is worse when DHT-R and E2-R increase; N = number of patients or tests done; P = tail probability (when in italics it is ≤ level of significance α = 0.05).

Table VIII Spearman rank correlations between amount of stromal cells and binding capacity of steroid hormone receptors.

	DHT-R			E2-R		
	r	N	P	r	N	P
group 1	−0.08	66	0.54	−0.05	60	0.58
group 2	−0.03	26	0.90	0.14	26	0.48
group 3	−0.17	19	0.47	0.46	19	*0.05*

r = correlation coefficient; a negative correlation means that response is worse when DHT-R and E2-R increase; N = number of patients or tests done; P = tail probability (when in italics it is ≤ level of significance α = 0.05).

Discussion

Recently, and during this meeting, several investigators have presented their data on receptor binding in human prostatic tissue [2, 3, 5, 8–13]. Different study methods were used, which may explain some of the differences in results between these studies. Investigators using agar gel electrophoresis mostly found no significant correlation between DHT-R binding and response to endocrine therapy [1, 5, 13] and the suggestion of our own preliminary results [18] had to be reassessed. Ekman, using metribolone (MT) as a ligand, claims an 80% response to endocrine therapy in patients with high DHT-R binding [8], but the possibility of cross-reactivity of MT to progesterone receptors cannot be excluded completely [14].

Most other methods used to determine receptor binding do not distinguish accurately between receptor binding and binding to plasma contaminants such as sex hormone binding globulin (SHBG), though in some of these studies correlations with response to endocrine therapy are mentioned [11, 12].

Even more significant are the problems of obtaining enough tissue material in prostatic cancer and the heterogeneity of this tissue. In most instances prostatic cancer tissue has to be obtained by repeated needle biopsies, a procedure not without a certain risk to the patient and not, therefore, very suitable for use in follow-up. Although we have shown that TUR material can be used for receptor studies [1], TUR is only acceptable in patients with signs of obstruction.

The exact amount of carcinoma present and the distribution of stromal and epithelial elements should, ideally, be known for each sample of tissue assayed for receptor binding. This is, however, not possible. The situation can be determined only approximately by morphometric analysis of tissue immediately adjacent. To our knowledge, there is no other way in which this problem can be overcome, though there is no doubt of its influence on the results of all studies.

In our material, after morphometric analysis, we found a significant negative correlation between the amount of carcinoma and E2-R values, together with a positive correlation between amount of stroma and E2-binding. In our opinion this suggests that the E2-R in question is located mainly in stromal tissue, an interesting finding in view of some of the other studies presented during this meeting [15–19].

However, the disappointing results mentioned above concerning correlation between cytoplasmic DHT-R and response to endocrine therapy, together with the problems of obtaining suitable tissue material and the heterogeneity of prostatic cancer tissue imply, in our view, that the assay of cytoplasmic steroid receptors is not a suitable tool for the routine clinical assessment of prognosis of response of prostatic cancer patients to endocrine therapy. Future investigations will probably be directed to determining whether the nuclear receptor assay procedure [20] or investigation of material obtained by aspiration biopsy can be developed into simple methods for routine clinical use.

Acknowledgements

This study was supported by grant U 74–23 of the KWF (Dutch Organization for Cancer Research). The statistical analysis was carried out by Drs

E. A. v. d. Velde of the Department of Medical Statistics of the University of Leiden, The Netherlands.

References

1. Dingjan, P. G. (1978): *Steroid receptors in humaan prostaatweefsel.* Thesis, Leiden.
2. Bashirelahi, N. and Armstrong, E. G. (1975): 17β-estradiol binding by human prostate. In: *Normal and Abnormal Growth of the Prostate,* chapter 36, p. 632. M. Goland, Ch. Thomas, Springfield.
3. Bashirelahi, N., O'Toole, J. H. and Young, J. D. (1976): A specific 17β-estradiol receptor in human benign hypertrophic prostate. *Biochem. Med., 15,* 254.
4. Hawkins, E. F., Nijs, M., Brassine, C. and Tagnon, H. J. (1975): Steroid receptors in the human prostate. I. Estradiol-17β-binding. *Steroids, 26,* 458.
5. Wagner, R. K. (1978): *Acta Endocrinol. Suppl. 218.*
6. Wagner, R. K. (1972): Characterization and assay of steroid hormone receptors and steroid binding serum proteins by agar gel electrophoresis at low temperature. *Hoppe Seyler's Z. Physiol. Chem., 353,* 1235.
7. de Voogt, H. J. and Dingjan, P. G. (1978): Steroid receptors in human prostatic tissue, a preliminary evaluation. *Urol. Res., 6,* 151.
8. Ekman, P. (1978): *Steroid receptors in the human prostate.* Thesis, Stockholm.
9. Ghanadian, R., Auf, G., Chisholm, C. D. and O'Donoghue, E. P. N. (1978): Receptor proteins for androgens in prostatic disease. *Br. J. Urol., 50,* 567.
10. Menon, M., Tananis, C. E., McLoughlin, M. G., Lippman, M. E. and Walsh, P. C. (1977): The measurement of androgen receptors in human prostatic tissue utilizing sucrose density centrifugation and a protamine precipitation assay. *J. Urol., 117,* 309.
11. Menon, M., Tananis, C. E., McLoughlin, M. G. and Walsh, P. C. (1977): Androgen receptors in human prostatic tissue: a review. *Cancer Treat. Rep. 61,* 265.
12. Mobbs, B. G., Johnson, I. E. and Connolly, J. G. (1980): Androgen receptors and treatment of prostatic cancer. This volume, p. 225.
13. Voigt, K. D. and Krieg, M. (1978): Biochemical endocrinology of prostatic tumours. *Curr. Top. Exp. Endocrinol., 3.*
14. Menon, M., Tananis, C. E., Hicks, L. L., Hawkins, E. F., McLoughlin, M. G. and Walsh, P. C. (1978): Characterization of the binding of a potent synthetic androgen, methyltrienolone, to human tissues. *J. Clin. Invest., 61,* 150.
15. Bashirelahi, N., Young Jr., J. D., Sidh, S. M. and Sanefuji, H. (1980): Androgen, oestrogen and progestogen and their distribution in epithelial and stromal cells of human prostate. This volume, p. 240.
16. Bruchovsky, N., Rennie, P. S. and Wilkin, R. P. (1979): New aspects of androgen action in the prostate: Stromal localization of 5α-reductase, nuclear abundance dihydrotestosterone and binding of receptor to linker DNA. This volume, p. 57.
17. Bard, D. R., Lasnitzki, I. and Mizuno, T. (1979): Induction of the rat prostate by androgens in vitro and testosterone metabolism of isolated urogenital epithelium and stroma. This volume, p. 41.
18. Romijn, J. C., Oishi, K., Mulder, E., Schweikert, H. U., Schroeder, F. H. and Bolt-de Vries, J. (1979): Steroid metabolism and androgen receptors in epithelium of human prostate. This volume, p. 134.
19. Schweikert, H. U., Hein, H. J. and Schroeder, F. H. (1979): Androgen metabolism in cultured human fibroblasts from benign prostatic hyperplasia, prostatic carcinoma and non-genital skin. This volume, p. 126.
20. Lieskovsky, G. and Bruchovsky, N. (1979): Assay of nuclear androgen receptor in human prostate. *J. Urol., 121,* 54.

Discussion

R. Ghanadian (London, UK): In one of your tables I noticed a figure of

2,600 fmol/mg protein for oestrogen receptor. Do you have an explanation for this exceptionally high amount of receptor protein? Is there a technical problem of the method involved?

H. J. de Voogt: The oestrogen receptor values in our study ranged from 0–15,507 fmol/mg, which means that there were some very high values indeed. For that reason we also gave the median, which ranged between 50 and 380.

One of the possible reasons for the very high values was that we skipped the dextran coated charcoal treatment, as we observed that in this way also receptor-bound steroids could be removed. However, in certain cases there is an overlap then between specific receptor-bound and albumin-bound (non specific) steroids, which might account for some of the high values.

As we found very low and negative values as well, I think that in the overall picture of our study it did not influence the point we wanted to make.

H. A. van Gilse (Rotterdam, The Netherlands): Could you answer the question of not treating prostate cancer with endocrine treatment, if no receptors were present, already now, or only after laboratory methods are standardized and more is exactly known of the value of receptor estimations (since an overall 60% remission rate in metastatic prostate cancer is a rather good result compared with, e.g., a 30% in breast cancer).

H. J. de Voogt: Much as I should like to be able to answer that question already now, I must say that in my opinion it is not yet possible. It is not only a question of standardization and simplification of our methods, but also our understanding of what steroids actually do in prostatic tissue, and prostatic cancer in particular, is still deficient.

General Discussion

M. E. Harper (Cardiff, United Kingdom): May I make a comment on our experience with organ culture. In organ culture it is easy to identify individual cell types, because of their well-established morphological characteristics, and to observe their proportional responses to hormones. In separated cells morphological identification is difficult. Often they take on disguises in terms of their enzyme content and activity. There is also the problem of selecting clones which may be or may not be hormone responsive.

I also have a question: How were prostate samples obtained? Were they from open prostatectomy or trans-urethral resection (TUR)? I feel very strongly that TUR specimens are of little use. We have measured various biochemical parameters in the same prostatic cancer specimens obtained by cold punch and TUR techniques. The endogenous androgen content is 5 to 10 times higher using the former method. Benign prostatic hyperplasia (BPH) samples obtained by open prostatectomy also have concentrations 5 times greater than those obtained by TUR. If we turn to quite different fields, the polyamines, the content of these compounds and the enzymes involved in their synthesis are very much higher in these open operative than in TUR specimens. One could cite many more examples such as platin activity in tissue culture, etc.

N. Bruchovsky (Edmonton, Canada): Samples were obtained at the time of open retropubic prostatectomy. Immediately upon removal of the gland from the patient the hyperplastic nodules were dissected from the periurethral zone and frozen at $-80°C$ within 15–20 minutes. No TUR specimens were included in our study.

M. Krieg (Hamburg, Federal Republic of Germany): Carcinoma samples were obtained during the course of open perineal cryosurgery. BPH samples were obtained during open prostatectomy.

We have also had bad experiences with TUR specimens. In no case so far could a receptor protein be demonstrated.

H. J. van der Molen (Rotterdam, The Netherlands): Does anybody have information on how the parameters which have been discussed this afternoon (receptor levels, steroid levels, steroid metabolism) could be or are responsible for BPH or prostatic carcinoma, or on how they change after treatment?

M. E. Harper: Concerning the relevance of measuring hormone levels, steroid metabolism and hormone receptors, these parameters can only be studied in patients with prostatic hyperplasia once tumours are established. We have been studying an animal model for BPH, the hamster BIO 87.2 strain which develops this tumour spontaneously in middle age. Because of its short life span it has been possible to study the endogenous androgen concentration and steroid activities before development, during development and when the tumour is established. Our results show that only when you have the tumour established are the increased levels of androgens and enzymes seen. Comparison with control animals has also been undertaken.

H. A. van Gilse (Rotterdam, The Netherlands): In our Society for Endocrine-related Cancer, workers on distinct tumours, the normal tissue relating to which serves particular and distinct purposes (breast, uterus, prostate, kidney), have found that the same hormones may act in different ways on malignant cells originating in these tissues. Comparison of these differences may lead to better insight in the essence of hormonal influences on certain cancers.

Concluding remarks

F. H. Schröder
Institute of Urology, Erasmus University, Rotterdam, The Netherlands

Dear friends,

After two days of first class presentations and extensive discussion it is impossible to give a short and still concise summary of what has been said about steroid receptors and steroid metabolism related to prostatic cancer. Being primarily a clinician, I should prefer to state and stress once again what should be achieved in this field in the near future. Finally, I shall try to make some suggestions how our continuous efforts may be coordinated in a more fruitful manner.

Prostatic carcinoma is the second to third most frequent malignant tumour in the age groups of males involved. It is estimated that about 60% of these tumours are diagnosed in late stages beyond a chance of total removal or curative radiotherapy [1]. It is in the interest of this large group that an optimal form of systemic treatment should be established which could consist of endocrine or chemotherapeutic management.

For this group, being mainly concerned with endocrinology, the following questions should be of major interest:

1. Is the pathogenesis of prostatic carcinoma related to steroid hormones and, if so, what are the mechanisms? Can carcinoma of the prostate be prevented?
2. What, precisely, are the mechanisms of endocrine dependence? How are growth and function of the prostatic cancer cell regulated?
3. What are the reasons for prostatic cancers becoming hormone independent? Can this process be manipulated?
4. Can the results of endocrine management be predicted? Can applicable parameters be used for pre-treatment selection of patients?
5. What is the function of the prostate as an endocrine organ? Is its steroid metabolism involved in the regulation of growth and function of the tumour cell?
6. Can mechanisms which may be found in the future be used for growth control? Which substances may be useful?
7. Is there immunological control of growth of prostatic carcinoma and are the immunological properties related to the endocrinological ones?

As this meeting and the recent literature have shown there is an enormous increase of knowledge and of experimental possibilities in this field. Many of the questions mentioned above have been partially answered, and their complete answer can be foreseen for the near future. This process could be made smoother and quicker by a better coordination of research efforts. Some obvious examples have become evident during the discussions of our congress.

There was, for example, agreement that the finding of an estradiol receptor in BPH tissue by some groups and of no estradiol receptor by some others is probably based on technical differences. It is annoying if the results of incubation experiments are not comparable because of longer or shorter incubation times used or because of other, easily exchangeable technical variations used in different laboratories. Such problems could be minimized by having more regular contact with the group actively involved in research in this field. Therefore the organizers of this meeting and a group of participants proposed the foundation of a 'European Society of Experimental Urological Oncology and Endocrinology'; they were happy to learn that this plan has the support of the vast majority of participants of this symposium.

Before closing, I should like to state that the pending problems can only be solved by biologically oriented interdisciplinary research. The parameters to be studied cannot be handled by any single specialty.

To close I should like to express our gratitude to the Schering AG of the Netherlands for the rare, unselfish sponsorship which made this Symposium possible, and to the team from Excerpta Medica for the outstanding organization which made this meeting a success and a pleasure for every participant.

Reference

1. Whitmore, W. F. (1973): The natural history of prostatic cancer. *Cancer 32*, 1104.

Index of authors